Sport and Exercise Pharmacology

Stan Reents, PharmD
Gold Standard Multimedia, Inc.
Tampa, FL

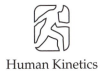

Human Kinetics

Library of Congress Cataloging-in-Publication Data

Reents, Stan, 1954-
   Sport and exercise pharmacology / Stan Reents.
      p.   cm.
   Includes bibliographical references.
   ISBN 0-87322-937-1
   1. Doping in sports. 2. Drug interactions. 3. Exercise--Physiological aspects. I. Title.

RC1230 .R43 2000
615'.1'088796--dc21

00-021137

ISBN: 0-87322-937-1

Acquisitions Editor: Michael S. Bahrke, PhD; **Managing Editor:** Cynthia McEntire; **Assistant Editor:** John Wentworth; **Copyeditor:** John Mulvihill; **Proofreader:** Pamela S. Johnson; **Permission Manager:** Heather Munson; **Graphic Designer:** Fred Starbird; **Graphic Artist:** Kathleen Boudreau-Fuoss; **Cover Designer:** Jack W. Davis; **Illustrator:** Sharon Smith; **Printer:** Versa Press

Printed in the United States of America   10 9 8 7 6 5 4 3 2 1

Human Kinetics
Web site: http://www.humankinetics.com/

United States: Human Kinetics, P.O. Box 5076, Champaign, IL 61825-5076
1-800-747-4457
e-mail: humank@hkusa.com

Canada: Human Kinetics, 475 Devonshire Road Unit 100, Windsor, ON N8Y 2L5
1-800-465-7301 (in Canada only)
e-mail: humank@hkcanada.com

Europe: Human Kinetics, P.O. Box IW14, Leeds LS16 6TR, United Kingdom
+44 (0)113-278 1708
e-mail: humank@hkeurope.com

Australia: Human Kinetics, 57A Price Avenue, Lower Mitcham, South Australia 5062
(08) 82771555
e-mail: liahka@senet.com.au

New Zealand: Human Kinetics, P.O. Box 105-231, Auckland Central
09-523-3462
e-mail: humank@hknewz.com

Contents

Credits

Figures

Figure 1.1 Adapted, by permission, from F.H.H. Leenen, 1980, "Effects of cardioselective and non-cardioselective beta-blockade on dynamic exercise performance in mildly hypertensive men," *Clinical Pharmacology and Therapeutics* 28 (1): 12-21.

Figure 1.2 Adapted from *American Journal of Cardiology*, Vol. 54, P.A. Ades, H.L. Brammell, J.H. Greenberg, and L.D. Horwitz, "Effect of beta-blockade and intrinsic sympathomimetic activity on exercise performance," Page No. 1337-1342, Copyright (1984), with permission from Excerpta Medica Inc.

Figure 1.3 Adapted, by permission, from P.A. Ades, 1987, "Cardiac effects of beta-adrenoceptor blockade with intrinsic sympathomimetic activity during submaximal exercise," *British Journal of Clinical Pharmacology* 24: 325.

Figure 1.4 Adapted, by permission, from R. Fagard, J. Staessen, L. Thijs, and A. Amery, 1993, "Influence of antihypertensive drugs on exercise capacity," *Drugs* 46 (supp. 2): 33.

Figure 1.5 Adapted from *American Journal of Cardiology*, Vol. 54, P.A. Ades, H.L. Brammell, J.H. Greenberg, and L.D. Horwitz, "Effect of beta-blockade and intrinsic sympathomimetic activity on exercise performance," Page No. 1337-1342, Copyright (1984), with permission from Excerpta Medica Inc.

Figure 1.6 Adapted, by permission, from P. Arner, E. Kriegholm, P. Engfeldt, and J. Bolinder, 1990, "Adrenergic regulation of lipolysis *in situ* at rest and during exercise," *Journal of Clinical Investigation* 85: 895.

Figure 1.7 Adapted, by permission, from K. Laustiola, A. Uusitalo, T. Koivula, A. Sovijarvi, E. Seppala, T. Nikkari, and H. Vapaatalo, 1983, " Divergent effects of atenolol, practolol and propranolol on the peripheral metabolic changes induced by dynamic exercise in healthy men," *European Journal of Clinical Pharmacology* 25: 296.

Figure 1.8 Adapted, by permission, from J. Cleroux, P. Van Nguyen, A.W. Taylor, and F.H.H. Leenen, 1989, "Effects of beta-1 vs. beta-1 plus beta-2 blockade on exercise endurance and muscle metabolism in humans," *Journal of Applied Physiology* 66 (2): 552.

Figure 1.9 Adapted, by permission, from J. Cleroux, P. Van Nguyen, A.W. Taylor, and F.H.H. Leenen, 1989, "Effects of beta-1 vs. beta-1 plus beta-2 blockade on exercise endurance and muscle metabolism in humans," *Journal of Applied Physiology* 66 (2): 550.

Figure 2.1 Adapted, by permission, from B.J. Freund, E.M. Shizuru, G.M. Hashiro, and J.R. Claybaugh, 1991, "Hormonal, electrolyte, and renal responses to exercise are intensity dependent," *Journal of Applied Physiology* 70 (2): 904.

Figure 2.2 Adapted, by permission, from B.J. Freund, E.M. Shizuru, G.M. Hashiro, and J.R. Claybaugh, 1991, "Hormonal, electrolyte, and renal responses to exercise are intensity dependent," *Journal of Applied Physiology* 70 (2): 904.

Figure 2.3 Adapted, by permission, from W.F. Brechue and J.M. Stager, 1990, "Acetazolamide alters temperature regulation during submaximal exercise," *Journal of Applied Physiology* 69 (4): 1405.

Figure 2.4 Adapted, by permission, from E.R. Nadel, S.M. Fortney, and C.B. Wenger, 1980, "Effect of hydration state on circulatory and thermal regulations," *Journal of Applied Physiology* 49: 718.

Figure 2.5 Adapted, by permission, from L.E. Armstrong, D.L. Costill, and W.J. Fink, 1985, "Influence of diuretic-induced dehydration on competitive running performance," *Medicine and Science in Sports and Exercise* 17 (4): 456-461.

Figure 2.6 Adapted, by permission, from L.E. Armstrong, D.L. Costill, and W.J. Fink, 1985, "Influence of diuretic-induced dehydration on competitive running performance," *Medicine and Science in Sports and Exercise* 17 (4): 456-461.

Figure 3.1 Adapted, by permission, from J.D. MacDougall, D. Tuxen, D.G. Sale, J.R. Moroz, and J.R. Sutton, 1985, "Arterial blood pressure response to heavy resistance exercise," *Journal of Applied Physiology* 58 (3): 788.

Credits

Figure 8.6 Adapted, by permission, from J.S. Volek, N.D. Duncan, S.A. Mazzetti, R.S. Staron, M. Putukian, A.L. Gomez, D.R. Pearson, W.J. Fink, and W.J. Kraemer, 1999, "Performance and muscle fiber adaptations to creatine supplementation and heavy resistance training," *Medicine and Science in Sports and Exercise* 31 (8): 1147-1156.

Figure 8.7 Adapted, by permission, from J.S. Volek, N.D. Duncan, S.A. Mazzetti, R.S. Staron, M. Putukian, A.L. Gomez, D.R. Pearson, W.J. Fink, and W.J. Kraemer, 1999, "Performance and muscle fiber adaptations to creatine supplementation and heavy resistance training," *Medicine and Science in Sports and Exercise* 31 (8): 1147-1156.

Figure 9.2 Adapted, by permission, from B. Ekblom, 1996, "Blood doping and erythropoietin. The effects of variation in hemoglobin concentration and other r elated factors on physical performance," *American Journal of Sports Medicine* 24: S41.

Figure 9.3 Adapted, by permission, from I.Casoni, G. Ricci, E. Ballarin, C. Borsetto, G. Grazzi, C. Guglielmini, F. Manfredini, G. Mazzoni, M. Patrecchini, E. De Paoli Vitali, et al., 1993, "Hematological indices of erythropoietin administration in athletes," *International Journal of Sports Medicine* 14 (6): 310.

Figure 10.1 Adapted, by permission, from A. Head, P.M. Jakeman, M.J. Kendall, R. Cramb, and S. Maxwell, 1993, "The impact of a short course of three lipid lowering drugs on fat oxidation during exercise in healthy volunteers," *Postgraduate Medical Journal* 69: 199. Courtesy BMJ Publishing Group.

Figure 10.2 Adapted, by permission, from A. Head, P.M. Jakeman, M.J. Kendall, R. Cramb, and S. Maxwell, 1993, "The impact of a short course of three lipid lowering drugs on fat oxidation during exercise in healthy volunteers," *Postgraduate Medical Journal* 69: 200. Courtesy BMJ Publishing Group.

Figure 10.3 Adapted, by permission, from A. Head, P.M. Jakeman, M.J. Kendall, R. Cramb, and S. Maxwell, 1993, "The impact of a short course of three lipid lowering drugs on fat oxidation during exercise in healthy volunteers," *Postgraduate Medical Journal* 69: 201. Courtesy BMJ Publishing Group.

Figure 11.1 Adapted, by permission, from A. Danon, S. Ben-Shimon, and Z. Ben-Zvi, 1986, "Effect of exercise and heat exposure on percutaneous absorption of methyl salicylate," *European Journal of Clinical Pharmacology* 31: 50.

Figure 11.3 Adapted, by permission, from S.M. Hasson, J.C. Daniels, J.G. Devine, B.R. Niebuhr, S. Richmond, P.G. Stein, and J.H. Williams, 1993, "Effects of ibuprofen use on muscle soreness, damage, and performance: A preliminary investigation," *Medicine and Science in Sports and Exercise* 25 (1): 12.

Figure 11.4 Adapted, by permission, from S.M. Hasson, J.C. Daniels, J.G. Devine, B.R. Niebuhr, S. Richmond, P.G. Stein, and J.H. Williams, 1993, "Effects of ibuprofen use on muscle soreness, damage, and performance: A preliminary investigation," *Medicine and Science in Sports and Exercise* 25 (1): 12.

Figure 11.5 Adapted, by permission, from J.R. Lisse, K. MacDonald, M.E. Thurmond-Anderle, J.E. Fuchs, Jr., 1991, "A double-blind, placebo-controlled study of acetylsalicylic acid (ASA) in trained runners," *Journal of Sports Medicine and Physical Fitness* 31: 563.

Figure 12.1 Adapted, by permission, from L.D. Bowers, 1998, "Athletic drug testing," *Clinics in Sports Medicine* 17 (2): 307.

Figure 12.2 Adapted, by permission, from D.S. King, R.L. Sharp, M.D. Vukovich, G.A. Brown, T.A. Reifenrath, N.L. Uhl, and K.A. Parsons, 1999, "Effect of oral androstenedione on serum testosterone and adaptations to resistance training in young men," *JAMA* 281: 2023.

Figure 12.3 Adapted, by permission, from D.S. King, R.L. Sharp, M.D. Vukovich, G.A. Brown, T.A. Reifenrath, N.L. Uhl, and K.A. Parsons, 1999, "Effect of oral androstenedione on serum testosterone and adaptations to resistance training in young men," *JAMA* 281: 2024

Figure 12.4 Adapted, by permission, from D.S. King, R.L. Sharp, M.D. Vukovich, G.A. Brown, T.A. Reifenrath, N.L. Uhl, and K.A. Parsons, 1999, "Effect of oral androstenedione on serum testosterone and adaptations to resistance training in young men," *JAMA* 281: 2024

Figure 12.5 Adapted, by permission, from R. Beneke and S.P. von Duvillard, 1996, "Determination of maximal lactate steady state response in selected sports events," *Medicine and Science in Sports and Exercise* 28 (2): 261-246.

Figure 13.1 Adapted, by permission, from R.D. Wemple, D.R. Lamb, and K.H. McKeever, 1997, "Caffeine vs. caffeine-free sports drink: Effects on urine production at rest and during prolonged exercise," *International Journal of Sports Medicine* 18 (1): 44.

Figure 13.2 Adapted, by permission, from R.D. Wemple, D.R. Lamb, and K.H. McKeever, 1997, "Caffeine vs. caffeine-free sports drink: Effects on urine production at rest and during prolonged exercise," *International Journal of Sports Medicine* 18 (1): 42.

Figure 13.3 Adapted, by permission, from T.E. Graham, E. Hibbert, and P. Sathasivam, 1998, "Metabolic and exercise endurance effects of coffee and caffeine ingestion," *Journal of Applied Physiology* 85 (3): 885.

Figure 13.4 Adapted, by permission, from W.J. Pasman, M.A. van Baak, A.E. Jeukendrup, and A. de Haan, 1995, "The effect of different dosages of caffeine on endurance performance time," *International Journal of Sports Medicine* 16 (4): 227.

Figure 13.5 Adapted, by permission, from T.E. Graham and L.L. Spriet, 1991, "Performance and metabolic responses to a high caffeine dose during prolonged exercise," *Journal of Applied Physiology* 71 (6): 2294.

Figure 13.6 Adapted, by permission, from T.E. Graham and L.L. Spriet, 1995, "Metabolic catecholamine, and exercise performance responses to various doses of caffeine," *Journal of Applied Physiology* 78 (3): 872.

Figure 13.7 Adapted, by permission, from P.J. van der Merwe, H.G. Luus, and J.G. Barnard, 1992, "Caffeine in sport. Influence of endurance exercise on the urinary caffeine concentration," *International Journal of Sports Medicine* 13 (1): 75.

Figure 15.1 Adapted, by permission, from C.G. Cigarroa, J.D. Boehrer, E. Brickner, E.J. Eichhorn, and P.A. Grayburn, 1992, "Exaggerated pressor response to treadmill exercise in chronic cocaine abusers with left ventricular hypertrophy," *Circulation* 86 (1): 228.

Tables

Table 1.3 Adapted, by permission, from K. Laustiola, A. Uusitalo, T. Koivula, A. Sovijarvi, E. Seppala, T. Nikkari, and H. Vapaatalo, 1983, " Divergent effects of atenolol, practolol and propranolol on the peripheral metabolic changes induced by dynamic exercise in healthy men," *European Journal of Clinical Pharmacology* 25: 294.

Table 2.3 Adapted, by permission, from L.E. Armstrong, D.L. Costill, and W.J. Fink, 1985, "Influence of diuretic-induced dehydration on competitive running performance," *Medicine and Science in Sports and Exercise* 17 (4): 456-461.

Table 2.4 Adapted, by permission, from J.E. Caldwell, E. Ahonen, and U. Nousiainen, 1984, "Differential effects of sauna-, diuretic-, and exercise-induced hypohydration," *Journal of Applied Physiology* 57 (4): 1020.

Table 3.3 Adapted, by permission, from N.F. Gordon, J.P. van Rensburg, D.L. Kawalsky, H.M. Russell, C.P. Celliers, and D.P. Myburgh, 1986, "Effect of acute calcium slow-channel antagonism on the cardiorespiratory response to graded exercise testing," *International Journal of Sports Medicine* 7 (5): 254-258, GEORG THIEME VERLAG.

Table 3.4 Adapted, by permission, from T.W. Chick, A.K. Halperin, and E.M. Gacek, 1988, "The effect of antihypertensive medications on exercise performance: A review," *Medicine and Science in Sports and Exercise* 20 (5): 447-454.

Table 3.5 Adapted, by permission, from F. Carré, R. Handschuh, J. Beillot, J. Dassonville, P. Rochcongar, P.H. Guivarc'h, and Y. Lessard, 1992, "Effects of captopril chronic intake on the aerobic performance and muscle strength of normotensive trained subjects," *International Journal of Sports Medicine* 13 (4): 310.

Table 3.6 Adapted, by permission, from A. Cohen-Solal, S. Baleynaud, T. Laperche, C. Sebag, and R. Gourgon, 1993, "Cardiopulmonary response during exercise of a beta 1-selective beta-blocker (atenolol) and a calcium-channel blocker (diltiazem) in untrained subjects with hypertension," *Journal of Cardiovascular Pharmacology* 22 (1): 35.

Table 5.4 Adapted, by permission, from S.L. Dodd, S.K. Powers, I.S. Vrabas, D. Criswell, S. Stetson, and R. Hussain, 1996, "Effects of clenbuterol on contractile and biochemical properties of skeletal muscle," *Medicine and Science in Sport and Exercise* 28 (2): 669-676.

Table 6.2 Adapted, by permission, from D.M. Crist, G.T. Peake, P.A. Egan, and D.L. Waters, 1988, "Body composition response to exogenous GH during training in highly conditioned adults," *Journal of Applied Physiology* 65 (2): 581.

Table 6.3 Adapted, by permission, from K.E. Yarasheski, J.A. Campbell, K. Smith, M.J. Rennie, J.O. Holloszy, and D.M. Bier, 1992, "Effect of growth hormone and resistance exercise on muscle growth in young men," *American Journal of Physiology* 262: E264.

Table 7.1 Adapted, by permission, from D.A. Smith and P.J. Perry, 1992, "The efficacy of ergogenic agents in athletic competition. Part I: Androgenic-anabolic steroids." *Annals of Pharmacotherapy* 26: 521.

Table 7.3 Reprinted, by permission, from M.H. Williams, 1998, *The Ergogenics Edge* (Champaign, IL: Human Kinetics), 127.

Table 8.1 Adapted, by permission, from L.M. Odland, J.D. MacDougall, M.A. Tarnopolsky, A. Elorriaga, and A. Borgmann, 1997, "Effect of oral creatine supplementation on muscle [PCr] and short-term maximum power output," *Medicine and Science in Sports and Exercise* 29 (2) 216-219.

Table 10.3 Adapted, by permission, from J.H. Wilmore and D.L. Costill, 1999, *Physiology of Sport and Exercise*, 2d ed. (Champaign, IL: Human Kinetics), 117.

Table 10.5 Adapted, by permission, from P.D. Thompson, P.A. Gadaleta, S. Yurgalevitch, E. Cullinane, and P.N. Herbert, 1991, "Effects of exercise and lovastatin on serum creatine kinase activity," *Metabolism* 40 (12): 1334.

Table 10.7 Adapted, by permission, from P.D. Thompson, A.M. Nugent, and P.N. Herbert, 1990, "Increases in creatine kinase after exercise in patients treated with HMG-CoA reductase inhibitors," *JAMA* 264: 2992.

Table 10.8 Adapted, by permission, from P.D. Thompson, P.A. Gadaleta, S. Yurgalevitch, E. Cullinane, and P.N. Herbert, 1991, "Effects of exercise and lovastatin on serum creatine kinase activity," *Metabolism* 40 (12): 1334.

Table 11.1 Adapted, by permission, from Human Kinetics, 1997, *Pharmacology for Athletic Trainers: Therapeutic Medications* (Champaign, IL: Human Kinetics).

Table 12.1 Adapted, by permission, from M.A. Hallmark, T.H. Reynolds, C.A. DeSouza, C.O. Dotson, R.A. Anderson, and M.A. Rogers, 1996, "Effects of chromium and resistive training on muscle strength and body composition," *Medicine and Science in Sports and Exercise* 28 (1): 143.

Table 13.1 Adapted, by permission, from S. Flinn, J. Gregory, L.R. McNaughton, S. Tristram, and P. Davies, 1990, "Caffeine ingestion prior to incremental cycling to exhaustion in recreational cyclists," *International Journal of Sports Medicine* 11 (3): 189.

Table 13.3 Adapted, by permission, from R.J. Fuentes, 1999, *Athletic Drug Reference '99* (Durham, NC: Clean Data/Glaxo Wellcome), 35.

Table 14.1 Adapted, by permission, from J.C. Wagner, 1991, "Enhancement of athletic performance with drugs: An overview," *Sports Medicine* 12 (4): 252.

Table 14.3 Adapted, by permission, from T. Reilly, 1988, Alcohol, anti-anxiety drugs and exercise. In *Drugs in Sport*, edited by D.R. Mottram (Champaign, IL: Human Kinetics), 141.

Table 15.1 Adapted, by permission, from J.V. Chandler and S.N. Blair, 1980, "The effect of amphetamines on selected physiological components related to athletic success," *Medicine and Science in Sports and Exercise* 12:65-69. Reprinted, by permission, from J.H. Wilmore and D.L. Costill, 1999, *Physiology of Sport and Exercise*, 2d ed. (Champaign, IL: Human Kinetics), 418.

Table 16.3 Adapted, by permission, from A. Must, J. Spadano, E.H. Coakley, A.E. Field, G. Colditz, and W.H. Dietz, 1999, "The disease burden associated with overweight and obesity," *JAMA* 282: 1526.

Table 16.5 Adapted, by permission, from B.S. Lewis and W.D. Lynch, 1993, "The effect of physician advice on exercise behavior," *Preventive Medicine* 22: 116.

Acknowledgments

The production of *Sport and Exercise Pharmacology* would not have been possible without the valuable assistance of several people who I would like to recognize:

Dean LaGalla, PharmD, for assisting with literature research;

Lester Bruns, PhD; Christine Crain, PharmD; Randy Hatton, PharmD; David Huang, MD; Larry Lopez, PharmD; Donald Mars, MD; and James Popp, MD, personal and professional colleagues who reviewed various chapters and provided valuable feedback and suggestions;

The staff at Human Kinetics, some of whom I have not met but I know have put a great deal of effort into this project, particularly Anne Heiles for shaping the manuscript; Cynthia McEntire for handling the myriad of details during the production process; Heather Munson for assisting with copyright permissions; and especially Mike Bahrke, PhD, who supervised the long project and answered my endless questions and provided support and encouragement during the process; and, last but not least, Rainer Martens for agreeing to take on this project. Thank you one and all for helping me bring this book to completion.

Finally, I would like to acknowledge certain members of my family, not necessarily because they assisted with the creation of this book, but because they finally committed themselves to quit smoking and start exercising. It is people like them to whom this book is dedicated.

Introduction

Some five years after the U.S. Public Health Service published *Healthy People 2000*, advocating health goals for the nation to achieve by the year 2000, McGinnis and Lee (1995) assessed progress toward getting more Americans to exercise regularly. They found that only 24% of Americans had adopted a regular practice of exercise. Recalling the surge in popularity of fitness centers in the 1980s, one might have expected substantially more people to be engaging in more active lifestyles. In 1994 alone an estimated $8.4 billion was spent on health club memberships in the United States, and these fitness centers make available to the general public a lot of expensive and elaborate equipment previously found only at training facilities for collegiate and professional athletes.

The lack of regular exercise by the general population has staggering health consequences. First, about 12% of deaths reported in the United States each year are attributable simply to a lack of regular physical activity (McGinnis and Foege 1993). McGinnis and Foege (1993) concluded that the combination of poor dietary and exercise habits was the second most prominent contributor to mortality (approximately 300,000 deaths) in the United States in 1990, just behind tobacco use, which claimed about 400,000 lives and just ahead of alcohol use, which took about 100,000 lives. The Cardiovascular Health Study, which evaluated over 5,000 subjects aged 65 and above, concluded that lack of moderate or vigorous exercise was a significant factor in their overall five-year mortality between 1990 and 1995 (Fried et al. 1998). At the other end of the age spectrum, children too seem headed toward a sedentary lifestyle, as watching television and playing computer games fills time that might be spent more actively.

Furthermore, the population is getting older, and the development of potent prescription drugs by pharmaceutical manufacturers has increased dramatically in the 1990s (see table 1). Thus, advanced age, a sedentary lifestyle, and the availability of newer, more potent drugs help explain why drug use is increasing among a significant portion of the population.

To better appreciate the magnitude of drug consumption, it is worth looking at how many drugs are available and how many people use those drugs. More than 100,000 drug products are approved for use in the United States alone. Retail pharmacies in this country dispensed nearly 2.2 billion prescriptions during 1992, according to the National Association of Chain Drug Stores (NACDS). This is the equivalent of

Table 1   New Chemical Entities (NCEs) Approved in the United States

Year	NCEs approved
1994	22
1995	28
1996	53
1997	39
1998	25
1999	25

Data source: U.S. Food and Drug Administration. [Online]. Available: http://www.fda.gov/cder [January 26, 2000].

eight prescriptions per person per year. In 1996 and 1997, roughly 2.3 billion prescriptions were filled; in 1998, the number jumped to 2.8 billion. Each individual spends roughly $50 per year on nonprescription drugs. Ron Ziegler, the president of NACDS, predicts that by 2005 an estimated 4 billion prescriptions will be dispensed annually. The following shows the total dollar amount spent on prescriptions per year:

1995: $50.2 billion

1996: $62.2 billion

1997: $74.3 billion

By the year 2008, the figure is expected to top $180 billion (Blank 1998). And these statistics don't include nonprescription, over-the-counter (OTC) drugs!

Several large surveys have shown that the elderly consume surprisingly large numbers of medications. Persons over age 65 constitute 12% of the population, but they take 25% of all prescription and OTC drugs (Lund and Duthie 1982; Magaziner and Cadigan 1989), and some elderly individuals consume as many as 17 drugs concurrently (Helling et al. 1987; May et al. 1982)! The three largest categories of drugs that the elderly consume are cardiovascular drugs, central nervous system agents, and analgesics or antirheumatics (Chrischilles et al. 1990; Helling et al. 1987; May et al. 1982). The elderly are likely to be taking multiple medications chronically, often including cardiovascular drugs and analgesics.

Age is not the only factor that determines rate of drug use. When elderly runners were compared to age-matched, community control subjects, Fries and colleagues (1994) found that the runners were leaner, reported joint symptoms less frequently, had fewer medical problems, and took fewer medications. Chrischilles and colleagues (1990) also found an inverse relationship between analgesic use and degree of physical functioning in elderly.

Still, otherwise healthy individuals and even elite athletes are consuming medications more regularly than one might assume. The weekend softball player may use an antihistamine for his or her allergic rhinitis. The cross-country skier may require an inhaler for exercise-induced bronchoconstriction. Even elite athletes may require medication for diabetes or asthma, and many are known to consume nonprescription analgesics and anti-inflammatory agents routinely for their aches and pains. McMahon and colleagues (1984) discovered that 17 of 32 marathon runners used either aspirin or nonsteroidal anti-inflammatory drugs around the time of running the race.

Not to be overlooked is the persistent desire of some elite athletes to use ergogenic substances. Despite more rigorous testing for banned substances, athletes continue to go to great lengths to use and abuse substances if these agents appear to be ergogenic. Many examples of this appeared in 1998 alone: Mark McGwire admitted to regularly using androstenedione and creatine during his chase for professional baseball's home run title; the Italian cycling team was caught with 400 vials of the hematinic agent erythropoietin at the Tour de France; and sprinter Florence Griffith Joyner died suddenly, reawakening rumors that she used growth hormone and other performance-enhancing agents.

The popularity of fitness has transcended the baby-boomer generation, and ever more people regard exercise as an essential component of a healthy lifestyle for all age groups. The general public receives health-related information from increasing numbers of sources: the evening news, travel magazines, food labels, and even stories in investment newspapers.

Many newcomers to the fitness scene, however, are deconditioned and may be consuming medications for chronic health ailments. Many wonder, "What risk does exercising bring to my taking medications?" Conversely, many athletes and trainers want to know the impact of various drugs on performance. Sadly, the implications of combining exercise with medication use are often unknown. This issue is not routinely investigated during the clinical testing of a drug prior to its approval by the Food and Drug Administration (FDA). Thus, for many prescription drugs, little to no data exist regarding combining strenuous exercise with drug therapy.

This book addresses several general questions. First, how do drugs and medications affect the physiology and performance of people who are exercising or actively engaged in sport? I examine not only drugs that are well known in sports medicine, such as anabolic steroids, growth hormone, erythropoietin, and creatine, but also some medications used in clinical medicine. Anyone involved in helping people engaged in sport and physical activity should not overlook the impact of therapeutic medications on an individual's ability to exercise.

Most physicians, athletic trainers, and other sports medicine personnel will encounter individuals wanting to exercise who are taking at least one, if not many, medications. There are many questions about how exercise and medications combine. For example, some antihypertensive drugs and some lipid-lowering drugs can adversely affect exercise duration. Should patients taking lovastatin avoid weightlifting since this drug has been associated with muscle injury? Does a marathoner risk additional gastrointestinal (GI) bleeding if she takes NSAIDs before a race? Should the hypertensive patient who is taking a diuretic avoid playing tennis in the hot sun? Further, under certain circumstances, caffeine, androstenedione, and some asthma drugs are banned from use during competition. Competitive athletes will want to know what drugs or supplements could be ergolytic so they can avoid them during training and competition.

The effect of exercise on drug action and, conversely, the effect of the drug on the body's response to exercise are generally poorly understood. These issues are not usually addressed during the preapproval phase of data collection on a new drug. In this book, I consider if additive risks can occur when individuals taking medications subject themselves to strenuous exercise.

Coming at the problem from a different direction, I look at the effects that exercise exerts on drug pharmacokinetics. *Pharmacokinetics* is defined as what the body does to the drug after it is ingested. *Pharmacology* can be defined as the reverse: what the drug does to the body. A change in a drug's pharmacokinetics can affect its pharmacologic action, and exercise may influence the efficacy and incidence of side effects of some drugs. Unfortunately, not enough is yet known in this area to present as complete a discussion as this topic deserves.

■ Why a Book on Pharmacology and Exercise?

Exercise pharmacology is a relatively young science. And like most developing fields or entities, this science's growth is exciting but uneven. Most of this book falls into two lines of thought: How does exercise affect the actions of drugs? How do drugs affect the physiology and performance of exercisers?

Before discussing various categories of drugs and agents in this light, however, I will discuss some of the limitations of the scientific literature on exercise pharmacology.

Better Clinical Research Is Needed

While good information is available on how drugs and exercise interact for some agents, such as beta-blockers or caffeine, the data are quite limited for many other agents. Consider, for example, the effect of epoetin alfa (erythropoietin) on performance in elite cyclists, or the effect on performance of some of the newer respiratory drugs that are used by individuals with exercise-induced bronchoconstriction. While several studies have documented an ergogenic effect of epoetin alfa in anemic hemodialysis patients (Robertson et al. 1990; Guthrie et al. 1993), there are very little data to document its effects in nonanemic elite cyclists. In the case of anabolic steroids, ethical issues prevent studying these agents in doses and in combinations that some athletes use.

The fact is that neither the effects of exercise on the pharmacologic action nor, conversely, the impact of the drug on the body's response to exercise have yet been well studied for many drugs. During clinical trials for a new drug, it is not typical to assess the impact of exercise on that drug's actions—that is, its pharmacokinetics. Furthermore, prior to its approval by the FDA, a drug may have been studied in as few as 1,000 subjects. Data on the combination of exercise with regular use of a particular drug are almost never known until *years after* the drug is approved. This is particularly significant in the case of antihypertensive drugs. Hypertension is pervasive in our society—and well over a hundred individual drugs are available to use in treating hypertension. If the Healthy People initiative succeeds in convincing more sedentary individuals to start exercising, then how these antihypertensive drugs affect exercise tolerance and overall performance becomes quite an important issue.

Moreover, it is important to study drugs and exercise because of potential complications in their interaction. For example, even though preclinical animal studies revealed that ciprofloxacin (a fluoroquinolone antibiotic) could cause cartilage lesions and arthropathy, the issue of tendon rupture in humans was not reported until years after the drug was formally approved. Prescribing fluoroquinolone antibiotics to tennis or racquetball players, aerobics instructors, gymnasts, basketball players, or any other athlete who jumps or abruptly changes direction might not be wise. Similarly, it was years after the popular and highly effective lipid-lowering drug lovastatin had been on the market that its role in myopathy was detected. It is as yet unclear if strenuous exercise exacerbates this problem.

Still another area that needs more research is nutritional supplements. These substances are not regulated as drugs; yet some athletes consume thousands of dollars' worth of these products every year. Much more research is needed on these products! And individuals must realize that these supplements may not contain the amount of particular ingredients printed on their labels.

Considering the number of these agents and other supplements available and consumed, the push to get more deconditioned Americans exercising, and the desire of athletes to use any product that will improve performance, questions, if not physical sequelae, are bound to arise about the interactions of exercise and drugs.

Study Design

The quality and soundness of study design is an important consideration when evaluating a drug for use and looking at its known impact on the response to exercise. For example, the ergolytic effect of beta-blocker therapy during submaximal exercise can be more pronounced after 5 to 6 months of drug administration than after the first month (van Baak et al. 1987). Mode of exercise and type of subjects chosen for the study also can influence interpretation of the results. Even when these variables are held constant, it may not be possible to extrapolate study results from one drug within a class to another (for example, the calcium-channel blockers).

In designing a study or in evaluating the usefulness of a study, the *type of exercise* that is selected is significant; it can influence what drug effects occur as the response. For example, androgenic-anabolic steroids can improve muscular strength (Bhasin et al. 1996), but they do not improve aerobic exercise performance. Sodium bicarbonate and creatine (Williams and Branch 1998) appear to be ergogenic only in situations requiring short bursts of energy; caffeine, on the other hand, is ergogenic only in sustained aerobic exercise. Ethanol impairs running performance in distances of 200 m and higher, but not in the 100 m dash, and the detrimental effects of diuretics on performance in middle-distance running are also proportional to effects on the distance run.

Another significant factor in setting up a study is the *intensity of exercise*. If endurance exercise is chosen as the mode of exercise, should it be maximal exercise or submaximal exercise? Renal responses to aerobic exercise, for instance, are intensity dependent (Freund et al. 1991). If one is interested in measuring the effects of exercise on the pharmacokinetics of a drug, then exercise intensity must be considered. Further, it is important to understand that employing maximal exercise may reveal an ergolytic or ergogenic drug effect not seen during submaximal exercise. Atenolol decreased oxygen uptake ($\dot{V}O_2$) during maximal exercise—but not during submaximal exercise (Derman, Sims, and Noakes 1992). Low-intensity treadmill walking revealed differences in cardiovascular effects between two types of beta-blockers, differences that were not seen at intensity levels approaching $\dot{V}O_2$max in another study (Martin et al. 1989).

Jesek et al. (1990) clearly state that differences in study design are why conflicting results have been seen when the effects of beta-blockers on lipolysis were assessed. They point out that exercise protocols in these studies fall into four general types:

1. steady-state submaximal exercise;
2. exercise to exhaustion at a fixed heart rate or a fixed percent of $\dot{V}O_2$max;
3. graded exercise tests where the work rate is increased at a specific interval until a predetermined limit is attained; and
4. a combination of steady-state and graded exercise tests in which subjects are exercised to exhaustion.

Yet another consideration is that the majority of the exercising population seldom exercise at a maximal level; thus, it can be difficult to extrapolate conclusions to the deconditioned population from studies that utilize subjects tested at maximal exercise.

Study Subjects

Clearly, it is important in evaluating the usefulness of a study or in planning its design to scrutinize the type of subjects that investigators choose to include. As examples, diabetic (Roy et al. 1989) and hypertensive (Chick, Halperin, and Gacek 1988) patients do not show the same cardiovascular responses to exercise as do normal subjects. Trained athletes rely more on free fatty acids (FFAs) as an energy substrate than untrained subjects do (Holloszy et al. 1977), and these trained subjects may be affected more by drugs that influence the process of lipolysis (Jesek et al. 1990). As mentioned in chapter 13, for example, when studying caffeine, the response will depend on whether naive or tolerant subjects are used. Because exercise is a recommended component of therapy for some disease states, and we want to know what impact exercise has on the actions of drugs, data must be generated in subjects who have the disease for which the drug is indicated (i.e., not normal volunteers). Regarding the complications of exercising while taking drugs, young, healthy volunteers may not be as susceptible to lovastatin-induced myopathy (Reust, Curry, and Guidry 1991) as are older males with hyperlipidemia (Thompson et al. 1991). And there is no sense or relevance in trying to extrapolate the effects of erythropoietin (epoetin alfa) in anemic dialysis patients to its effects on the athletic performance of elite (nonanemic) cyclists. These discrepancies underscore the risk of extrapolating data obtained from young, healthy subjects to other patient populations.

Sport and Exercise Pharmacology

Pharmacokinetic Issues

A further area that must be examined when interpreting the effects of drugs on the exercise response is their pharmacokinetics. Exercise specialists who are not well versed in drug pharmacokinetics should keep in mind that data generated from single-dose studies do not always predict what will happen during chronic dosing. The extremely long half-life of drugs such as amiodarone or astemizole means that several weeks of regular administration are necessary before the full effects of the drug can be expected.

In addition, some drugs have a delayed onset or a very short duration of action. The peak effects of caffeine on FFA concentrations, for example, occur about 3 to 4 hours after a dose, despite the fact that caffeine serum concentrations peak within 15 to 45 minutes after a dose. If study measurements are obtained either before or after the clinical effects of the drug are maximal, the investigators could miss a relevant effect. Conversely, the effects of epoetin alfa can last for a week after use of the drug is stopped. Thus, the timing of study measurements in relationship to the peak activity of the drug is an important variable in drug-exercise studies.

In summary, with many drug-exercise studies, additional data are needed before a clinician can evaluate the relevance for deconditioned subjects using a medication or for athletes who experiment with supplements to enhance performance. And additional data are needed for many individual types of therapeutic agents.

References

Bhasin, S., Storer, T.W., Berman, N., Callegari, C., Clevenger, B., Phillips, J., Bunnell, T.J., Tricker, R., Shirazi, A., and Casaburi, R. 1996. The effects of supraphysiological doses of testosterone on muscle size and strength in normal men. *N Engl J Med* 335:1-7.

Blank, C. 1998. *Hospital Pharmacist Report*, November, 54.

Chick, T.W., Halperin, A.K., and Gacek, E.M. 1988. The effect of antihypertensive medications on exercise performance: A review. *Med Sci Sports Exerc* 20:447-454.

Chrischilles, E.A., Lemke, J.H., Wallace, R.B., and Drube, G.A. 1990. Prevalence and characteristics of multiple analgesic drug use in an elderly study group. *J Am Geriatr Soc* 38:979-984.

Derman, W.E., Sims, R., and Noakes, T.D. 1992. The effects of antihypertensive medications on the physiological response to maximal exercise testing. *J Cardiovasc Pharmacol* 19(suppl 5):S122-S127.

Freund, B.J., Shizuru, E.M., Hashiro, G.M., and Claybaugh, J.R. 1991. Hormonal, electrolyte, and renal responses to exercise are intensity dependent. *J Appl Physiol* 70:900-906.

Fried, L.P., Kronmal, R.A., Newman, A.B., Bild, D.E, Mittelmark, M.B., Polak, J.F., Robbins, J.A., and Gardin, J.M. 1998. Risk factors for 5-year mortality in older adults. The Cardiovascular Health Study. *JAMA* 279:585-592.

Fries, J.F., Singh, G., Morfeld, D., Hubert, H.B., Lane, N.E., and Brown, B.W. 1994. Running and the development of disability with age. *Ann Intern Med* 121:502-509.

Guthrie, M., Cardenas, D., Eschbach, J.W., Haley, N.R., Robertson, H.T., and Evans, R.W. 1993. Effects of erythropoietin on strength and functional status of patients on hemodialysis. *Clin Nephrol* 39:97-102.

Helling, D.K., Lemke, J.H., Semla, T.P., Wallace, R.B., Lipson, D.P., and Cornoni-Huntley, J. 1987. Medication use characteristics in the elderly: The Iowa 65+ Rural Health Study. *J Am Geriatr Soc* 35:4-12.

Holloszy, J.O., Rennie, M.J., Hickson, R.C., Conlee, R.K., and Hagberg, J.M. 1977. Physiological consequences of the biochemical adaptations to endurance exercise. *Ann NY Acad Sci* 301:440-450.

Jesek, J.K., Martin, N.B., Broeder, C.E., Thomas, E.L., Wambsgans, K.C., Hofman, Z., Ivy, J.L., and Wilmore, J.H. 1990. Changes in plasma free fatty acids and glycerols during prolonged exercise in trained and hypertensive persons taking propranolol and pindolol. *Am J Cardiol* 66:1336-1341.

Lund, M.D., and Duthie, E.H. 1982. Drug usage in the elderly. *Wisconsin Med J* 81(8):21-25.

Magaziner, J., and Cadigan, D.A. 1989. Community resources and mental health of older women living alone. *J Aging Health* 1(1):35-49.

Martin, N.B., Broeder, C.E., Thomas, E.L., Wambsgans, K.C., Scruggs, K.D., Jesek, J.K., Hofman, Z., and Wilmore, J.H. 1989. Comparison of the effects of pindolol and propranolol on exercise performance in young men with systemic hypertension. *Am J Cardiol* 64:343-347.

May, F.E., Stewart, R.B., Hale, W.E., and Marks, R.G. 1982. Prescribed and nonprescribed drug use in an ambulatory elderly population. *South Med J* 75(5):522-528.

McGinnis, J.M., and Foege, W.H. 1993. Actual causes of death in the United States. *JAMA* 270:2207-2212.

McGinnis, J.M., and Lee, P.R. 1995. Healthy People 2000 at mid decade. *JAMA* 273:1123-1129.

McMahon, L.F., Ryan, M.J., Larson, D., and Fisher, R.L. 1984. Occult gastrointestinal blood loss in marathon runners. *Ann Intern Med* 100:846-847.

Reust, C.S., Curry, S.C., and Guidry, J.R. 1991. Lovastatin use and muscle damage in healthy volunteers undergoing eccentric muscle exercise. *West J Med* 154:198-200.

Robertson, H.T., Haley, N.R., Guthrie, M., Cardenas, D., Eschbach, J.W., and Adamson, J.W. 1990. Recombinant erythropoietin improves exercise capacity in anemic hemodialysis patients. *Am J Kidney Dis* 25:325-332.

Roy, T.M., Peterson, H.R., Snider, H.L., Cyrus, J., Broadstone, V.L., Fell, R.D., Rothchild, A.H., Samols, E., and Pfeifer, M.A. 1989. Autonomic influence on cardiovascular performance in diabetic subjects. *Am J Med* 87:382-388.

Thompson, P.D., Gadaleta, P.A., Yurgalevitch, S., Cullinane, E., and Herber, P.N. 1991. Effects of exercise and lovastatin on serum creatine kinase activity. *Metabolism* 40:1333-1336.

Van Baak, M.A., Bohn, R.O., Arends, B.G., van Hooff, M.E., and Rahn, K.H. 1987. Long-term antihypertensive therapy with beta-blockers: Submaximal exercise capacity and metabolic effects during exercise. *Int J Sports Med* 8:342-347.

Williams, M.H., and Branch, J.D. 1998. Creatine supplementation and exercise performance: An update. *J Am Coll Nutr* 17:216-234.

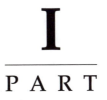

I

PART

Cardiopulmonary Agents

1

CHAPTER

Beta-Receptor Antagonists (Beta-Blockers)

■ *CASE*   Bill is a 59-year-old, deconditioned executive who is taking propranolol for hypertension. He tells you that he wants to start a new exercise program that includes jogging, and he asks for your advice about exercising while taking this medication. You wonder if the propranolol will affect his ability to exercise. What do you tell him?

■ *COMMENT*   Exercising while taking a "beta-blocker," as this drug is commonly called, presents a variety of issues to consider. Beta-blockers slow both resting and exercise heart rate, making it difficult to determine exercise intensity and target heart rate. Since these drugs lower blood pressure, the hypotensive effects of the drug may be additive to those produced by exercise itself. Beta-blockers can also affect energy metabolism and may, therefore, adversely affect exercise duration. Bill should not be discouraged from exercising. Instead, he should be counseled on these issues and monitored carefully during each exercise session. His physician may want to consider alternative choices of drug therapy for treating his hypertension.

Drugs known as beta-blockers antagonize beta-adrenergic (i.e., sympathetic) receptors found throughout the body. Clinically, these drugs are used to treat a variety of conditions, including hypertension, angina, cardiac arrhythmias, anxiety, tremor, and migraine headache. Thus, beta-blockers have a lucrative market and, as a result, drug companies have developed many beta-blocker compounds to satisfy this market (see table 1.1). Today, no fewer than 14 different beta-blockers have been approved for use in clinical medicine in the United States. Pharmaceutical companies have produced nearly every imaginable type of beta-blocker, and it is helpful to know what subgroup each one belongs to. Table 1.1 summarizes beta-blockers. The characteristics known as intrinsic sympathomimetic activity (ISA) and cardioselectivity are discussed later.

Unfortunately, beta-blockers exert ergolytic effects on exercise performance. Beta-blockers are more detrimental on exercise performance than other antihypertensive drugs in both hypertensive (Mooy et al. 1987; Thompson et al. 1989; Vanhees et al. 1991) and normotensive (Bouckaert, Lefebvre, and Pannier 1989; Derman, Sims, and Noakes 1992; Herbertsson and Fagher 1990) exercising subjects. As a result, experts in sports medicine suggest that patients with hypertension

Table 1.1   Beta-Blockers

	Cardioselective	Noncardioselective
With ISA*	Acebutolol[+]	Carteolol[++]
	(Celiprolol)	(Mepindolol)
	(Practolol)	(Oxprenolol)
		Penbutolol[+]
		Pindolol[+++]
Without ISA	Atenolol	Carvedilol
	Betaxolol	Labetalol
	Bisoprolol	Nadolol
	Metoprolol	Propranolol
		Sotalol
		Timolol

*ISA: intrinsic sympathomimetic activity
[+]minimal ISA
[++]moderate ISA
[+++]substantial ISA

Drugs listed in parentheses are not yet approved for use in the United States.

avoid this class of drug (van Baak 1994); but since beta-blockers have many cardiovascular and noncardiovascular uses, they are likely to be widely prescribed in clinical medicine for many years to come. Even though use of beta-blockers for the treatment of hypertension in the elderly has been discouraged (Messerli, Grossman, and Goldbourt 1998), the latest recommendations from the Joint National Committee on the Prevention, Detection, Evaluation, and Treatment of High Blood Pressure (National Institutes of Health [NIH] 1997) continue to recommend beta-blockers as a first-line agent for treating hypertension. Thus, it is likely you will encounter athletes who use beta-blockers. If you are a physician, you are likely to be counseling patients taking beta-blockers who want to exercise. Clinicians generally recommend drug categories other than beta-blockers when treating hypertension and prescribing an exercise regimen (Jacober and Sowers 1995). Other types of antihypertensive agents are discussed in chapter 3.

Commercially available beta-blockers can be subdivided into four categories, based on whether or not they possess intrinsic sympathomimetic activity and whether or not they are cardioselective. *Intrinsic sympathomimetic activity* (ISA) describes a beta-blocker's property of exerting low-level agonism (i.e., stimulation) at the receptor while simultaneously blocking the ability of endogenous catecholamines (e.g., epinephrine) to bind to the receptor. The agonist (i.e., sympathomimetic) properties of these beta-blockers are less significant, however, than their antagonist effects.

Beta-blockers having ISA are less potent agonists than either endogenous catecholamines or another class of drugs referred to as *beta-agonists* (see chapter 5). Because agonism by beta-blockers with ISA is mild, relative to their blocking ability, and because stimulation at the receptor is far less potent for these drugs than for true beta-agonists, these drugs are referred to as *beta-blockers with ISA* and not as beta-agonists. Clinically, beta-blockers with ISA are useful for patients who require high doses of the drug but develop bothersome bradycardia at these high doses. In sports medicine applications, the ISA property may benefit some athletes who have a low resting heart rate (HR) and require therapy with a beta-blocker.

A *cardioselective* beta-blocker is one that exerts its effects preferentially on the beta-1-receptor subtype more than on the beta-2 subtype. In the heart and kidney, beta-receptors are predominantly of the beta-1 subtype, whereas in the lung, arterioles, and gastrointestinal (GI) tract beta-receptors are mostly the beta-2-receptor subtype. In the heart, positive inotropic and chronotropic effects are mediated via stimulation at the beta-1 receptor. In the lung, however, stimulation of beta-2 receptors produces smooth muscle relaxation and bronchodilation. Antagonism at the bronchiolar beta-receptor inhibits bronchodilation.

Thus, a cardioselective beta-blocker has some advantage over a nonselective beta-blocker for patients with asthma, although most clinicians would probably avoid using any beta-blocker in patients with asthma. Beta-blockers also are typically avoided in patients with diabetes mellitus, since beta-blockers can mask the symptoms of hypoglycemia. The hydrolysis of muscle triglycerides as an energy source during prolonged exercise appears to be mediated by beta-2 receptors (Cleroux et al. 1989), thus representing another potential advantage of cardioselective agents over nonselective ones.

How Exercise Affects the Action of Beta-Blockers

Exercise affects both the pharmacokinetics and pharmacology of beta-blockers. Pharmacokinetics is the science of what the body does to the drug once it is introduced. Pharmacology is the science of what the drug does to the body. When the clearance (i.e., removal) of a drug from the circulation is highly dependent on blood flow to the organ responsible for removal (e.g., liver, kidney), we say that such a drug is "flow-limited." Exercise is one factor that can influence the clearance of some drugs, since blood flow to these organs decreases during exercise (Dossing 1985; Somani et al. 1990; van Baak 1990). Thus, exercise can influence the actions of some drugs. This may occur by influencing either their pharmacology or their pharmacokinetics. Beta-blockers that are flow-limited include the following:

acebutolol	metoprolol	sotalol
alprenolol	nadolol	timolol
atenolol	pindolol	
labetalol	propranolol	

Effects on Pharmacokinetics

Data on the effects of exercise on the clearance of beta-blockers are limited and contradictory. Some data (Arends et al. 1986; Frank, Somani, and Kohnle 1990) show that exercise decreases propranolol half-life and area-under-the-curve, but that clearance itself is not affected, despite the fact that hepatic blood flow (measured by indocyanine green clearance) decreases. Both studies evaluated the effects of exercise on single doses of propranolol. When the effects of 16 weeks of aerobic training on propranolol pharmacokinetics were assessed, no differences were seen (Panton et al. 1995). Van Baak, Mooij, and Schiffers (1992) found that 25 minutes of exercise at 70% maximum aerobic power (Wmax) decreased volume of distribution for propranolol, but not for atenolol. In addition to decreases in blood flow to organs responsible for clearance, changes in factors such as bioavailability, protein binding, bile flow, state of hydration, and perhaps other factors may explain the variable effects on propranolol clearance. What impact these observations should have on the clinical response to any of the beta-blockers is unclear. Somani (1996) has thoroughly reviewed the scientific literature regarding the effects of exercise on drug pharmacokinetics; however, van Baak puts the issue in perspective:

> The chance of a clinically relevant effect of exercise on the pharmacokinetics of a particular drug is largest in those with a steep dose-response curve, a narrow therapeutic index, a need for continuity of therapeutic effectiveness and a relatively short half-life, in combination with intensive exercise of long duration. (van Baak 1990, p. 32)

Effects on Pharmacology

Exercise affects the action of beta-blockers on several organ systems, primarily the cardiovascular and pulmonary systems. In this section we will look at the cardiovascular and the metabolic effects separately.

Cardiovascular Actions

Beta-blockers interfere with the sympathetic nervous system, while exercise stimulates sympathetic tone. Exercise induces a positive chronotropic and inotropic effect on the heart, whereas beta-blockers exert a negative chronotropic and inotropic effect.

Are the actions of these drugs abolished during exercise? In theory, exercise should potentiate the clinical effects of beta-blockers that are flow-limited, since the clearance of these drugs would decrease during acute exercise. But because the changes seen in beta-blocker pharmacokinetics with exercise are variable, it is impossible to predict the effect of exercise on the pharmacologic action of these drugs. In general, and unlike drugs known as digitalis glycosides, exercise does not override the negative chronotropic effects of beta-blockers on the heart in elite athletes (Anderson et al. 1985), in hypertensive patients (Martin et al. 1989), or even in patients with documented supraventricular arrhythmias (Huikuri, Koistenen, and Takkunen 1992). The effects of physical training did not compromise either the antihypertensive or the bradycardic response to high-dose atenolol in men with mild hypertension (Leenen et al. 1980).

Metabolic Actions

In clinical medicine, beta-blockers without ISA exert unfavorable changes in serum lipids. Beta-blockers with ISA properties (e.g., pindolol), however, exert neutral or slightly favorable effects on serum lipids (Houston 1989). Duncan and colleagues (1989) found that when hypertensive patients receiving beta-blockers were subjected to 20 weeks of exercise conditioning (the subjects walked or jogged 3 times a week), exercise training offset the detrimental effects of therapy with a non-ISA beta-blocker (propranolol) on lipoprotein metabolism and that the beneficial effects of therapy with an ISA+ beta-blocker (pindolol) did not seem to be synergistic. The beneficial effects of the ISA property seen in sedentary hypertensives disappeared when subjects were exercise trained. The effects of beta-blocker drugs on exercise metabolism have been thoroughly reviewed by Head (1999) and will be discussed in more detail below.

How Beta-Blockers Affect Exercisers

Many interrelated responses are innervated via the sympathetic system. The sympathetic nervous system mediates the fight-or-flight response. Thus, it should not be surprising that beta-blockers, drugs that interfere with a major division of the autonomic nervous system, affect many aspects of exercise physiology. For example, beta-blockers oppose the stimulatory actions of endogenous catecholamines (e.g., epinephrine, norepinephrine) at adrenergic beta-receptors. In addition, training-induced changes in plasma catecholamines are blunted during beta-blockade (Wolfel et al. 1990). Table 1.2 briefly summarizes the physiologic responses to beta-adrenergic stimulation.

The obvious conclusion one might draw is that beta-blockers produce physiologic effects that are exactly the opposite of those mediated via sympathetic stimulation. Yet this conclusion is not entirely accurate. For example, hepatic glycogenolysis and gluconeogenesis respond not only to neuronal pathways (i.e., epinephrine-mediated sympathetic stimulation) but also to hormonal stimuli (e.g., cortisol, growth hormone) (Kjaer 1995).

Recently researchers have identified a third subtype of beta-receptor (e.g., beta-3). Though many questions remain, the data indicate that beta-3 receptors may be involved in the development of obesity (Clement et al. 1995). A discussion of issues related to beta-3 receptors is not included because commercially available beta-blocking drugs aren't known to possess activity at this receptor.

The effects of beta-blockers on exercise physiology are diverse. This topic has been thoroughly reviewed by van Baak (1988, 1994) and Head (1999).

Table 1.2   Physiologic Responses to Beta-Adrenergic Stimulation

Organ	Response	Beta-receptor subtype
Heart	Positive chronotropic effect	Beta-1
	Positive inotropic effect	Beta-1
	Increased conduction velocity	Beta-1
	Increased automaticity	Beta-1
Lung	Bronchial smooth muscle relaxation	Beta-2
GI tract	Decreased mobility and tone	Beta-2
Liver	Stimulation of glycogenolysis and gluconeogenesis	Beta-2
Pancreas	Stimulation of glucagon secretion	Beta-2
Kidney	Increased renin secretion	Beta-1
Skeletal muscle	Increased contractility	Beta-2
	Stimulation of glycogenolysis	Beta-2
	Stimulation of triglyceride hydrolysis	Beta-2
	Intracellular potassium uptake	Beta-2
Adipose tissue	Stimulation of lipolysis	Beta-1

Beta-Blocker Effects on the Cardiovascular System

It is the job of the cardiovascular system, together with the respiratory system, to deliver oxygen to exercising muscles. Oxygen uptake at maximal exercise, or $\dot{V}O_2$max, is a measurement of aerobic work. Changes in $\dot{V}O_2$max are used to monitor the progression of fitness. Many investigators measure $\dot{V}O_2$max to assess the effects of drugs on the exercise response. $\dot{V}O_2$max, as determined by the Fick equation, is based on cardiac output and the difference in oxygen concentration between the arterial and venous pulmonary circulation:

$$\dot{V}O_2\text{max} = \text{COmax} \times (P_vO_2 - P_aO_2)\text{max}$$

Cardiac output, in turn, is calculated from heart rate and stroke volume:

$$CO = HR \times SV$$

Therefore, HR, SV, cardiac output, and $\dot{V}O_2$ are all parameters that can describe or affect oxygen utilization during exercise. The effect of drugs on exercise HR is important, if for no other reason than to monitor exercise intensity and determine the target HR. The data in this chapter, unless specifically indicated otherwise, were obtained from subjects with normal sinus rhythm.

Heart Rate

Heart rate is readily used as a barometer of exercise intensity and can be easily monitored by either the subject or an athletic trainer. According to the Karvonen formula (Karvonen, Kentala, and Mustala 1957), resting HR is used to derive target HR. In contrast, exercise HR is the basis for Borg's ratings of perceived exertion (RPE) scale (Borg 1970). In general, beta-blockers decrease both resting and exercise HR. Combining these medications with exercise can impact, either directly or indirectly, the specialist's ability to design and monitor an exercise regimen.

Resting heart rate. Resting HR is influenced mainly by the degree of tone of the parasympathetic and sympathetic nervous systems and the circulating levels of catecholamines. At rates lower than 100 beats/min, the sympathetic nervous system contributes relatively less to HR than does the parasympathetic system. A gradual decrease in vagal activity is responsible for the rise in HR up to about 100 beats/min. At this point, the levels of circulating norepinephrine rise and continue to increase as HR rises above 100 beats/min. This physiology is important to keep in mind when discussing how beta-blockers and other drugs affect exercise HR.

It is not surprising, then, that drugs with anticholinergic properties are most likely to affect resting HR, whereas drugs active at beta-adrenergic receptors affect both resting and exercise HR. It is worthwhile to consider differences in HRs between trained and untrained subjects, since, in general, elite athletes have a slower resting HR than untrained subjects. Leenen and colleagues (1980) also demonstrated these differences in hypertensive subjects (see figure 1.1).

Heart rate response may also vary among the different beta-blocker subtypes (see table 1.1). Beta-blockers with ISA do not decrease resting HR as much as beta-blockers without this property. Resting HR was lower in healthy normal volunteers (Ades et al. 1984), in hypertensive subjects (Martin et al. 1989), and in patients with stable angina (Magder et al. 1987) after being given a non-ISA beta-blocker (e.g., propranolol) than after being given a beta-blocker with ISA (e.g., pindolol).

The characteristic of beta-blockers with ISA producing less of a decrease in resting HR than beta-blockers without this property can be clinically significant in exercising patients who require beta-blocker therapy. It is well known that resting HR decreases as aerobic fitness improves. This is probably a compensatory response to the increase in SV and $\dot{V}O_2$ that occurs. Symptomatic bradycardia at rest developed in hypertensive patients, who subsequently participated in an aerobic

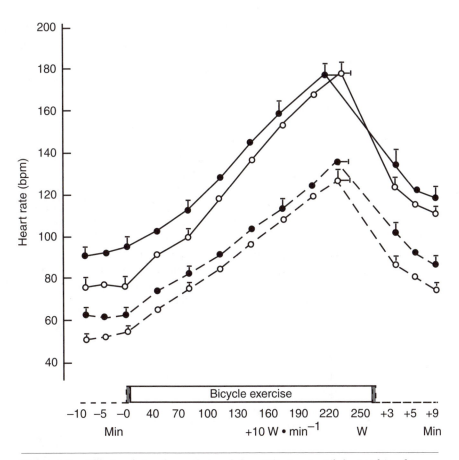

Figure 1.1   Effects of placebo and atenolol on HR at rest and during bicycle exercise to exhaustion in untrained and trained mildly hypertensive men. Values are mean ± *SEM*. ● = untrained group (*n* = 5); ○ = trained group (*n* = 7); —— = placebo; – – – = atenolol 100 mg.

Adapted from Leenen 1980.

conditioning program, stabilized on a non-ISA beta-blocker (i.e., atenolol). As fitness level improved, resting HR decreased in these subjects (Davies et al. 1989). Bradycardia may have been avoided if a beta-blocker with ISA properties (e.g., pindolol) had been used instead of atenolol, which does not possess ISA properties.

Exercise heart rate.   Compared with placebo, all types of beta-blockers, even in low doses, reduce HR during exercise. Since most subjects do not exercise at their $\dot{V}O_2$max, the exercise HR while receiving beta-blocker therapy rarely exceeds 120-130 beats/min, even when a beta-blocker with ISA properties is administered (Krumke et al. 1991). In elite runners, maximum HR is still lower while receiving beta-blockade compared to placebo (Anderson et al. 1985). However, differences exist among the various categories of beta-blockers. Regarding the property of ISA, ISA+ beta-blockers (e.g., pindolol) do not depress exercise HR as much as do non-ISA beta-blockers (e.g., propranolol), although this difference disappears as exercise intensity increases to high levels. These findings have also been observed in normotensive subjects during treadmill exercise to exhaustion (figure 1.2) (Ades et al. 1984) and during isometric exercise (Rapola et al. 1990), as well as in patients with hypertension (Martin et al. 1989). As exercise becomes more intense, the property of ISA becomes obscured, perhaps due to the heightened sympathetic tone (i.e., high circulating levels of catecholamines).

Conversely, the differences between cardioselective and noncardioselective beta-blockers on HR are seen mostly during maximal exercise. Sorensen, Jensen, and Faergeman (1991) postulated that, at lower levels of exercise, the HR increases in response to norepinephrine acting via beta-1 receptors. In contrast, at extreme levels of exercise the

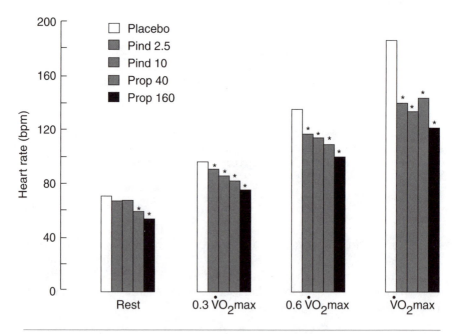

Figure 1.2   Changes in HR with pindolol (Pind) and propranolol (Prop) at rest and during exercise. * = $p < 0.05$ compared to placebo; $\dot{V}O_2$max = maximal oxygen consumption.

Adapted from Ades et al. 1984.

heart responds to epinephrine acting mainly via beta-2 receptors (Sorensen, Jensen, and Faergeman 1991). Since epinephrine stimulates both beta-1 and beta-2 receptors, the actions of epinephrine on the heart are inhibited less by cardioselective agents than by noncardioselective beta-blockers. In single-dose studies, cardioselective beta-blockers did not depress exercise HR as much as did noncardioselective beta-blockers. The difference ranged from 12 to 15 beats/min, but these differences were significant only at maximal exercise (see table 1.3) (Laustiola et al. 1983; Sorensen, Jensen, and Faergeman 1991). Cardioselective agents also suppress maximal exercise HR less than ISA-containing beta-blockers (Erikssen et al. 1982). When exercise is kept at 50% $\dot{V}O_2$max, no differences are seen on exercise HR between these types of beta-blockers (Lundborg et al. 1981). These studies were all short-term ones. When beta-blockers were administered for 5 to 6 months in hypertensive subjects, however, no differences were seen between a cardioselective agent (metoprolol), a drug with ISA activity (pindolol), and a non-cardioselective, non-ISA drug (propranolol) in effect on HR during cycling at 70% $\dot{V}O_2$max (van Baak et al. 1987).

In the setting of isometric exercise, the cardiovascular response during beta-blockade is variable (although the data are limited for this situation). Exercise HR was slightly less when a cardioselective beta-blocker without ISA (atenolol) was compared to a noncardioselective

Table 1.3   Effect of Beta-Blockade on Mean HR During Maximal Exercise

	Heart rate (beats/min)			
	Placebo	Atenolol	Practolol	Propranolol
After treatment at rest	67	59	71	63
Exercise				
30 minutes	132	102[b]	105[b]	100[b]
60 minutes	136	110[b]	109[b]	105[b]
Exhaustion	151	119[b, c]	113[b]	104[b]
Recovery				
15 minutes	86	72[a]	74[a]	63[b]
30 minutes	83	73[a]	72[a]	65[b]

Control value 67 indicates mean of pooled measurements at rest before treatment. $n = 6$; [a]$p < 0.05$; [b]$p < 0.01$ vs. placebo; [c]$p < 0.05$ vs. propranolol.

Adapted from Laustiola et al. 1983.

agent with ISA properties (mepindolol) during a 3 min sustained handgrip test (Fogari et al. 1982). Extrapolating these findings to subjects during heavy weightlifting exercise may be difficult since the handgrip test involves only a 30% maximal voluntary contraction. These authors also noted significant differences in the response to beta-blockade when short-term therapy was compared with long-term therapy (Fogari, Zoppi, and Orlandi 1985).

In short, although all beta-blockers suppress HR, distinctions do exist. These may appear only in specific settings, however: beta-blockers with the ISA property do not depress resting HR as much as other types of beta-blockers do, while cardioselective beta-blockers do not suppress maximal HR as much as noncardioselective types. Clinicians should note that short-term (i.e., 1 to 2 days) use of beta-blockers does not predict the cardiovascular response seen with long-term (i.e., 5 to 6 months) use (Fogari, Zoppi, and Orlandi 1985; van Baak et al. 1987). Although there is a correlation between HR reductions and decreases in $\dot{V}O_2$ (van Baak 1994), the effects of beta-blockers on HR do not predict their effect on either running performance (Kaiser 1982) or mobilization of energy substrates (Head, Maxwell, and Kendall 1997).

■ *Monitoring Exercise Intensity During Beta-Blockade*

The athletic trainer needs to understand how beta-blockers affect the determination of target HR, since these drugs affect both resting and exercise HR. Responses to beta-blockade may vary slightly, depending on the specific characteristics of the beta-blocker. For example, at rest the ISA properties are apparent, although the maximal HR is where the cardioselectivity property is most apparent.

Using the Karvonen formula, the target HR for a 55-year-old patient (with a resting HR of 90) who is exercising at 70% intensity is 142. However, the target HR becomes 130 if the resting HR is only 50, as might be seen in a patient taking a beta-blocker. Even though the lower resting HR is accounted for by the Karvonen formula, the target HR may still be higher than the subject can attain while receiving a beta-blocker. Even at $\dot{V}O_2$max, maximum HRs higher than 120 to 130 beats/min during beta-blockade are uncommon in either normotensive (Ades et al. 1984, 1989; Cleroux et al. 1989) or hypertensive subjects (Cohen-Solal et al. 1993; Leenen et al. 1980; Martin et al. 1989). In subjects taking beta-blocker drugs, it appears that RPE values remain a good indicator of workload intensity, keeping in mind that noncardioselective beta-blockers increase RPE more than cardioselective agents (Eston et al. 1996).

Cardiac Output

Regarding the effects different types of beta-blockers have on exercise cardiac output, the data are conflicting. Perhaps this is explained by differences between hypertensive and normotensive subjects (van Baak, Koene, and Verstappen 1988) or differences among types of beta-blockers. Subjects taking pindolol (noncardioselective and ISA+) were compared with ones taking propranolol (noncardioselective and without ISA) at different exercise intensities. During low-intensity exercise (2 h walks at 25% and 45% of $\dot{V}O_2$max), researchers did not find differences in the effects of the two beta-blockers (Broeder et al. 1993). On the other hand, during submaximal exercise at 70% $\dot{V}O_2$max, cardiac output during exercise in the presence of pindolol was not different from placebo but was significantly lower in the presence of propranolol (see figure 1.3) (Ades 1987). In another study, hypertensive and normotensive subjects who took atenolol for 3 days reduced exercise cardiac output, compared to baseline (van Baak, Koene, and Verstappen 1988). Scruggs and colleagues (1991) showed that beta-blockade had no effect on cardiac output at various intensities of submaximal exercise, regardless of whether normotensives or hypertensives were studied, and regardless of whether ISA+ agents were used or not. Given these data, it is impossible to draw firm conclusions regarding the effects of beta-blockers on cardiac output during exercise.

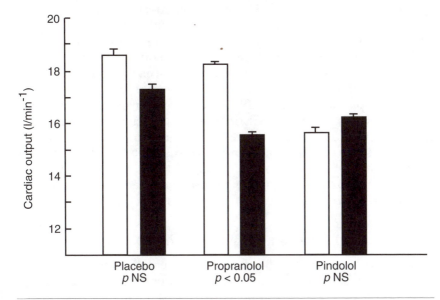

Figure 1.3   Cardiac output (mean ± *SE* mean) during submaximal exercise (0.7 percent $\dot{V}O_2$max). □ = predrug; ■ = on drug.

Adapted from Ades 1987.

Blood Pressure

It is beyond the scope of this discussion to summarize the effects of beta-blockers on blood pressure (BP). Beta-blockers of all types reduce the rate-pressure product during exercise (Caruso et al. 1986), and clinicians consider the hemodynamic profile of beta-blockers during exercise to be less favorable than that of other antihypertensive agents (Houston 1989; Jacober et al. 1995) despite the fact that the guidelines from the Sixth Joint National Committee on the Prevention, Evaluation, and Treatment of High Blood Pressure (JNC VI) continue to recommend beta-blockers as first-line therapy (NIH 1997). Variables such as dose, types of subjects, and concomitant disease states and/or drug therapy can all affect the BP response during beta-blocker administration. Duration of drug therapy is also an important variable: both exercise BP (Fogari, Zoppi, and Orlandi 1985) and exercise performance (van Baak et al. 1987) are more dramatically affected after several months of beta-blocker therapy than at the beginning. Finally, exercise BP and peripheral vascular resistance are higher in hypertensive subjects than in normotensives (van Baak, Koene, and Verstappen 1988).

When hypertensive subjects exercised on a bicycle ergometer at 70% $\dot{V}O_2$max after 6 months of treatment with a cardioselective (metoprolol), noncardioselective (propranolol), or beta-blockade with an ISA (pindolol) agent, no differences were seen among drugs in the effect on resting and exercise BP (van Baak et al. 1987). When isometric handgrip was used as the exercise, both a cardioselective, non-ISA (atenolol) agent (Orlandi and Fogari 1983) and a noncardioselective, ISA+ (mepindolol—not available in the U.S.) agent (Fogari et al. 1982) suppressed the rise in BP in patients with essential hypertension; however, the response during the first month of drug therapy differed from that seen after 6 months (Fogari, Zoppi, and Orlandi 1985). Antihypertensives of the angiotensin-converting enzyme (ACE) inhibitor and calcium-channel blocker groups appear to attenuate the pressor response to sustained handgrip more effectively than beta-blockers (Cleroux et al. 1994). These findings may be difficult to extrapolate to weightlifting: brachial artery BPs during heavy weightlifting have been documented to rise as high as 480/350 in one bodybuilder during leg press (MacDougall et al. 1985)!

Beta-Blocker Effects on Pulmonary Physiology

It is well known that beta-blockers can exacerbate asthma, and these drugs should be avoided in athletes who suffer from exercise-induced bronchoconstriction. This issue is discussed in more detail in the bronchodilators chapter (see chapter 5). What happens to lung function when nonasthmatics exercise while taking beta-blockers? Although data are limited, it appears that exercise intensity may influence determining the effect of beta-blockers on pulmonary physiology during exercise. At $\dot{V}O_2$max, neither atenolol (cardioselective) (Cohen-Solal et al. 1993; Gordon 1985) nor propranolol (noncardioselective) (Petersen et al. 1983) affected pulmonary physiology. However, when subjects exercised at 60% $\dot{V}O_2$max, both atenolol and propranolol depressed peak expiratory flow rate and tidal volume, which were compensated for by an increase in respiratory rate (McLeod et al. 1985). A similar response to atenolol was seen in trained athletes when tested at 70% $\dot{V}O_2$ and $\dot{V}O_2$max; at 70% of $\dot{V}O_2$max, atenolol was associated with a significantly higher minute ventilation than was a placebo (McLenachan et al. 1991). These data are relevant for all persons, since the majority of us do not exercise at $\dot{V}O_2$max. It is also noteworthy that cardioselective beta-blockers—which are supposedly less likely to have adverse pulmonary effects than noncardioselective agents—still exerted detrimental effects on pulmonary physiology.

Beta-Blocker Effects on Oxygen Uptake

Beta-blockers can exert detrimental effects on cellular oxygen uptake ($\dot{V}O_2$) during exercise. Fagard and colleagues (1993) have nicely summarized the acute effects of these drugs on $\dot{V}O_2$ (see figure 1.4). According to these data, regardless of whether the beta-blocker was cardioselective or possessed intrinsic sympathomimetic properties, or whether the subject population comprised hypertensives or normotensives, the general trend was a reduction in $\dot{V}O_2$max during beta-blocker therapy. The change in peak $\dot{V}O_2$ ranged from –22% to +2% (see figure 1.4).

Do the properties of cardioselectivity or ISA offer any advantages over beta-blockers that do not possess these properties? In a study of elite runners, $\dot{V}O_2$max was suppressed more by a noncardioselective agent (propranolol) than by a cardioselective agent (atenolol), though both types of beta-blockers exerted detrimental effects on $\dot{V}O_2$ relative to placebo (Anderson et al. 1985). However, in another study, neither propranolol nor metoprolol affected $\dot{V}O_2$ during a dynamic treadmill exercise test after 48 hours of drug administration in normal volunteers. The authors concluded that there is no advantage to cardioselective beta-blockade over noncardioselective agents on $\dot{V}O_2$ (Sklar et al. 1982). Since most subjects, particularly the types of individuals who require chronic beta-blockade therapy, do not exercise at their peak aerobic capacity, it is important to consider the effects of these drugs at lower exercise intensities.

Beta-blockers with ISA properties do not appear to offer any advantage over non-ISA agents with regard to effects on $\dot{V}O_2$. Pindolol (ISA+) has been compared to propranolol (non-ISA) in several different populations. No differences were seen at any exercise intensity in normal

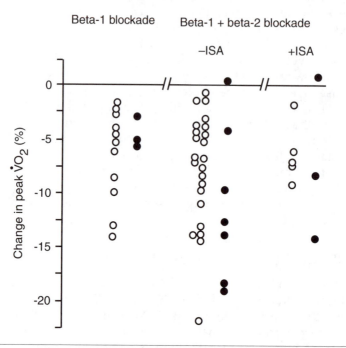

Figure 1.4   Change in V̇O₂max in normal subjects (○) or in hypertensive patients (●) in several studies. Three groups of beta-blockers were used: beta-1-receptor blockers and noncardioselective beta-blockers with or without ISA.

Adapted from Fagard et al. 1993.

volunteers (see figure 1.5) (Ades et al. 1984) or in hypertensive patients (Martin et al. 1989).

Effects of Beta-Blockers on Training

Beta-blockers suppress exercise HR and cardiac output and interfere with epinephrine-mediated fat oxidation; though the degree to which these effects occur depends on the specific beta-blocker in question. According to Fagard and colleagues, "It appears that the beta-blocker-induced reduction in maximal HR is not completely compensated for by the increase in stroke volume and/or peripheral oxygen extraction" (p. 33). Since beta-blockers exert detrimental effects on both the cardiovascular and the metabolic system during exercise, is it possible to achieve a training effect in persons who take these drugs chronically? Considering the importance of the sympathetic nervous system to the exercise response, it would not be surprising if sympatholytic drugs—and beta-

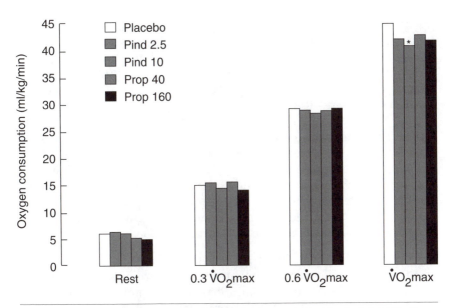

Figure 1.5   Changes in total body oxygen consumption with pindolol (Pind) and propranolol (Prop) at rest and during exercise. * = $p < 0.05$ compared to placebo; $\dot{V}O_2$max = maximal oxygen consumption.

Adapted from Ades et al. 1984.

blockers are sympatholytics—exert detrimental effects on the body's ability to adapt to chronic physiologic exertion.

■ Can a Training Effect Be Achieved While Taking Beta-Blockers?

Van Baak reviewed this topic and concluded that beta-blockers "may" exert a negative effect on trainability (van Baak 1988, 1994). Since the cardioselectivity property of beta-blockers is clinically significant at maximal levels of exercise (i.e., cardioselective agents suppress maximal HR less than noncardioselective agents), are there corresponding differences between different types of beta-blockers on the training effect?

With regard to exercise performance, in general, noncardioselective beta-blockers impair performance to a greater degree than cardioselective agents (Cleroux et al. 1989; McLeod, Kraus, and Williams 1984; Wilmore et al. 1985). Thus, it seems that a training effect would likewise be impaired more by noncardioselective agents.

(continued)

Savin and colleagues reviewed this topic and identified several factors that may explain why different investigators recorded different effects of beta-blockers on training: initial fitness level of subjects studied; degree of beta-blockade (i.e., doses used); altitude; successful blinding; and training intensity (Savin et al. 1985). Savin and colleagues found that, in general, training can still occur in the presence of long-term beta-blocker therapy—even when the beta-blocker is a noncardioselective agent—despite the capacity of these drugs to diminish exercise capacity acutely (Savin et al. 1985). One should be cautious, however, about comparing results obtained in sedentary subjects or patients with heart disease to those obtained in elite athletes. Patients with coronary artery disease—beta-blockers are routinely prescribed for these patients—cannot attain $\dot{V}O_2$max.

Conflicting data exist. When otherwise healthy sedentary volunteers were given beta-blocker therapy and trained for 6 weeks (Savin et al. 1985) or 15 weeks (Wilmore et al. 1985), $\dot{V}O_2$max improved in subjects receiving cardioselective (atenolol) or noncardioselective (propranolol) agents. Wilmore and colleagues found that, although a training-induced increase in $\dot{V}O_2$max was seen in both groups while still taking active drug, the degree of improvement in $\dot{V}O_2$max was lower in the propranolol (noncardioselective) group than in the atenolol (cardioselective) group. This distinction disappeared when measurements of $\dot{V}O_2$max were repeated 1 week after drug therapy was discontinued (Wilmore et al. 1985). Still other investigators found that the noncardioselective beta-blockers nadolol (Wolfel et al. 1986) and propranolol (Hiatt et al. 1984) prevented any training-induced increase in $\dot{V}O_2$ in healthy volunteers. Muscle biopsies have revealed that despite the occurrence of detrimental effects of beta-blockade on exercise conditioning, adaptive changes in skeletal muscle oxidative enzymes and capillary supply still occur (Wolfel et al. 1986). For reasons that are unclear, the full effects of training while receiving noncardioselective agents (e.g., nadolol, propranolol) are not fully realized until several days after the medication has been discontinued (Sweeney, Fletcher, and Fletcher 1989; Wilmore et al. 1985); but because beta-blockers are generally used to treat chronic conditions, this finding seems irrelevant in the clinical setting. It does not appear that the ISA property of pindolol offers any unique advantage over noncardioselective beta-blockers; increases in $\dot{V}O_2$max are equivalent with both drug types in hypertensive subjects (Duncan et al. 1990).

It is important to consider that most subjects who require beta-blocker therapy are not likely to be elite athletes and, thus, are not likely to exercise at $\dot{V}O_2$max. At 60% $\dot{V}O_2$max, $\dot{V}O_2$ remained relatively constant when beta-blockers were administered during 15 weeks of training (Wilmore et al. 1985).

While the cardiovascular effects of beta-blockers during exercise are somewhat predictable, a firm relationship between these effects and the impact on performance is not always observed. This is explained by the fact that beta-blockers exert dramatic effects on exercise metabolism (discussed in the next section) as well as on the cardiovascular system.

Effects of Beta-Blockers on Metabolism

In this section we will discuss the effects of beta-blockers on exercise metabolism. This is an important issue in cardiac patients who are often receiving these drugs chronically. Eagles and Kendall (1997) demonstrated that beta-blockers exert detrimental effects on exercise metabolism and performance even during sustained walking. Turcotte, Richter, and Kiens (1995) and Head (1999) have reviewed this topic; so only a short summary of the metabolic issues relevant to beta-blocker pharmacology is included here. The effects of beta-blockers on exercise performance are discussed in more detail later in this chapter.

Effects of Beta-Blockers on Lipid Metabolism During Exercise

Adipose tissue is the most important energy store in mammals (Turcotte, Richter, and Kiens 1995). In humans, 10% to 25% of body weight is adipose tissue. Thus, a 70 kg person has some 63,000 to 157,500 kcal available as fat, compared to only several hundred kcal available from carbohydrate stores (i.e., glycogen).

Lipolysis of adipose tissue is mainly controlled by catecholamines (i.e., epinephrine), parathormone (PTH), and thyroid-stimulating hormone (TSH). Insulin is the major hormone responsible for inhibition of lipolysis. During prolonged exercise, lipolysis of adipose tissue is controlled by beta-adrenergic stimulation. Lipolysis of adipose tissue triglycerides releases FFAs and glycerol. Glycerol is the better estimate of adipose tissue lipolytic rate, since it cannot be reutilized by the adipocyte; glycerol appears in the blood only as a product of lipolysis (Turcotte, Richter, and Kiens 1995; Franz et al. 1983).

The fact that oxidation of plasma FFAs does not match estimates of total lipid oxidation during prolonged exercise suggests that the difference is made up from oxidation of muscle triglycerides (Turcotte, Richter, and Kiens 1995). Even when nonesterified fatty acids were supplied exogenously via intravenous infusion of lipids, endurance deficits while receiving beta-blockers were still present (van Baak, Mooij, and Wijnen 1993). But lipids in general are not the sole source of energy during exercise, particularly when exercise intensity rises above 50% to 60% $\dot{V}O_2$max (Hargreaves 1995, 42). Further, as exercise intensity increases, muscle glycogenolysis increases. Several factors may explain this, one of which is increased circulating concentrations of epinephrine.

Since epinephrine and insulin are both involved in the utilization of fat and carbohydrate during exercise metabolism, and because beta-blockers can affect the activity of both of these hormones, one can readily see how these drugs might exert dramatic effects on exercise metabolism (see figure 1.6).

The effects of beta-blockade on lipid metabolism are more dramatic than their effects on carbohydrate metabolism during exercise (Cleroux et al. 1989; van Baak et al. 1987). Beta-blockade can significantly reduce both FFA and glycerol mobilization from adipose stores (Cleroux et al. 1989; Jesek et al. 1990; Lundborg et al. 1981). This lack of fats as substrates forces the body into relying more heavily on carbohydrates for energy during endurance exercise. Since carbohydrate reserves are less plentiful than fat reserves, subjects who exercise while taking beta-blockers may experience fatigue earlier than those not receiving these drugs.

Do the ancillary properties of ISA or cardioselectivity that differentiate beta-blockers make any difference on lipid metabolism during exercise? Many investigations in healthy volunteers have shown that noncardioselective beta-blockers exert more detrimental effects on lipid metabolism during exercise than do cardioselective agents (Cleroux et al. 1989; Lundborg et al. 1981; van Baak, Mooij, and Wijnen 1993; Verstappen and van Baak 1987), although even cardioselective agents are detrimental when compared to placebo (Head et al. 1994; van Baak et al. 1985). Laustiola and colleagues (1983) compared the effects of practolol (cardioselective, ISA+), atenolol (cardioselective, no ISA), and propranolol (noncardioselective, no ISA). Propranolol appeared to exert the most detrimental effect on both plasma FFAs and on exercise

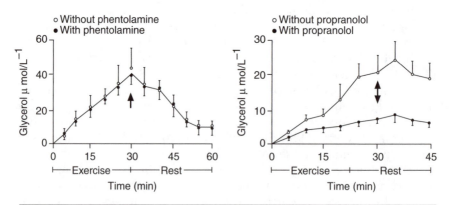

Figure 1.6 Effect of adrenoceptor blockade on exercise-induced glycerol levels in dialysates of abdominal subcutaneous adipose tissue.

Adapted from Arner et al. 1990.

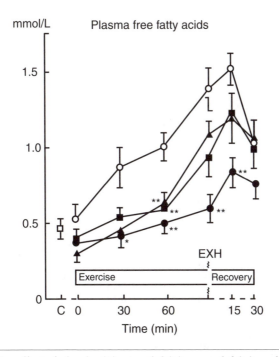

Figure 1.7   The effect of placebo (○), atenolol (▲), practolol (■), and propranolol (●) on exercise-induced changes in plasma free fatty acids. Control (□) indicates mean of pooled values of samples collected at rest before treatment. Values are mean ± *SEM*, *n* = 6. * = *p* < 0.05; ** = *p* < 0.01 vs. placebo.

Adapted from Laustiola et al. 1983.

duration (see figure 1.7). The ISA property of some beta-blockers does not appear to substantially offset the detrimental effects of beta-blockers on lipid metabolism during exercise (Head, Maxwell, and Kendall 1997; Jesek et al. 1990; Krumke et al. 1991; Laustiola et al. 1983; van Baak et al. 1987). These data suggest a cardioselective agent might be preferable to a noncardioselective agent during endurance exercise. Head has reviewed this topic recently (Head 1999).

In an elegant and well-designed study, Cleroux and colleagues demonstrated that utilization of muscle triglycerides might be the pivotal metabolic step delineating why differences are seen with different types of beta-blockers. Muscle triglyceride utilization during cardioselective (i.e., beta-1 only) blockade occurred at a faster rate than during placebo, whereas noncardioselective (i.e., beta-1, beta-2) blockade completely prevented it (see figure 1.8). Since both drugs appeared to impair rises in FFA and glycerol levels equally, the authors concluded that muscle triglyceride utilization is mediated by beta-2 stimulation, while adipose tissue lipolysis is mediated by beta-1 stimulation (Cleroux et al. 1989). These data support a skeletal muscle effect as the explanation, more than they do inhibition of adipose tissue lipolysis for the detrimental effects of beta-blockade on lipid metabolism during exercise. When atenolol was compared with sustained-release metoprolol, both cardioselective beta-blockers, more detrimental effects were seen with atenolol. The authors explained this as due to more profound beta-blockade by atenolol and loss of some degree of beta-1-receptor specificity compared to the more moderate and even pharmacodynamics of the sustained-release metoprolol (Eagles and Kendall 1997). Extrapolating these data into practical terms, cardioselective beta-blockers are preferable to noncardioselective agents to minimize the detrimental effects on exercise endurance.

It is important to consider (a) exercise intensity and (b) duration of drug therapy when evaluating the effects of beta-blockers on exercise metabolism. Substrate utilization changes as exercise intensity changes (Hargreaves 1995). In all the studies of beta-blockers discussed above, only one group of investigators evaluated drug therapy for longer than 1 week. When beta-blockade is given continuously for 6 months to hypertensive subjects who were exercised to exhaustion at 70% $\dot{V}O_2$max, the differences between the various types of beta-blockers on lipid metabolism tended to disappear. Plasma glycerol and nonesterified fatty acid concentrations were decreased by noncardioselective beta-blockade (e.g., propranolol), cardioselective beta-blockade (e.g.,

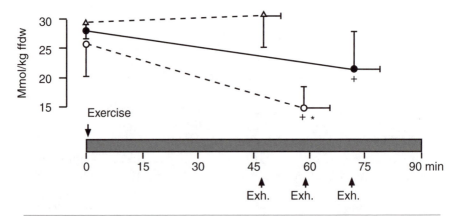

Figure 1.8 Muscle concentrations of triglycerides at rest and at exhaustion after 1 week of placebo, beta-1 cardioselective blockade with atenolol, or noncardioselective beta-blockade with nadolol. Values are mean ± *SEM*, $n = 8$. + = $p < 0.05$ vs. rest ($t = 0$). * = $p < 0.05$ vs. PLAC. ● = placebo; ○ = atenolol; △ = nadolol.

Adapted from Cleroux et al. 1989.

metoprolol), and during ISA+ beta-blockade (e.g., pindolol) during exercise. Plasma glucose was reduced at the end of the exercise test during propranolol treatment only. However, exercise duration was impaired by all three types of beta-blockers (van Baak et al. 1987). Even during simple walking, beta-blockers can impair exercise metabolism (Eagles and Kendall 1997).

Blood Glucose and Muscle Glycogen

Glycogenolysis in skeletal muscle is mediated by epinephrine via stimulation of beta-2 receptors. While the relationship between serum glucose (i.e., hypoglycemia) and fatigue (Boyle et al. 1995; Felig et al. 1982; Krumke et al. 1991) is questionable, there does appear to be a relationship between glycogen stores and fatigue. In patients with essential hypertension, detrimental effects of beta-blockers on carbohydrate metabolism and exercise performance were seen even after 6 months of chronic administration (van Baak et al. 1987). Thus, the effects of beta-blockers on carbohydrate metabolism are also important.

When subjects cycled to exhaustion at 70% $\dot{V}O_2$max, muscle glycogen content declined in both placebo and beta-blocked subjects, but the decline was significantly greater for the placebo group than for the propranolol group (van Baak et al. 1995). When propranolol was compared to atenolol, blood glucose was lower during propranolol administration than during atenolol administration (McLeod, Kraus, and Williams 1984). When atenolol was compared to a pure beta-2-receptor antagonist, more detrimental effects on glucose metabolism were seen after beta-2 blockade than after beta-1 blockade (Hespel et al. 1986). These data imply that beta-2 blockade impairs mobilization of glycogen stores during exercise, producing, in turn, lower serum glucose values. Van Baak has thoroughly reviewed this issue and concluded that muscle glycogenolysis is unaffected by beta-blockade at submaximal exercise, but that the maximal glycogenolytic rate at high exercise intensities can be impaired (van Baak 1988).

Table 1.4 provides a summary of how beta-blockers affect exercise physiology.

How Beta-Blockers
Affect Exercise Performance

So far, we have discussed several general distinctions among beta-blockers in exercise:

- Cardioselective beta-blockers (e.g., atenolol and others) suppress maximum HR less than noncardioselective agents.

Table 1.4　Effects of Beta-Blockers on Exercise Physiology

Physiologic parameter	Type of beta-blocker responsible
Cardiovascular	
Resting HR	Decreased by all types; decreased less by ISA+ agents than by non-ISA beta-blockers
Exercise HR	Decreased by all types; decreased less by cardio-selective agents than by noncardioselective agents
Cardiac output	Conflicting data exist; exercise CO either decreases or remains unchanged during beta-blockade
$\dot{V}O_2$max	Decreased acutely by all types; increases in response to training can still occur during chronic use
Metabolic	
Adipose tissue lipolysis	Impaired by all types of beta-blockers
Muscle TG utilization	Impaired most by noncardioselective agents
Glycogenolysis	Impaired most by noncardioselective agents
Serum potassium	Post-exercise levels higher with noncardioselective agents

- Acutely, beta-blockers of all types reduce $\dot{V}O_2$max (mean reduction of 6-14% in both healthy subjects and patients with cardiovascular disease) (Head 1999). Although the training effect of regular exercise is suppressed most by nonselective agents (McLeod, Kraus, Williams 1984), it is still possible for subjects taking beta-blockers chronically to improve their fitness level as a result of an exercise program.
- Cardioselective beta-blockers interfere with utilization of energy substrates less than noncardioselective agents during exercise.

With these points in mind, what is the overall impact of beta-blockers on exercise performance?

　　To evaluate the effects of beta-blockers on exercise performance, you will want to consider several distinct issues. To start with, it is useful to distinguish the drugs' effects on maximal exercise and effects on submaximal exercise, which have shown differences in reactions (McLenachan et al. 1991). The impact of beta-blockade on maximal aerobic power output and $\dot{V}O_2$max is moderate; the typical decrease is 5-10%. The effects on submaximal endurance performance are much more substantial; here the typical decreases are roughly 40% decline in time to exhaustion for noncardioselective agents (e.g., nadolol, propranolol, timolol) and a 20% decline for beta-1 cardioselective agents like atenolol and metoprolol (van Baak 1994).

Second, it is important not to extrapolate findings conducted among normal volunteers to subjects with hypertension. Hypertensive subjects usually have a substantially reduced exercise capacity compared with age-matched controls (Lim et al. 1996). That said, van Baak, Koene, and Verstappen (1988) found to the contrary that the response to atenolol was similar in hypertensive and normotensive subjects.

Finally, although beta-blockers are detrimental to aerobic exercise performance, they are beneficial in shooting events—and for this reason they are considered banned substances. Van Baak has reviewed beta-blockers in sports (van Baak 1988).

Normotensive Subjects

In normotensive, healthy volunteers, beta-blockers generally exert negative effects on aerobic exercise performance; noncardioselective types (e.g., nadolol, propranolol) exert more detrimental effects than do the cardioselective types (e.g., atenolol, metoprolol). During cycle ergometry to exhaustion, for example, cardioselective beta-blockers reduce exercise performance by 14% to 23%, and noncardioselective agents reduce it by roughly twice that (see figure 1.9 and table 1.5) (Cleroux et al. 1989; Lundborg et al. 1981; van Baak, Mooij, and Wijnen 1993; van Baak et al. 1995). This difference may be due to a combination of metabolic actions (i.e., impaired muscle triglyceride utilization, impaired glycogenolysis, impaired adipose lipolysis, disruption of potassium homeostasis) and cardiovascular actions (i.e., decreased cardiac output, decreased $\dot{V}O_2$), or perhaps even to a central nervous system effect. Although differences between specific beta-blockers are seen in exercise duration, these differences are not seen in subjective symptoms of breathlessness or fatigue in tests where subjects are exercised to exhaustion (Sorensen, Jensen, and Faergeman 1991).

Hypertensive Subjects

After hypertensive subjects received either atenolol or propranolol for 1 week, neither drug was found to affect maximum workload during cycle ergometry, despite these beta-blockers' documented circulatory and metabolic effects (Leenen et al. 1980). The high doses used in this study may have masked any distinctions typically seen between cardioselective and noncardioselective agents. In another study, different types of beta-blockers were administered regularly for 5 to 6 months to subjects with hypertension. When these subjects were then exercised at 70% $\dot{V}O_2$max, exercise times were found to be significantly reduced by

Sport and Exercise Pharmacology

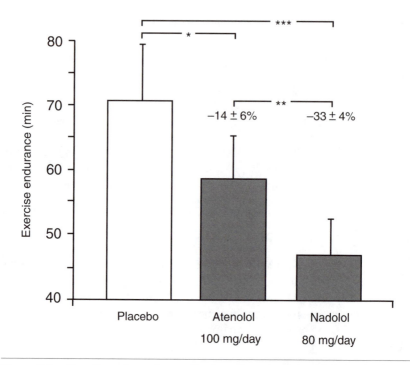

Figure 1.9 Duration of exercise until exhaustion after 1 week of placebo, beta-1 cardioselective blockade with atenolol, or noncardioselective beta-blockade with nadolol. Values are mean ± *SEM*, $n = 8$. * = $p < 0.05$; ** = $p < 0.01$; *** = $p < 0.001$.
Adapted from Cleroux et al. 1989.

all types of beta-blockers (i.e., metoprolol, pindolol, propranolol) (van Baak et al. 1987).

In hypertensive patients, beta-blockers exert more detrimental effects on exercise performance than do other types of antihypertensive drugs, including alpha-blockers such as doxazosin (Gillin et al. 1989), transdermal clonidine (Davies et al. 1989), ACE inhibitors (van Baak et al. 1991), and calcium-channel blockers (Mooy et al. 1987). These drugs are reviewed in chapter 3 in this book.

While beta-blockers are ergolytic in aerobic events, they are actually beneficial in riflery and other shooting events (Kruse et al. 1986; Siitonen, Sonck, and Janne 1977). They have the ability to slow HR and reduce skeletal muscle tremor. Pistol shooting performance improved by 13.4% during beta-blockade. This was attributed to decreased hand tremor, not any effect on HR (Kruse et al. 1986). Beta-blockers do not appear to affect either auditory or visual reaction time (Kostis and Rosen 1987); nor have any beneficial effects on strength, power, or muscular endurance been found (Tesch 1985).

Table 1.5 Duration of Exercise to Exhaustion

Subject	Exercise duration (minutes)		
	Placebo (b.i.d.)	Propranolol (80 mg b.i.d.)	Metoprolol (100 mg b.i.d.)
1	188	128	131
2	148	83	125
3	145	90	124
4	130	70	92
5	126	63	128
6	175	92	100
Mean	152	88	117
± SEM	± 10	± 9	± 6
Reduction vs. placebo (%)		42%	
			23%

Exercise was performed for 30 minute intervals followed by 10 minutes rest on an ergometer bicycle at about 50% VO_2max up to exhaustion.

Reproduced with permission from P. Lundborg, H. Astrom, C. Bengtsson, E. Fellenius, H. von Schenck, L. Svensson, and U. Smith, 1981, *Clinical Science*, 61, 299-305. © the Biochemical Society and the Medical Research Society.

Avoiding Potential Complications

The biggest concern regarding the use of beta-blockers in combination with exercising is that they might have detrimental effects on performance in aerobic exercise. This issue appears to be most significant for noncardioselective agents. Limited data indicate that beta-blockers, particularly noncardioselective types, can increase sweat loss during sustained aerobic exercise in heat (Gordon 1985). For sports medicine specialists, therapy with a beta-blocker of any type will confound the ability to calculate and achieve target exercise HR. Finally, beta-blockers can cause significant bradycardia at rest in highly fit individuals, particularly with agents that do not possess ISA properties.

NCAA and USOC Status

All beta-blockers are banned by the National Collegiate Athletic Association (NCAA) for use during riflery or shooting events. These drugs slow HR and reduce tremor, thus providing users with an advantageous effect in shooting events. The U.S. Olympic Committee (USOC) has a similar ban, but tests for them only in certain events: archery, biathlon, bobsled, diving, equestrian, fencing, gymnastics, luge, modern pentathlon, sailing, freestyle skiing, and synchronized swimming (Fuentes and Rosenberg 1999).

Guidelines for Athletic Trainers

Clearly, beta-blockers are undesirable for athletes or individuals wishing to engage in endurance exercise. However, for some subjects, there may be no other choice of drug therapy. When you work with these subjects, keep the following factors in mind:

- These drugs affect both resting and exercise HRs; target exercise HR may not be attainable in subjects taking beta-blockers.
- While a training effect can occur in subjects chronically taking beta-blockers, a poor correlation exists between HR and exercise performance.
- Beta-blockers do not appear to affect temperature regulation, but propranolol has been shown to increase total sweat loss. Since hypertensive patients are typically instructed to maintain a low-sodium diet, fluid replacement with high-sodium beverages might be unwise in these subjects.
- Note that beta-blockers are banned from some types of athletic competition.

Guidelines for Physicians

There are many issues of detrimental effects regarding beta-blockers (i.e., decreased exercise performance, decreased HR, etc.), despite the fact that the JNC VI committee recommended beta-blockers as first-line therapy for the treatment of hypertension (NIH 1997). Some clinicians (Houston 1989; Messerli, Grossman, and Goldbourt 1998) do not support routine use of these drugs in the management of hypertension. In treating hypertensive subjects who wish to exercise, select another type of antihypertensive drug whenever possible. When a beta-blocker must be prescribed for subjects who wish to participate in endurance exercise, consider the following points:

- Cardioselective agents are preferable to those in the propranolol (e.g., noncardioselective, non-ISA) group.
- A cardioselective beta-blocker that has ISA properties should be considered in subjects who have an already low resting HR, who are

fit, or who are beginning a sustained training phase that might lead to a lowered resting HR as fitness improves.

• Several weeks of therapy may be required to observe the full metabolic effects of these drugs on exercise metabolism.

• Even though regular exercise may not alleviate the need for drug therapy in subjects with hypertension, many other benefits of exercise (i.e., increased musculoskeletal health, decreased atherosclerosis, psychological enhancements) can be realized. Handing out a prescription for a drug should not preclude encouraging the patient to exercise.

References

Ades, P.A. 1987. Cardiac effects of beta-adrenoceptor blockade with intrinsic sympathomimetic activity during submaximal exercise. *Br J Clin Pharmacol* 24:29S-33S.

Ades, P.A., Brammell, H.L., Greenberg, J.H., and Horwitz, L.D. 1984. Effect of beta-blockade and intrinsic sympathomimetic activity on exercise performance. *Am J Cardiol* 54:1337-1341.

Ades, P.A., Wolfel, E.E., Hiatt, W.R., Fee, C., Rolfs, R., Brammell, H.L., and Horwitz, L.D. 1989. Exercise haemodynamic effects of beta-blockade and intrinsic sympathomimetic activity. *Eur J Clin Pharmacol* 36:5-10.

Anderson, R.L., Wilmore, J.H., Joyner, M.J., Freund, B.H., Hartzell, A.A., Todd, C.A., and Ewy, G.A. 1985. Effects of cardioselective and nonselective beta-adrenergic blockade on the performance of highly trained runners. *Am J Cardiol* 55:149D-154D.

Arends, B.G., Bohm, R.O., van Kemenade, J.E., Rahn, K.H., and van Baak, M.A. 1986. Influence of physical exercise on the pharmacokinetics of propranolol. *Eur J Clin Pharmacol* 31:375-377.

Arner, P., Kriegholm, E., Engfeldt, P., and Bolinder, J. 1990. Adrenergic regulation of lipolysis *in situ* at rest and during exercise. *J Clin Invest* 85:893-898.

Borg, G.A.V. 1970. Perceived exertion as an indicator of somatic stress. *Scand J Rehabil Med* 2:92-98.

Bouckaert, J., Lefebvre, R., and Pannier, J.L. 1989. Effects of diltiazem and atenolol on exercise performance in man. *J Sports Med* 29:240-244.

Boyle, P.J., Kempers, S.F., O'Connor, A.M., and Nagy, R.J. 1995. Brain glucose uptake and unawareness of hypoglycemia in patients with insulin-dependent diabetes mellitus. *N Engl J Med* 333(26):1726-1731.

Broeder, C.E., Thomas, E.L., Martin, N.B., Hofman, Z., Jesek, J.K., Scruggs, K.D., Wambsgans, K.C., and Wilmore, J.H. 1993. Effects of propranolol and pindolol on cardiac output during extended periods of low-intensity physical activity. *Am J Cardiol* 72:1188-1195.

Caruso, F.S., Berger, B.M., Darragh, A., Weng, T., and Vukovich, R. 1986. Effect of celiprolol, a new beta-1 alpha-2 blocker, on the cardiovascular response to exercise. *J Clin Pharmacol* 26:32-38.

Clement, K., Vaisse, C., Manning, B.S., Basdevant, A., Guy-Grand, B., Ruiz, J., Silver, K.D., Shuldiner, A.R., Froguel, P., and Strosberg, A.D. 1995. Genetic variation in the beta-3-adrenergic receptor and an increased capacity to gain weight in patients with morbid obesity. *N Engl J Med* 333(6):352-354.

Cleroux, J., Beaulieu, M., Kouame, N., and Lacourciere, Y. 1994. Comparative effects of quinapril, atenolol, and verapamil on blood pressure and forearm hemodynamics during handgrip exercise. *Am J Hypertens* 7:566-570.

Cleroux, J., Van Nguyen, P., Taylor, A.W., and Leenen, F.H.H. 1989. Effects of beta-1 vs. beta-1 plus beta-2 blockade on exercise endurance and muscle metabolism in humans. *J Appl Physiol* 66:548-554.

Cohen-Solal, A., Baleynaud, S., Laperche, T., Sebag, C., and Gourgon, R. 1993. Cardiopulmonary response during exercise of a beta-1-selective beta-blocker (atenolol) and a calcium-channel blocker (diltiazem) in untrained subjects with hypertension. *J Cardiovasc Pharmacol* 22:33-38.

Davies, S.F., Graif, J.L., Husebye, D.G., Maddy, M.M., McArthur, C.D., Path, M.J., O'Connell, M.B., Iber, C., and Davidman, M. 1989. Comparative effects of transdermal clonidine and oral atenolol on acute exercise performance and response to aerobic conditioning in subjects with hypertension. *Arch Intern Med* 149:1551-1556.

Derman, W.E., Sims, R., and Noakes, T.D. 1992. The effects of antihypertensive medications on the physiologic response to maximal exercise testing. *J Cardiovasc Pharmacol* 19(suppl 5): S122-S127.

Dossing, M. 1985. Effect of acute and chronic exercise on hepatic drug metabolism. *Clin Pharmacokinet* 10:426-431.

Duncan, J.J., Vaandrager, H., Farr, J.E., Kohl, H.W., and Gordon, N.F. 1989. Effect of intrinsic sympathomimetic activity on serum lipids during exercise training in hypertensive patients receiving chronic beta-blocker therapy. *J Cardiopulmonary Rehabil* 9:110-114.

Duncan, J.J., Vaandrager, H., Farr, J.E., Kohl, H.W., and Gordon, N.F. 1990. Effect of intrinsic sympathomimetic activity on the ability of hypertensive patients to derive a cardiorespiratory training effect during chronic beta-blockade. *Am J Hypertens* 3:302-306.

Eagles, C.J., and Kendall, M.J. 1997. The effects of combined treatment with beta-1 selective receptor antagonists and lipid-lowering drugs on fat metabolism and measures of fatigue during moderate intensity exercise: A placebo-controlled study in healthy subjects. *Br J Clin Pharmacol* 43:291-300.

Erikssen, J., Thaulow, E., Mundal, R., Opstad, P., and Nitter-Hauge, S. 1982. Comparison of beta-adrenoceptor blockers under maximal exercise (pindolol vs. metoprolol vs. atenolol). *Br J Clin Pharmacol* 13(suppl 2):201S-209S.

Eston, R., and Connolly, D. 1996. The use of rating of perceived exertion for exercise prescription in patients receiving beta-blocker therapy. *Sports Med* 21:176-190.

Fagard, R., Staessen, J., Thijs, L., and Amery, A. 1993. Influence of anti-hypertensive drugs on exercise capacity. *Drugs* 46(suppl 2):32-36.

Felig, P., Cherif, A., Minagawa, A., and Wahren, J. 1982. Hypoglycemia during prolonged exercise in normal men. *N Engl J Med* 306:895-900.

Fogari, R., Marchesi, E., Bellomo, G., Parini, A., and Corradi, L. 1982. Effects of different beta-receptor antagonists on handgrip in essential hypertension. *Int J Clin Pharmacol Ther Toxicol* 20:551-553.

Fogari, R., Zoppi, A., and Orlandi, C. 1985. Time-related effects of chronic atenolol treatment on cardiovascular responses to handgrip. *Int J Clin Pharmacol Ther Toxicol* 23:83-88.

Frank, S., Somani, S.M., and Kohnle, M. 1990. Effect of exercise on propranolol pharmacokinetics. *Eur J Clin Pharmacol* 39:391-394.

Franz, I.W., Lohmann, F.W., Koch, G., and Quabbe, H.J. 1983. Aspects of hormonal regulation of lipolysis during exercise: Effects of chronic beta-receptor blockade. *Int J Sports Med* 4(1):14-20.

Fuentes, R.J., and Rosenberg, J.M. 1999. *Athletic drug reference '99*. Durham, NC: Clean Data.

Gillin, A.G., Fletcher, P.J., Horvath, J.S., Hutton, B.F., Bautovich, G.J., and Tiller, D.J. 1989. Comparison of doxazosin and atenolol in mild hypertension, and effects of exercise capacity, hemodynamics and left ventricular function. *Am J Cardiol* 63:950-954.

Gordon, N.F. 1985. Effect of selective and nonselective beta-adrenoceptor blockade on thermoregulation during prolonged exercise in heat. *Am J Cardiol* 55:74D-78D.

Hargreaves, M., ed. 1995. *Exercise metabolism*. Champaign, IL: Human Kinetics.

Head, A. 1999. Exercise metabolism and beta-blocker therapy: An update. *Sports Med* 27:81-96.

Head, A., Maxwell, S., and Kendall, M.J. 1997. Exercise metabolism in healthy volunteers taking celiprolol, atenolol, and placebo. *Br J Sports Med* 31:120-125.

Head, A., Maxwell, S., Kendall, M.J., and Eagles, C. 1994. Exercise metabolism in healthy volunteers taking atenolol, high and low doses of metoprolol CR/ZOK, and placebo. *Br J Clin Pharmacol* 38:499-504.

Herbertsson, P., and Fagher, B. 1990. Effects of verapamil and atenolol on exercise tolerance in 5,000 m cross-country running: A double-blind cross-over study in normal humans. *J Cardiovasc Pharmacol* 16:23-27.

Hespel, P., Lijnen, P., Vanhees, L., Fagard, R., Fiocchi, R., Moerman, E., and Amery, A. 1986. Differentiation of exercise-induced metabolic responses during selective beta 1- and beta 2-antagonism. *Med Sci Sports Exerc* 18:186-191.

Hiatt, W.R., Marsh, R.C., Brammell, H.L., Fee, C., and Horwitz, L.D. 1984. Effect of aerobic conditioning on the peripheral circulation during chronic beta-adrenergic blockade. *J Am Coll Cardiol* 4:958-963.

Houston, M.C. 1989. New insights and new approaches for the treatment of essential hypertension: Selection of therapy based on coronary heart disease risk factor analysis, hemodynamic profiles, quality of life, and subsets of hypertension. *Am Heart J* 117:911-951.

Huikuri, H.V., Koistenen, J., and Takkunen, J.T. 1992. Efficacy of intravenous sotalol for suppressing inducibility of supraventricular tachycardias at rest and during isometric exercise. *Am J Cardiol* 69:498-502.

Jacober, S.J., and Sowers, J.R. 1995. Exercise and hypertension. *JAMA* 273:1965.

Jesek, J.K., Martin, N.B., Broeder, C.E., Thomas, E.L., Wambsgans, K.C., Hofman, Z., Ivy, J.L., and Wilmore, J.H. 1990. Changes in plasma free fatty acids and glycerols during prolonged exercise in trained and hypertensive persons taking propranolol and pindolol. *Am J Cardiol* 66(19):1336-1341.

Kaiser, P. 1982. Running performance as a function of the dose-response relationship to beta-adrenoceptor blockade. *Int J Sports Med* 3:29-32.

Karvonen, M.J., Kentala, E., and Mustala, O. 1957. The effects of training heart rate: A longitudinal study. *Annales Medicinae Experimentalis et Biologiae Fenniae* 35:307-315.

Kjaer, M. 1995. Hepatic fuel metabolism during exercise. In *Exercise metabolism*, edited by M. Hargreaves. Champaign, IL: Human Kinetics.

Kostis, J.B., and Rosen, R.C. 1987. Central nervous system effects of beta-adrenergic blocking drugs: The role of ancillary properties. *Circulation* 75:204-212.

Krumke, W., Mader, A., Michael, H., Giannetti, B.M., and Hollmann, W. 1991. An examination of the hemodynamic and metabolic effects of carteolol during different workloads on a bicycle ergometer. *Int J Sports Med* 12:548-556.

Kruse, P., Ladefoged, J., Nielsen, U., Paulev, P.E., and Sorensen, J.P. 1986. Beta-blockade used in precision sports: Effect on pistol shooting performance. *J Appl Physiol* 61:417-420.

Laustiola, K., Uusitalo, A., Koivula, T., Sovijarvi, A., Seppala, E., Nikkari, T., and Vapaatalo, H. 1983. Divergent effects of atenolol, practolol and propranolol on the peripheral metabolic changes induced by dynamic exercise in healthy men. *Eur J Clin Pharmacol* 25:293-297.

Leenen, F.H.H., Coenen, C.H.M., Zonderland, M., and Maas, A.H.J. 1980. Effects of cardioselective and nonselective beta-blockade on dynamic exercise performance in mildly hypertensive men. *Clin Pharmacol Ther* 28:12-21.

Lim, P.O., MacFadyen, R.J., Clarkson, P.B.M., and MacDonald, T.M. 1996. Impaired exercise tolerance in hypertensive patients. *Ann Intern Med* 124(1 pt 1):41-55.

Lundborg, P., Astrom, H., Bengtsson, C., Fellenius, E., von Schenck, H., Svensson, L., and Smith, U. 1981. Effect of beta-adrenoceptor blockade on exercise performance and metabolism. *Clin Sci* 61:299-305.

MacDougall, J.D., Tuxen, D., Sale, D.G., Moroz, J.R., and Sutton, J.R. 1985. Arterial blood pressure response to heavy resistance exercise. *J Appl Physiol* 58:785-790.

Magder, S., Sami, M., Ripley, R., and Lisbona, R. 1987. Comparison of the effects of pindolol and propranolol on exercise performance in patients with angina pectoris. *Am J Cardiol* 59:1289-1294.

Martin, N.B., Broeder, C.E., Thomas, E.L., Wambsgans, K.C., Scruggs, K.D., Jesek, J.K., Hofman, Z., and Wilmore, J.H. 1989. Comparison of the effects of pindolol and propranolol on exercise performance in young men with systemic hypertension. *Am J Cardiol* 64:343-347.

McLenachan, J.M., Grant, S., Ford, I., Henderson, E., and Dargie, H.J. 1991. Submaximal, but not maximal, exercise testing detects differences in the effects of beta-blockers during treadmill exercise: A study of celiprolol and atenolol. II. *Am Heart J* 121(2 pt 2):691-696.

McLeod, A.A., Knopes, K.D., Shand, D.G., and Williams, R.S. 1985. Beta-1 selective and non-selective beta-adrenoceptor blockade, anaerobic threshold and respiratory gas exchange during exercise. *Br J Clin Pharmacol* 19:13-20.

McLeod, A.A., Kraus, W.E., and Williams, R.S. 1984. Effects of beta-1 selective and nonselective beta-adrenoceptor blockade during exercise conditioning in healthy adults. *Am J Cardiol* 53:1656-1661.

Messerli, F.H., Grossman, E., and Goldbourt, U. 1998. Are beta-blockers efficacious as first-line therapy for hypertension in the elderly? *JAMA* 279:1903-1907.

Mooy, J., van Baak, M., Bohm, R., Does, R., Petri, H., van Kemanade, J., and Rahn, K.H. 1987. The effects of verapamil and propranolol on exercise tolerance in hypertensive patients. *Clin Pharmacol Ther* 41:490-495.

National Institutes of Health. 1997. *The sixth report of the Joint National Committee on the Prevention, Detection, Evaluation, and Treatment of High Blood Pressure.* U.S.

Department of Health and Human Services, NIH Publication no. 98-4080, November.

Orlandi, C., and Fogari, R. 1983. Effect of chronic atenolol therapy on the cardiovascular response to handgrip in hypertensive patients. *Clin Ther* 5:632-637.

Panton, L.B., Guillen, G.J., Williams, L., Graves, J.E., Vivas, C., Cediel, M., Pollock, M.L., Garzarella, L., Krumerman, J., Derendorf, H., and Lowenthal, D.T. 1995. The lack of effect of aerobic exercise training on propranolol pharmacokinetics in young and elderly adults. *J Clin Pharmacol* 35:885-894.

Petersen, E.S., Whipp, B.J., Davis, J.A., Huntsman, D.J., Brown, H.V., and Wasserman, K. 1983. Effects of beta-adrenergic blockade on ventilation and gas exchange during exercise in humans. *J Appl Physiol* 54:1306-1313.

Rapola, J.M., Pellinen, T.J., Koskinen, P., Toivonen, L., and Nieminen, M.S. 1990. Hemodynamic effects of pindolol and atenolol at rest and during isometric exercise: A noninvasive study with healthy volunteers. *Cardiovasc Drugs Ther* 4:737-743.

Savin, W.M., Gordon, E.P., Kaplan, S.M., Hewitt, B.F., Harrison, D.C., and Haskell, W.L. 1985. Exercise training during long-term beta-blockade treatment in healthy subjects. *Am J Cardiol* 55:101D-109D.

Scruggs, K.D., Martin, N.B., Broeder, C.E., Hofman, Z., Thomas, E.L., Wambsgans, K.C., and Wilmore, J.H. 1991. Stroke volume during submaximal exercise in endurance-trained normotensive subjects and in untrained hypertensive subjects with beta blockade (propranolol and pindolol). *Am J Cardiol* 67(5):416-421.

Siitonen, L., Sonck, T., and Janne, J. 1977. Effect of beta-blockade on performance: Use of beta-blockade in bowling and in shooting competitions. *J Int Med Res* 5:349-356.

Sklar, J., Johnston, G.D., Overlie, P., Gerber, J.G., Brammell, H.L., Gal, J., and Nies, A.S. 1982. The effects of a cardioselective (metoprolol) and a nonselective (propranolol) beta-adrenergic blocker on the response to dynamic exercise in normal men. *Circulation* 65:894-899.

Somani, S.M., ed. 1996. *Pharmacology in exercise and sports.* Boca Raton, FL: CRC Press.

Somani, S.M., Gupta, S.K., Frank, S., and Corder, C.N. 1990. Effect of exercise on disposition and pharmacokinetics of drugs. *Drug Dev Res* 20:251-275.

Sorensen, E.V., Jensen, H.K., and Faergeman, O. 1991. Comparison of the effects of xamoterol, atenolol and propranolol on breathlessness, fatigue and plasma electrolytes during exercise in healthy volunteers. *Eur J Clin Pharmacol* 41:51-55.

Sweeney, M.E., Fletcher, B.J., and Fletcher, G.F. 1989. Exercise testing and training with beta-adrenergic blockade: Role of the drug washout period in "unmasking" a training effect. *Am Heart J* 118(5 pt 1):941-946.

Tesch, P.A. 1985. Exercise performance and beta-blockade. *Sports Med* 2:389-412.

Thompson, P.D., Cullinane, E.M., Nugent, A.M., Sady, M.A., and Sady, S.P. 1989. Effect of atenolol or prazosin on maximal exercise performance in hypertensive joggers. *Am J Med* 86(suppl 1B):104-109.

Turcotte, L.P., Richter, E.A., and Kiens, B. 1995. Lipid metabolism during exercise. In *Exercise metabolism*, edited by M. Hargreaves. Champaign, IL: Human Kinetics.

van Baak, M.A. 1988. Beta-adrenergic blockade and exercise: An update. *Sports Med* 5:209-225.

van Baak, M.A. 1990. Influence of exercise on the pharmacokinetics of drugs. *Clin Pharmacokinet* 19:32-43.

van Baak, M.A. 1994. Hypertension, beta-adrenoceptor blocking agents and exercise. *Int J Sports Med* 15:112-115.

van Baak, M.A., Bohm, R.O., Arends, B.G., van Hooff, M.E., and Rahn, K.H. 1987. Long-term antihypertensive therapy with beta-blockers: Submaximal exercise capacity and metabolic effects during exercise. *Int J Sports Med* 8:342-347.

van Baak, M.A., de Haan, A., Saris, W.H., van Kordelaar, E., Kuipers, H., and van der Vusse, G.J. 1995. Beta-adrenoceptor blockade and skeletal muscle energy metabolism during endurance exercise. *J Appl Physiol* 78(1): 307-313.

van Baak, M.A., Jennen, W., Muijtjens, A., and Verstappen, F.T. 1985. Effects of acute and chronic metoprolol administration during submaximal and maximal exercise. *Int J Sports Med* 6:347-352.

van Baak, M.A., Koene, F.M., and Verstappen, F.T. 1988. Exercise haemodynamics and maximal exercise capacity during beta-adrenergic blockade in normotensive and hypertensive subjects. *Br J Clin Pharmacol* 25:169-177.

van Baak, M.A., Koene, F.M., Verstappen, F.T.J., and Tan, E.S. 1991. Exercise performance during captopril and atenolol treatment in hypertensive patients. *Br J Clin Pharmacol* 32:723-728.

van Baak, M.A., Mooij, J.M., and Schiffers, P.M.H. 1992. Exercise and the pharmacokinetics of propranolol, verapamil, and atenolol. *Eur J Clin Pharmacol* 43:547-550.

van Baak, M.A., Mooij, J.M., and Wijnen, J.A. 1993. Effect of increased plasma nonesterified fatty acid concentrations on endurance performance during beta-adrenoceptor blockade. *Int J Sports Med* 14:2-8.

Vanhees, L., Fagard, R., Lijnen, P., and Amery, A. 1991. Effect of antihypertensive medication on endurance exercise capacity in hypertensive sportsmen. *J Hypertens* 9:1063-1068.

Verstappen, F.T., and van Baak, M.A. 1987. Exercise capacity, energy metabolism, and beta-adrenoceptor blockade. Comparison between a beta-1-selective and a non-selective beta blocker. *Eur J Appl Physiol* 56:712-718.

Wilmore, J.H. 1988. Exercise testing, training, and beta-adrenergic blockade. *Phys Sports Med* 16:45-51.

Wilmore, J.H., Ewy, G.A., Fruend, B.J., Hartzell, A.A., Jilka, S.M., Joyner, M.J., Todd, C.A., Kinzer, S.M., and Pepin, E.B. 1985. Cardiorespiratory alterations consequent to endurance exercise training during chronic beta-adrenergic blockade with atenolol and propranolol. *Am J Cardiol* 55:142D-148D.

Wolfel, E.E., Hiatt, W.R., Brammell, H.L., Carry, M.R., Ringel, S.P., Travis, V., and Horwitz, L.D. 1986. Effect of selective and nonselective beta-adrenergic blockade on mechanisms of exercise conditioning. *Circulation* 74:664-674.

Wolfel, E.E., Hiatt, W.R., Brammell, H.L., Travis, V., and Horwitz, L.D. 1990. Plasma catecholamine responses to exercise after training with beta-adrenergic blockade. *J Appl Physiol* 68:586-593.

2

CHAPTER

Diuretics

■ *CASE*   Danny is a college wrestler who has a big match on Saturday. Like most wrestlers, he wants to make sure he wrestles in the lowest weight category possible. To accomplish this, many wrestlers exercise while wearing rubber suits or sit in saunas attempting to lose weight through increased perspiration. Danny claims to have found an easier way to drop weight: he has confiscated the diuretic furosemide (Lasix) from his father's prescription bottle. He tells his teammates, "If it's okay for my dad to take, it's safe for wrestlers." Danny claims, having taken the drug once already, that it won't hurt him. What do you tell him?

■ *COMMENT*   First, all diuretics are banned substances for athletic competition. Also, it is important to stress to Danny that diuretics can impair athletic performance. Potent diuretics like furosemide can cause very serious side effects, including changes in electrolyte balance and impairment of the body's cooling mechanism. Since furosemide is a relatively short-lived drug, Danny may be reassured to know that if he stops taking the drug now, it should be undetectable in his urine within 1 to 2 days. Any one of these things is reason enough for Danny never again to experiment with diuretics!

Diuretics are substances that increase the clearance (removal) of water from the body via the kidneys. While diuretics are commonly prescribed in clinical medicine, they are also encountered in sports. Although it is not inconceivable that an elite athlete would have a bona fide medical need (e.g., hypertension) for a diuretic, most athletes who take diuretics are using them illicitly. In 1992, the International Olympic Committee reported that, after anabolic steroids, stimulants, and narcotics, diuretics were the fourth most common drug group abused by athletes (Benzi 1994). Athletes in sports such as wrestling, boxing, or judo may abuse diuretics to drop weight quickly. Some female gymnasts and ballet dancers also abuse diuretics to help maintain a low body weight. Athletes even use diuretics at times to mask the detection of other banned substances in urine samples (Delbeke and Debackere 1991). Bodybuilders are known to take diuretics in hopes of better accentuating muscle definition and body tone (Al-Zaki and Talbot-Stern 1996).

In clinical medicine, physicians commonly prescribe diuretics to treat hypertension and other cardiovascular disorders. Because of the drugs' low cost and proven benefit in reducing cardiovascular morbidity and mortality, the Joint National Committee on the Detection, Evaluation, and Treatment of High Blood Pressure (JNC) has repeatedly endorsed using thiazide diuretics as a first-line therapy for hypertension (National Institutes of Health 1997). This endorsement by the JNC is based on results from numerous long-term clinical trials that demonstrated a reduction in both cerebrovascular and cardiovascular morbidity with the use of diuretics in the management of hypertension. Nevertheless, there is controversy in the medical community regarding the role of diuretics as antihypertensive agents. Reasons given for using other drugs in place of diuretics in the treatment of hypertension include undesirable metabolic effects and lack of positive effect on reducing left ventricular hypertrophy; but Moser has summarized why these concerns with diuretics are unfounded (1998). Reports of the use of diuretics for the treatment of hypertension range from only 8% of new prescriptions for antihypertensives (Siegel and Lopez 1997) to as high as 47.5% (Psaty et al. 1995).

Diuretics are commonly organized into five groups (see table 2.1). Of these drugs, *loop diuretics* are the most potent. These diuretics produce substantial fluid losses very rapidly; they can also lead to significant depletion of minerals such as sodium, chloride, potassium, and magnesium. *Potassium-sparing diuretics* are a class that researchers developed to offset the substantial electrolyte loss from the loop diuretics. *Thiazide diuretics* are milder diuretics used in the treatment of hypertension. Many patients with hypertension take a thiazide diuretic, either alone or in combination with another antihypertensive drug. The *carbonic anhydrase inhibitors* are used clinically in the treatment of glaucoma; aceta-

Table 2.1   Diuretic Subgroups

Thiazide diuretics	Furosemide (Lasix)
Bendroflumethiazide (Naturetin)	Torsemide (Demadex)
Benzthiazide (Exna)	**Potassium-sparing diuretics**
Chlorothiazide (Diuril)	Amiloride (Midamor)
Chlorthalidone (Hygroton)	Spironolactone (Aldactone)
Cyclothiazide (Anhydron)	Triamterene (Dyrenium)
Hydrochlorothiazide (HCTZ) (Esidrex, HydroDIURIL)	**Osmotic diuretics**
	Glycerin (Osmoglyn)
Hydroflumethiazide (Saluron)	Isosorbide (Ismotic)
Methyclothiazide (Enduron)	Mannitol (Osmitrol)
Metolazone (Mykrox, Zaroxolyn)	Urea (Ureaphil)
Polythiazide (Renese)	**Carbonic anhydrase inhibitors**
Quinethazone (Hydromox)	Acetazolamide (Diamox)
Trichlormethiazide (Metahydrin, Naqua)	Dichlorphenamide (Daranide)
Loop diuretics	Methazolamide (Neptazane)
Bumetanide (Bumex)	
Ethacrynic acid (Edecrin)	

zolamide has proved helpful in preventing high-altitude mountain sickness (AMS) (Larson et al. 1982), and skiers or mountain climbers sometimes make legitimate use of the drug. The *osmotic diuretics*, rarely used, are included in the table only for completeness. Some substances (e.g., caffeine, demeclocycline, ethanol [alcohol], and lithium) that are not technically classified as diuretics nevertheless can cause a diuretic-like response. Some of these are discussed in later chapters.

How Exercise Affects the Action of Diuretics

Exercise affects both the pharmacology and pharmacokinetics of diuretics, and it is important for practitioners to be aware of these significant effects. We know more about the effects of exercise on the pharmacology of diuretics than on their pharmacokinetics.

Effects on Pharmacology

At the most simplistic level, exercise acutely induces a negative water balance, and long-term, regular exercise lowers blood pressure. These actions would be predicted to augment the pharmacologic properties of diuretics. Three days of exercise training did not reverse the hypovolemic effects of combined hydrochlorothiazide-triamterene diuresis in healthy untrained males (Zappe, Helyar, and Green 1996). Exercise induces many other metabolic effects that may influence specific actions of diuretics. For example, exercise causes an acute shift of intracellular potassium into the intravascular space (Young et al. 1992). This could potentiate the kaliuretic effects of most diuretics; however, epinephrine and norepinephrine concentrations also rise during exercise (Young et al. 1992), and these catecholamines drive potassium ions back into the intracellular space. Also, thiazide diuretics have been associated with insulin resistance, while exercise promotes a directly opposite action. The effect of thiazide diuretics on insulin resistance, however, appears to be minor (Moser 1998).

At the level of the nephron, exercise can both complement and antagonize the effects of diuretics.

Effects on Pharmacokinetics

Only limited data are available. We know that sustained aerobic exercise decreases renal and hepatic blood flow; so we may conclude that the clearance of "flow-limited" diuretics will decrease during sustained exercise. Such diuretics include chlorothiazide, chlorthalidone, hydrochlorothiazide, and triamterene (Somani 1996). All of these except chlorthalidone have a fairly short elimination half-life (i.e., 1.5-4.0 h). Thus, 1 h (or more) of sustained aerobic exercise could significantly affect the pharmacokinetics of these diuretics. The clinical significance of exercise-induced decreases in the clearance of a given diuretic, however, is uncertain.

How Diuretics Affect Exercisers

Diuretics exert a variety of effects on the exercise physiology of exercisers, but most of these concern the consequences of volume depletion and electrolyte loss. Exercise and diuretic use can each independently cause fluid loss and electrolyte loss.

How do these factors affect renal physiology (table 2.2)? Freund and colleagues (1991) found that renal and hormonal responses to exercise varied depending on exercise intensity. Urine flow, glomerular filtration rate (GFR), and osmotic clearance were only modestly altered by cycling at 25% and 40% of $\dot{V}O_2$max; however, all were significantly decreased at 60% and 80% of $\dot{V}O_2$max (see figures 2.1 and 2.2). Plasma concentrations of atrial natriuretic peptide (ANP), renin, and aldosterone all

Table 2.2 Effects of Exercise and Diuretics on Renal Physiology

	GFR	Urine output	PRA	Aldo
Exercise @ 25% $\dot{V}O_2$max	i	nc	i	i
Exercise @ 80% $\dot{V}O_2$max	D	D	I	I
Thiazide diuretics	D	D	I	I
Loop diuretics	nc	I	I	I
Spironolactone	nc	i	I	I
Other potassium-sparing agents	nc	i	I	I

i = insignificant increase
I = significant increase
nc = no change
D = decrease
GFR = glomerular filtration rate
PRA = plasma renin activity
Aldo = aldosterone

increased as exercise intensity increased. Antidiuretic hormone, how-ever, decreased during low-intensity exercise but increased with high-intensity exercise.

Diuretic Effects on Metabolism

Diuretics have many metabolic effects. The ones most relevant to exercise and sports medicine are discussed here.

Thermoregulation

Subjected to a hot environment, a resting human's skin blood flow may approach 8 L/min (Johnson 1986). During exercise, temperatures within skeletal muscle exceed core temperatures within several minutes. Skin blood flow during exercise is a dynamic interplay between a *vasoconstrictive* process that shunts blood to exercising muscle and a *vasodilatory* response that mediates temperature control via radiation. The demands of increased skin blood flow are met by an increase in cardiac output and redistribution of blood flow from other regions. Temperature regulation is compromised when adaptive increases in skin blood flow are impaired. Thermoregulatory control of skin blood flow has been reviewed by Johnson (1986) and Kenney and Johnson (1992)

While performing heavy exercise in hot conditions, more than 1 L of sweat per hour per square meter of body surface area can be lost

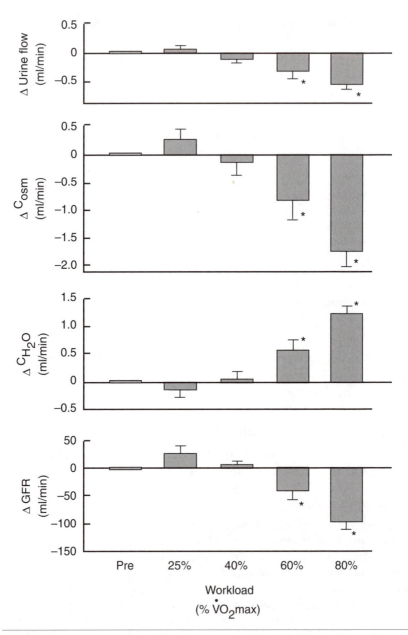

Figure 2.1 Changes in urine flow, osmotic clearance (C_{osm}), free water clearance (C_{H_2O}), and glomerular filtration rate (GFR). Values are mean ± *SEM* of 8 subjects. * = significant difference from preexercise value (p 0.05). Pr eexercise values: urine flow, 0.76 ± 0.05 ml/min; C_{osm}, 2.3 ± 0.1 ml/min; C_{H_2O}, 1.5 ± 0.1 ml/min; GFR, 127.3 ± 4.2 ml/min.

Adapted from Freund et al. 1991.

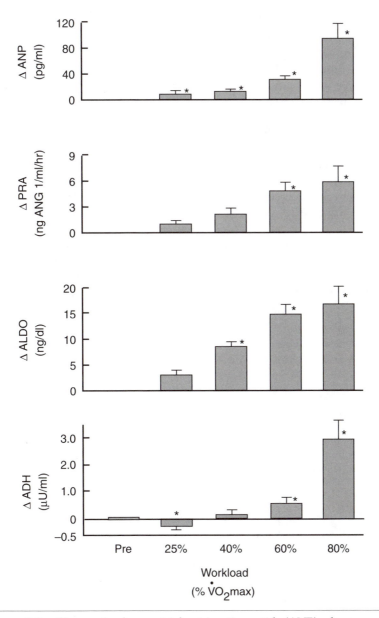

Figure 2.2 Changes in plasma atrial natriuretic peptide (ANP), plasma renin activity (PRA), plasma aldosterone (Aldo), and plasma vasopressin (ADH). Values are mean ± *SEM* of 8 subjects. ANG I, angiotensin I. * = significant difference from preexercise value (p 0.05). Pr eexercise values: ANP, 15.0 ± 0.9 pg · ml; PRA, 1.8 ± 0.1 ng ANG I · ml^{-1} · h^{-1}; Aldo, 10.0 ± 1.0 ng · dl; ADH, 0.78 ± 0.08 μU/ml.

Adapted from Freund et al. 1991.

(Wilmore and Costill 1994). Hypohydration exerts a detrimental effect on the cardiovascular and thermoregulatory systems of the body during exercise. This is why it is important for athletes to consume adequate amounts of fluids before and during prolonged exercise, particularly in hot conditions. Hypovolemia compromises venous return to the heart. To maintain cardiac output and blood pressure, heart rate (HR) increases and peripheral arterioles vasoconstrict. This response is favored over thermoregulation. Exercising under hot conditions compromises the heat transfer from core to periphery; blood flow is shunted away from the periphery in favor of the central circulation to maintain stroke volume (SV) and venous return. Nadel and colleagues (1979) have demonstrated that an SV of 100 ml/beat or lower impairs peripheral circulation. Exercise-induced dehydration, which leads to decreased circulating blood volume, contributes to increased HR (secondary to decreased venous return) and increased body temperature (secondary to decreased cutaneous blood flow) (Fortney et al. 1981). Both acetazolamide (Brechue and Stager 1990), a mild diuretic, and furosemide (Claremont et al. 1976), a potent diuretic, can exert detrimental effects on skin blood flow during exercise (see figure 2.3).

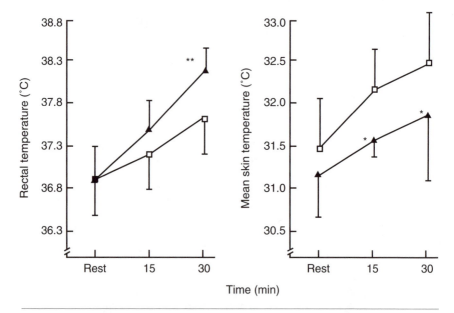

Figure 2.3 Thermoregulatory data: □ = placebo; ▲ = ACZ. * = significantly different from placebo trial, $p < 0.003$; ** = significant difference within trial as well as difference from placebo trial.

Adapted from Brechue and Stager 1990.

Further, despite a decrease in plasma volume (PV), subjects who exercise continue to perspire, thus adding to diuretic-induced fluid losses (Claremont et al. 1976). Sweat rates as high as 2-3 L/h have been observed, but these rates cannot be sustained for very long (Wilmore and Costill 1994). Dehydrated subjects are really at a disadvantage even before exercise begins. The clinical effects of diuretics on the exercise response will later be discussed in detail under "Avoiding Potential Complications."

Potassium Homeostasis

During exercise, potassium ions move from intracellular sites to extracellular sites (Young et al. 1992). Extracellular potassium is apparently taken up by other sites and then released to return to original intracellular sites after exercise ceases (Sjogaard 1986). Catecholamines, acting at the beta-2 receptor, facilitate intracellular re-uptake of these potassium ions (Clausen 1983; Young et al. 1992). Animal and human data show that onset of muscle fatigue has been associated with a decrease in intracellular potassium and decreases in resting membrane potential in exercising muscle (Sjogaard 1986). Not surprisingly, since all diuretics, except the potassium-sparing agents, increase kaliuresis, diuretics accelerate the depletion of intracellular potassium, another dimension of the detrimental effects these agents may have, depending on exercise duration.

Cardiovascular Actions

Despite the combined effects of exercise and diuretics on potassium balance, the frequency of cardiac arrhythmias did not increase in patients with hypertension; however, these data were generated in Veterans Administration patients (Papademetriou, Notargiacomo, and Freis 1989), who may not be representative of the triathlete who exercises longer and harder. Quite some time ago, a study showed that high school wrestlers who were hypohydrated—without the use of diuretics—subsequently demonstrated a higher exercise HR while cycling at 65% $\dot{V}O_2max$ (Allen, Smith, and Miller 1977). One might expect that *diuretic-induced hypohydration* would produce similar results; the data, however, are variable, depending on the duration of use and the exercise intensity. For example, compared with being on placebo, hypertensive patients stabilized on thiazide diuretics (i.e., not hypohydrated) did not demonstrate differences in exercise HR during maximum exercise (DeQuattro et al. 1985). In normotensives, HR during exercise at 35% $\dot{V}O_2$ after a single dose of furosemide was higher compared to the euvolemic state (Claremont et al. 1976). In a more recent study, three doses of acetazolamide did not significantly increase subjects' exercise HR at 70% $\dot{V}O_2$ despite a substantial decrease in PV and SV (Brechue and Stager 1990). Nor did two doses affect exercise HR under either normoxic or hypoxic conditions during submaximal exercise at 75% $\dot{V}O_2$max or during maximal exercise in normotensive volunteers (Stager et al. 1990). One explanation might be that the acute effects of diuretics on exercise HR are seen at lower exercise intensities but not at higher intensities or during maximal exercise. It is well known that PV returns to near normal during chronic therapy with thiazide diuretics. So it does not make sense, therefore, to extrapolate data generated in patients with hypertension who take diuretics month after month to the use of single doses by athletes (e.g., wrestlers, 4 h prior to a match).

Despite differences in potency among various diuretics, their acute effects on PV are remarkably similar. A single, 40 mg oral dose of the potent loop diuretic furosemide reduced PV prior to exercise testing 7.1% to 12.3% in young healthy male runners (Armstrong, Costill, and Fink 1985), and doses of 1.7 mg/kg reduced PV 14.1% in weightlifters, wrestlers, and boxers (Caldwell, Ahonen, and Nousiainen 1984). Carbonic anhydrase inhibitors and thiazide diuretics are weaker diuretics than loop diuretics (e.g., furosemide). Still, acetazolamide (250 mg taken orally every 6 h for 3 doses) reduced PV by 9.1% in untrained males prior to exercise testing (Brechue and Stager 1990); 4 days of hydrochlorothiazide-triamterene produced a decrease in PV of 11% in conditioned males (Nadel, Fortney, and Wenger 1980). Despite the decreases seen in PV, changes in plasma osmolality do not occur during exercise while taking diuretics (Brechue and Stager 1990; Nadel, Fortney, and Wenger 1980).

Diuretic-induced decreases in PV affect both the acute and the long-term physiologic responses to aerobic exercise. When exercise is intense and ambient temperature is high, the tone of peripheral blood vessels favors maintenance of venous return over heat dissipation (Nadel et al. 1979; Wilmore and Costill 1994). This is a critical physiological relationship. Acute decreases in PV, of 11% to 13%, have been associated with decreases in SV (Brechue and Stager 1990; Nadel, Fortney, and Wenger 1980), cardiac output (Nadel, Fortney, and Wenger 1980), and $\dot{V}O_2$max (Caldwell, Ahonen, and Nousiainen 1984), although dehydration appears to affect cardiac output more than it affects $\dot{V}O_2$ (Allen, Smith, and Miller 1977; Wilmore and Costill 1994). When euvolemic subjects exercised for 30 min in hot conditions, SV declined from a baseline of 125 ml/beat to 93 ml/beat within 30 min. Corresponding values after pretreatment with 4 days of hydrochlorothiazide-triamterene were 100 ml/beat at the beginning of exercise and 80 ml/beat after 30 min of exercise (Nadel, Fortney, and Wenger 1980). Figure 2.4 represents the combined effects of exercise and diuretic administration on SV.

Regular exercise stimulates influx of water into the intravascular space. The response to exercise is substantially greater than the response to chronic heat exposure (Convertino, Greenleaf, and Bernauer 1980; Wilmore and Costill 1994). Exercise-induced hypervolemia may be

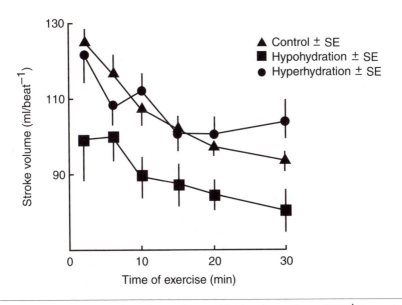

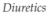

Figure 2.4   Cardiac stroke volume during 30 min of exercise at 55% $\dot{V}O_2$max in a 35 °C environment in three conditions of body hydration. Values are mean ± *SEM* from duplicate runs on each of 4 subjects in each condition.

Adapted from Nadel, Fortney, and Wenger 1980.

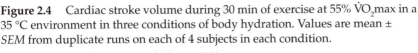

secondary to, among other mechanisms, increased aldosterone receptor sensitivity (Convertino 1991). Thus, diuretics, particularly spironolactone, which is a specific antagonist of aldosterone, will interfere with this normal, physiologic adaptation to long-term, regular exercise.

Pulmonary Actions and Effects on Oxygen Uptake

With the exception of acetazolamide, little is known regarding the effects of diuretics on pulmonary function during exercise. While all diuretics exert metabolic effects, acetazolamide specifically inhibits carbonic anhydrase, part of the acid-base regulation system. Carbonic anhydrase inhibitors induce a sodium bicarbonate diuresis. It is therefore impossible to separate the effects of carbonic anhydrase inhibitors on pulmonary function from their effects on cellular metabolism. Acetazolamide has been shown to impair CO_2 elimination during exercise (Scheuermann et al. 1999), but also impaired CO_2 efflux from inactive muscle (Kowalchuk et al. 1994). In acute mountain sickness (AMS), acetazolamide increases alveolar oxygenation. Mountain climbers who received daily acetazolamide had higher arterial oxygen pressures and lower arterial carbon dioxide pressures than those who received placebo (Bradwell et al. 1986). But the cellular/metabolic effects of acetazolamide may override its pulmonary effects; several groups of investigators have shown acetazolamide inhibits oxygen uptake during maximal exercise ($\dot{V}O_2$max) (Kowalchuk et al. 1992; Stager et al. 1990). Additional pulmonary effects of acetazolamide during exercise have been reported by Schoene and colleagues (1983).

Regarding the loop diuretic furosemide, tidal volume, minute ventilation, and respiratory exchange ratio at aerobic threshold decreased after furosemide administration in Finnish athletes during indoor cycling. Although O_2 pulse and $\dot{V}O_2$max also decreased after furosemide administration in this study, the impact of these findings are uncertain (Caldwell, Ahonen, and Nousiainen 1984). Conversely, other clinical data indicate that inhaled furosemide can protect a subject against exercise-induced bronchoconstriction (Munyard, Chung, and Bush 1995). Thus, furosemide appears to exert both detrimental and beneficial actions on the pulmonary response to exercise.

The process of rapid weight loss secondary to dehydration that wrestlers undergo to make weight has been shown to acutely reduce $\dot{V}O_2$ during a treadmill test (Webster, Rutt, and Weltman 1990). Earlier data from Allen and colleagues showed that dehydration, induced by fluid restriction and exercise, with or without rapid rehydration, did not affect oxygen uptake ($\dot{V}O_2$) in high school wrestlers during cycling at 65% $\dot{V}O_2$max, but the exercise test lasted for only 8 to 10 min in this study (Allen, Smith, and Miller 1977).

Variable effects on $\dot{V}O_2$ have been observed during exercise after diuretic administration. Single, 40 mg doses of furosemide had no effect on $\dot{V}O_2$max in healthy volunteers during treadmill running (Armstrong, Costill, and Fink 1985) or cycle ergometry (Baum, Essfeld, and Stegemann 1986), even though treadmill running performance and running times on the track were impaired (see figure 2.5). However, when higher doses of furosemide (1.7 mg/kg) were given to male Finnish athletes prior to cycle ergometry, $\dot{V}O_2$max was significantly decreased from baseline (Caldwell, Ahonen, and Nousiainen 1984).

The effects of acetazolamide on $\dot{V}O_2$ are seen only during maximal exercise (Kowalchuk et al. 1992; Schoene et al. 1983; Stager et al. 1990). Under normoxic conditions, 3 doses of acetazolamide 250 mg did not affect $\dot{V}O_2$ during submaximal exercise at 70% $\dot{V}O_2$ (Brechue and Stager 1990), but did decrease $\dot{V}O_2$max during progressive cycling to exhaustion (Schoene et al. 1983). Conversely, under hypoxic conditions, $\dot{V}O_2$ was improved with acetazolamide pretreatment (Schoene et al. 1983).

How Diuretics Affect Exercise Performance

In general, hypohydration impairs exercise performance (Caldwell, Ahonen, and Nousiainen 1984). However, while certain physiologic

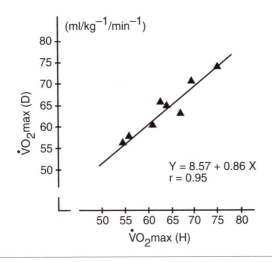

Figure 2.5 The relationship between hydrated (H) and dehydrated (D) V̇O₂max values measured during treadmill trials.

Adapted from Armstrong, Costill, and Fink 1985.

measurements are worsened by acute dehydration (Rankin, Ocel, and Craft 1996; Webster, Rutt, and Weltman 1990), overall performance in wrestlers may (Wroble and Moxley 1998) or may not (Horswill et al. 1994) be adversely affected. Likewise, diuretics produce ergolytic effects on exercise performance. Readers should note that most reports describing the effects of diuretics on athletic performance are based on either single doses or short-term administration; no data on long-term therapy exists (Fagard et al. 1993). However, single doses and short-term administration mimics the manner in which wrestlers and other athletes wishing to cut weight quickly use or abuse these drugs. Several authors have previously reviewed the topic of diuretics and exercise performance (Caldwell 1987; Fagard et al. 1993).

Effects on Aerobic Performance

Over 15 years ago, acute administration of the potent loop diuretic furosemide was shown to impair distance-running performance (Armstrong, Costill, and Fink 1985) and cycle ergometer performance (Caldwell, Ahonen, and Nousiainen 1984) in healthy athletes. A single, 40 mg oral dose of furosemide taken 5 h before exercise testing impaired both treadmill and track running. Treadmill running until volitional exhaustion decreased from 12.17 ± 0.33 min to 11.45 ± 0.35 min, a significant difference. Table 2.3 and figure 2.6 give data of how performances on the track were affected.

Table 2.3   Acute Effects of Furosemide on Athletic Performance

Distance	Mean track running time (minutes)	
	Euvolemic	Hypovolemic
1500 m	4.71 ± 0.16	4.87 ± 0.51 (not significant)
5000 m	18.22 ± 0.85	19.53 ± 0.93 ($p < 0.05$)
10,000 m	38.87 ± 1.73	41.49 ± 1.73 ($p < 0.05$)

Adapted from Armstrong, Costill, and Fink 1985.

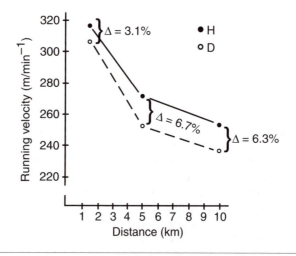

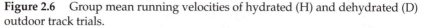

Figure 2.6   Group mean running velocities of hydrated (H) and dehydrated (D) outdoor track trials.

Adapted from Armstrong, Costill, and Fink 1985.

In another study of furosemide, sauna- and diuretic-induced methods resulted in only a slightly (i.e., roughly 1 kg) greater weight loss, but a 10- to 15-fold greater drop in PV when compared to exercise-induced weight loss. Decreases in $\dot{V}O_2$max and workload while cycling were proportionally decreased in the sauna and diuretic groups (see table 2.4). In this study, the diuretic regimen consisted of furosemide administered as a total amount of 1.7 mg/kg in two divided doses beginning 16 h prior to exercise testing (Caldwell, Ahonen, and Nousiainen 1984). Thus, hypohydration, regardless of etiology, can impair aerobic performance.

Table 2.4   Effect of Exercise-, Sauna-, and Diuretic-Induced Acute Hypohydration on Cycle Ergometer Performance

	Exercise	Sauna	Furosemide
Weight change (kg)	−2.3 ± 0.8*	−3.5 ± 0.8*	−3.1 ± 0.8*
Plasma volume change (%)	−0.9	−10.3*	−14.1*
$\dot{V}O_2$max (ml · kg · min)[a]	0.2 ± 3.0	−1.3 ± 4.4*	−2.8 ± 4.3*
Workload (W)[a]	−15.6 ± 22.3*	−15.1 ± 28.5*	−26.9 ± 28.7*
$\dot{V}O_2$max (ml · kg · min)[m]	1.1 ± 3.7	−2.3 ± 4.3*	−4.5 ± 4.3*
Workload (W)[m]	−6.9 ± 15.8*	−22.8 ± 17.4*	−21.3 ± 17.7*

* significantly worse than control group (not shown)
[a] = at anaerobic threshold
[m] = at maximal exercise
Adapted from Caldwell, Ahonen, and Nousiainen 1984.

Sometimes acetazolamide, a mild diuretic, is used legitimately to prevent AMS. Its effects on performance, similar to its effects on $\dot{V}O_2$, depend on the altitude. At sea level (Heigenhauser, Sutton, and Jones 1980) and under normoxic conditions (Schoene et al. 1983; Stager et al. 1990), short-term administration of acetazolamide may impair aerobic performance. Under hypoxic conditions, acetazolamide may decrease the time to exhaustion during submaximal exercise (Stager et al. 1990). However, with mountaineers given acetazolamide daily during a 10-day ascent to 4846 meters, the drug minimized the normal decline in aerobic work capacity that occurs when hikers ascend in altitude (Bradwell et al. 1986). Although physiologic adaptations to the diuretic effects of acetazolamide are known to occur within several days, the acid-base changes that the drug induces persist, which may explain the contradictory results in these studies.

Effects on Muscular Performance

Diuretics and profuse sweating can each adversely affect performance. For example, researchers found that thermal dehydration (i.e., a 4% decrease in body weight and 12% to 13% decrease in PV) in male college students was associated with a decrease in muscle endurance (isotonic and isometric) time of roughly 30%. However, even after rehydration back to baseline body weight, isometric and isotonic muscular performance remained significantly worse compared with baseline (Torranin, Smith, and Byrd 1979). Wrestlers who exercised while wearing a rubberized sweat suit to drop weight quickly were shown to have poorer performance in measurements of upper-body strength (Webster, Rutt, and Weltman 1990). It is important to inform wrestlers and boxers who attempt to make weight by sweating profusely or taking diuretics shortly before weigh-in of the possible detrimental effects of this strategy on performance.

Effects on Sport Performance

Thus, diuretics exert ergolytic actions on both aerobic and muscular performance. Only limited data, however, describe the effects of diuretics on overall athletic performance (see Caldwell 1987). Acute administration of diuretics decreases middle-distance running performance by about 7% (Armstrong, Costill, and Fink 1985) and decreases cycling workload substantially (Caldwell, Ahonen, and Nousiainen 1984). The effects on wrestlers' performance have generally been studied using exercise as the cause of hypohydration as opposed to diuretics, with no clear relationship noted (Horswill et al. 1994; Wroble and Moxley 1998). But it appears diuretic-induced hypohydration causes greater detrimental effects on athletic performance than exercise-induced methods (Caldwell, Ahonen, and Nousiainen 1984). Hypohydration, even when subjects were rehydrated prior to testing, markedly compromised parameters of muscle endurance. In addition, diuretics disrupt potassium homeostasis and thermoregulation (see later discussion). These factors must be weighed against the desire to achieve rapid weight loss. Athletes and coaches must realize that the detrimental effects of diuretics are greater than any perceived benefit.

Avoiding Potential Complications

One major potential risk of diuretic abuse by athletes is impaired thermoregulation. Skeletal muscle temperature exceeds core temperature within the first 5 min of aerobic exercise (Saltin, Gagge, and Stolwijk 1968). Thermal dehydration (Greenleaf and Castle 1971; Horstman and Horvath 1972), phlebotomy of 10% of blood volume (Fortney et al. 1981), and diuretic dehydration (Claremont et al. 1976; Nadel, Fortney, and Wenger 1980) have all been shown to impair thermoregulatory capacity. Greenleaf and Castle (1971) found that rectal temperatures during exercise increased 0.1 °C for every 1% loss in body weight due to hypohydration. However, phlebotomy or thermally induced hypohydration may not adequately represent diuretic-induced hypohydration. Phlebotomy removes cells in addition to volume, while thermally induced hypohydration produces a hypernatremic, hyperosmotic plasma, in contrast to diuresis, which produces a slightly hyponatremic, isosmotic plasma (Nadel, Fortney, and Wenger 1980). Exercise-induced hypohydration is also not a good model, since the lingering effects of physical stress may confound measurements of work performance during the testing phase.

Hypovolemia initiates cardiovascular adjustments during exercise that attempt to preserve circulating blood volume (to maintain venous return, cardiac output, and blood pressure) at the expense of the ability to regulate body temperature, a process requiring peripheral vasodilation (Claremont et al. 1976; Nadel, Fortney, and Wenger 1980). Cutaneous circulation (and heat transfer from core to periphery) is compromised when SV is reduced to 100 ml/beat or less during exercise in the heat (Nadel et al. 1979). Wilmore and Costill have thoroughly reviewed this topic in their text *Physiology of Sport and Exercise* (1994).

In addition to causing impaired peripheral vasodilation (radiation cooling), loss of PV disrupts thermoregulation through the decrease in sweating (evaporative cooling). At 35% $\dot{V}O_2$max, sweat rate was not compromised by diuretic administration (Claremont et al. 1976), for example; but at 70% $\dot{V}O_2$max, whole body sweat loss was decreased by 23% (Brechue and Stager 1990). Due to several mechanisms, therefore, the loss of PV impairs the normal vasodilatory response to exercise.

■ Electrolyte Imbalances: A Case of Diuretic Abuse in a Bodybuilder

A 24-year-old male bodybuilder called for an ambulance, complaining of lightheadedness, diffuse muscle cramps, and spasms. He also complained of lethargy, nausea, vomiting, and difficulty in swallowing. He denied chest pain, shortness of breath, abdominal pain, or diarrhea.

In the emergency department, vitals were temp 35 °C, RR 16, HR 116, and BP 106/93. His EKG showed sinus rhythm, tall and peaked T-waves, and a normal QRS complex. Laboratory data revealed sodium 133 mEq/L, potassium 8.2 mEq/L, chloride 93 mEq/L, CO_2 29 mEq/L, BUN 59 mg/dl, creatinine 2.5 mg/dl, glucose 146 mg/dl, magnesium 2.6 mg/dl, CPK 486 IU/L. Urine specific gravity was 1.016. Urine myoglobin was negative.

Initial questioning revealed that the patient had taken anabolic steroids in the past but not recently. He had been urinating frequently over the past 36 h, and he admitted to using multiple diuretics to reduce his body weight in preparation for a competition. He admitted to ingesting a mixture of 1 mg bumetanide twice daily,

(continued)

25 mg spironolactone 3 times daily, and 5 doses of KCl 20 mEq over the preceding 36 h.

He was treated for hyperkalemia with calcium chloride, intravenous dextrose and insulin, sodium bicarbonate, and Kayexalate. Over the next 24 h he became asymptomatic, with all lab values returning to normal. He confirmed to the nursing staff that he would continue his drug use; however, when contacted 5 months later, he denied any drug use (Al-Zaki and Talbot-Stern 1996).

All diuretics except the potassium-sparing group cause kaliuresis. In one study, administering a mean dose of 55 mg/day of hydrochlorothiazide produced hypokalemia in 17 of 20 hypertensive patients (DeQuattro et al. 1985). However, these doses were higher than the currently recommended dose of hydrochlorothiazide in the treatment of hypertension. If loop diuretics, which are more potent diuretics, are abused, the incidence of hypokalemia is still a concern. Hypokalemia, in turn, can lead to earlier muscle fatigue (Sjogaard 1986); in the setting of exercise-induced increases in circulating catecholamines, it may predispose subjects to ventricular ectopy (DeQuattro et al. 1985; Young et al. 1992).

Still another complication involves the combination of diuretics and exercising: photosensitivity. Thiazide diuretics are derivatives of sulfonamides. Dermatologic reactions are uncommon, but photosensitivity has been reported with use both of sulfonamides and of thiazide diuretics. Thus, this is another reason for subjects who must take thiazide diuretics to avoid exercising outdoors during midday hours.

In summary, the risks of exercising while taking diuretics include

• hyperthermia/heat exhaustion;
• decreased exercise duration;
• photosensitivity if exercising outdoors (thiazide diuretics);
• muscle cramps and/or cardiac arrhythmias secondary to electrolyte shifts/losses; and
• disqualification from competition.

NCAA and USOC Status

All diuretics are banned from athletic competition by both the NCAA and the USOC. Diuretics can dilute the normal concentrations of substances excreted in the kidneys. Thus, some athletes abuse diuretics, hoping to mask detection of other performance-enhancing drugs in a urine specimen. Diuretics are also banned because they can artificially reduce body weight, a consideration in such sports as wrestling, boxing, and judo.

Guidelines for Athletic Trainers

As we have discussed, athletic trainers may encounter diuretics in wrestlers who abuse these drugs in order to drop weight quickly or in deconditioned clients who wish to exercise while being treated for hypertension. It is important to counsel such people with whom you work about these drugs being banned substances, about their potentially serious side effects, and about their detrimental effects on endurance performance. The deconditioned hypertensive client who seeks the services of an athletic trainer poses a particular dilemma. While it would be inappropriate to tell such a person under the care of a physician to stop taking medicine for hypertension, the athletic trainer should make the client aware that diuretics adversely affect exercise duration and should encourage the client to discuss this issue with the prescribing physician. As you work with individuals who are using diuretics, keep the following factors in mind:

- Diuretics are banned substances; athletes should not use them in competition. Be suspicious of an athlete's use of diuretics if he or she does not have hypertension.
- Rapid dehydration, even if corrected prior to competition, has detrimental effects on performance.
- Be aware that persons with hypertension have significantly impaired exercise tolerance, irrespective of whether they are using diuretics (Lim et al. 1996). You should counsel people you work with about this effect. Because of this impaired tolerance and the fact that diuretics impair exercise performance, set conservative performance expectations for these individuals.
- Discourage people who are taking diuretics from exercising in high ambient temperatures or while wearing vinyl or rubber sweat suits. Dehydration impairs temperature regulation. Individuals can overheat quickly.
- Individuals taking diuretics will still perspire during exercise, thus exaggerating diuretic-induced fluid losses. Fluid intake is important, but replacement of fluid losses with mineral-containing (i.e., sodium, potassium) sport drinks should be done cautiously, since the client may also be on a potassium supplement or a potassium-sparing diuretic; hyperkalemia is a potentially serious medical problem.
- Thiazide diuretics have been associated with photosensitivity; encourage the client to wear sunscreen if he or she plans any outdoor midday exercise.

Guidelines for Physicians

It is important for a physician to balance the JNC guidelines recommending diuretics for first-line therapy in the treatment of hypertension against the detrimental effects these drugs have on exercise physiology. The medical community continues to endorse these drugs because of their proved benefit in reducing the risk of coronary heart disease and stroke in older adults (Moser 1998); and other factors (i.e., moderate cost, good compliance) argue strongly in favor of prescribing diuretics for patients with hypertension. Since exercise is a recommended part of the management of hypertension, physicians should consider the interaction between diuretics and exercise when treating the hypertensive patient.

Physicians should keep in mind the following issues:

- Hypertensive patients have significantly impaired exercise tolerance, irrespective of whether they are using diuretics (Lim et al. 1996).
- Exercise induces acute shifts in body potassium (Young et al. 1992), and these changes may contribute to exercise-induced tachyarrhythmias. Diuretic-induced electrolyte loss could exacerbate these changes.
- No data regarding the combined effects of long-term diuretic use and exercise exist.
- Many antihypertensive drugs now can be administered once daily that do not interfere with exercise duration, though these agents are generally more expensive than thiazide diuretics.
- Thiazide diuretics have been associated with photosensitivity; if diuretics must be prescribed, the patient should be encouraged to wear sunscreen if he or she plans any outdoor midday exercise.

In summary, prescribing diuretics to "weekend athletes" would seem to be undesirable for a variety of reasons. Because of detrimental effects of diuretics on exercise performance, alternative antihypertensive agents should be considered if the goal is to get more of the sedentary population to start exercising routinely.

References

Allen, T.E., Smith, D.P., and Miller, D.K. 1977. Hemodynamic response to submaximal exercise after dehydration and rehydration in high school wrestlers. *Med Sci Sports* 9:159-163.

Al-Zaki, T., and Talbot-Stern, J. 1996. A bodybuilder with diuretic abuse presenting with symptomatic hypotension and hyperkalemia. *Am J Emerg Med* 14:96-98.

Armstrong, L.E., Costill, D.L., and Fink, W.J. 1985. Influence of diuretic-induced dehydration on competitive running performance. *Med Sci Sports Exerc* 17:456-461.

Baum, K., Essfeld, D., and Stegemann, J. 1986. The influence of furosemide on heart rate and oxygen uptake in exercising man. *Eur J Appl Physiol* 55:619-623.

Benzi, G. 1994. Pharmacoepidemiology of the drugs used in sports as doping agents. *Pharmacol Res* 29:13-26.

Bradwell, A.R., Coote, J.H., Milles, J.J., Dykes, P.W., Forster, P.J.E., Chesner, I., and Richardson, N.V. 1986. Effect of acetazolamide on exercise performance and muscle mass at high altitude. *Lancet* 1(8488):1001-1005.

Brechue, W.F., and Stager, J.M. 1990. Acetazolamide alters temperature regulation during submaximal exercise. *J Appl Physiol* 69:1402-1407.

Caldwell, J.E. 1987. Diuretic therapy and exercise performance. *Sports Med* 4:290-304.

Caldwell, J.E., Ahonen, E., and Nousiainen, U. 1984. Differential effects of sauna-, diuretic-, and exercise-induced hypohydration. *J Appl Physiol* 57:1018-1023.

Claremont, A.D., Costill, D.L., Fink, W., and Van Handel, P. 1976. Heat tolerance following diuretic induced dehydration. *Med Sci Sports* 8:239-243.

Clausen, T. 1983. Adrenergic control of Na+-K+-homeostasis. *Acta Med Scand* 672(suppl):111-115.

Convertino, V.A. 1991. Blood volume: its adaptation to endurance training. *Med Sci Sports Exerc* 23:1338-1348.

Convertino, V.A., Greenleaf, J.E., and Bernauer, E.M. 1980. Role of thermal and exercise factors in the mechanism of hypervolemia. *J Appl Physiol* 48:657-664.

Delbeke, F.T., and Debackere, M. 1991. The influence of diuretics on the excretion and metabolism of doping agents. Part VI: Pseudoephedrine. *Biopharm Drug Dispos* 12:37-48.

DeQuattro, V., deGrau, A., Foti, A., Kim, S.J., DeQuattro, E., and Allen, J. 1985. Effects of exercise on blood pressure, plasma catecholamines, potassium and the electrocardiogram after diuretic and neural-blocking therapy for moderate hypertension. *Am J Cardiol* 56:39D-45D.

Fagard, R., Staessen, J., Thijs, L., and Amery, A. 1993. Influence of antihypertensive drugs on exercise capacity. *Drugs* 46(suppl 2):32-36.

Fortney, S.M., Nadel, E.R., Wenger, C.B., and Bove, J.R. 1981. Effect of acute alterations of blood volume on circulatory performance in humans. *J Appl Physiol* 50:292-298.

Freund, B.J., Shizuru, E.M., Hashiro, G.M., and Claybaugh, J.R. 1991. Hormonal, electrolyte, and renal responses to exercise are intensity dependent. *J Appl Physiol* 70:900-906.

Greenleaf, J.E., and Castle, B.L. 1971. Exercise temperature regulation in man during hypohydration and hyperhydration. *J Appl Physiol* 30:847-853.

Heigenhauser, G.J.F., Sutton, J.R., and Jones, N.L. 1980. Ventilation and carbon dioxide output during exercise: Effects of glycogen depletion and carbonic anhydrase inhibition. *Med Sci Sports Exerc* 12:123.

Horstman, D.H., and Horvath, S.M. 1972. Cardiovascular and temperature regulatory changes during progressive dehydration and euhydration. *J Appl Physiol* 33(4):446-450.

Horswill, C.A., Scott, J.R., Dick, R.W., and Hayes, J. 1994. Influence of rapid weight gain after the weigh-in on success in collegiate wrestlers. *Med Sci Sports Exerc* 26:1290-1294.

Johnson, J.M. 1986. Nonthermoregulatory control of human skin blood flow. *J Appl Physiol* 61:1613-1622.

Kenney, W.L., and Johnson, J.M. 1992. Control of skin blood flow during exercise. *Med Sci Sports Exerc* 24:303-312.

Kowalchuk, J.M., Heigenhauser, G.J., Sutton, J.R., and Jones, N.L. 1992. Effect of acetazolamide on gas exchange and acid-base control after maximal exercise. *J Appl Physiol* 72:278-287.

Kowalchuk, J.M., Heigenhauser, G.J., Sutton, J.R., and Jones, N.L. 1994. Effect of chronic acetazolamide administration on gas exchange and acid-base control after maximal exercise. *J Appl Physiol* 76:1211-1219.

Larson, E.B., Roach, R.C., Schoene, R.B., and Hornbein, T.F. 1982. Acute mountain sickness and acetazolamide. Clinical efficacy and effect on ventilation. *JAMA* 248:328-332.

Lim, P.O., MacFadyen, R.J., Clarkson, P.B.M., and MacDonald, T.M. 1996. Impaired exercise tolerance in hypertensive patients. *Ann Intern Med* 124(1 pt 1):41-55.

Moser, M. 1998. Why are physicians not prescribing diuretics more frequently in the management of hypertension? *JAMA* 279:1813-1816.

Munyard, P., Chung, K.F., and Bush, A. 1995. Inhaled frusemide and exercise-induced bronchoconstriction in children with asthma. *Thorax* 50:677-679.

Nadel, E.R., Cafarelli, E., Roberts, M.F., and Wenger, C.B. 1979. Circulatory regulation during exercise in different ambient temperatures. *J Appl Physiol* 46:430-437.

Nadel, E.R., Fortney, S.M., and Wenger, C.B. 1980. Effect of hydration state on circulatory and thermal regulations. *J Appl Physiol* 49:715-721.

National Institutes of Health. 1997. *The sixth report of the Joint National Committee on the Prevention, Detection, Evaluation, and Treatment of High Blood Pressure.* U.S. Department of Health and Human Services, NIH Publication no. 98-4080, November.

Papademetriou, V., Notargiacomo, A., and Freis, E.D. 1989. Diuretic therapy and exercise in patients with systemic hypertension. *J Hypertens Suppl* 7(6):S248-249.

Psaty, B.M., Koepsell, T.D., Yanez, N.D., Smith, N.L., Manolio, T.A., Heckbert, S.R., Borhani, N.O., Gardin, J.M., Gottdiener, J.S., Rutan, G.H., et al. 1995. Temporal patterns of antihypertensive medication use among older adults, 1989 through 1992. An effect of the major clinical trials on clinical practice? *JAMA* 273(18):1436-1438.

Rankin, J.W., Ocel, J.V., and Craft, L.L. 1996. Effect of weight loss and refeeding diet composition on anaerobic performance in wrestlers. *Med Sci Sports Exerc* 28:1292-1299.

Saltin, B., Gagge, A.P., and Stolwijk, J.A.J. 1968. Muscle temperature during submaximal exercise in man. *J Appl Physiol* 25:679-688.

Scheuermann, B.W., Kowalchuk, J.M., Paterson, D.H., and Cunningham, D.A. 1999. VCO_2 and VE kinetics during moderate- and heavy-intensity exercise after acetazolamide administration. *J Appl Physiol* 86:1534-1543.

Schoene, R.B., Bates, P.W., Larson, E.B., and Pierson, D.J. 1983. Effect of acetazolamide on normoxic and hypoxic exercise in humans at sea level. *J Appl Physiol* 55:1772-1776.

Siegel, D., and Lopez, J. 1997. Trends in antihypertensive drug use in the United States. Do the JNC V recommendations affect prescribing? *JAMA* 278:1745-1748.

Sjogaard, G. 1986. Water and electrolyte fluxes during exercise and their relation to muscle fatigue. *Acta Physiol Scand* 128(suppl 556):129-136.

Somani, S.M., ed. 1996. *Pharmacology in exercise and sports*. Boca Raton, FL: CRC Press.

Stager, J.M., Tucker, A., Cordain, L., Engebretsen, B.J., Brechue, W.F., and Matulich, C.C. 1990. Normoxic and acute hypoxic exercise tolerance in man following acetazolamide. *Med Sci Sports Exerc* 22:178-184.

Torranin, C., Smith, D.P., and Byrd, R.J. 1979. The effect of acute thermal dehydration and rapid rehydration on isometric and isotonic endurance. *J Sports Med Phys Fitness* 19:1-9.

Webster, S., Rutt, R., and Weltman, A. 1990. Physiologic effects of a weight loss regimen practiced by college wrestlers. *Med Sci Sports Exerc* 22:229-234.

Wilmore, J.H., and Costill, D.L. 1994. *Physiology of sport and exercise*. Champaign, IL: Human Kinetics.

Wroble, R.R., and Moxley, D.P. 1998. Acute weight gain and its relationship to success in high school wrestlers. *Med Sci Sports Exerc* 30:949-951.

Young, D.B., Srivastava, T.N., Fitzovich, D.E., Kivlighn, S.D., and Hamaguchi, M. 1992. Potassium and catecholamine concentrations in the immediate post exercise period. *Am J Med Sci* 304:150-153.

Zappe, D.H., Helyar, R.G., and Green, H.J. 1996. The interaction between short-term exercise training and a diuretic-induced hypovolemic stimulus. *Eur J Appl Physiol* 72:335-340.

3
CHAPTER

Other Antihypertensive Agents

■ *CASE*   Bill, the hypertensive executive described in the case study at the beginning of chapter 1, plans to begin exercising. You rule out beta-blockers and diuretics, which would be undesirable antihypertensive agents for someone like Bill who wishes to exercise. You know that beta-blockers and diuretics can be poor choices for many people with hypertension, despite the endorsement of these drugs by the Sixth Joint National Committee (JNC VI) on Prevention, Detection, Evaluation, and Treatment of High Blood Pressure. But with more than a hundred antihypertensive drugs or drug combinations on the market, which one should you select? And are the effects of drugs and exercise on blood pressure additive?

■ *COMMENT*   Fortunately, many different categories of drugs are potential alternatives. For hypertensive individuals who wish to exercise, angiotensin-converting enzyme (ACE) inhibitors, calcium-channel blockers, and alpha-blockers are all preferable to either beta-blockers or diuretics. You should consider coexisting medical conditions that Bill might have, since it may be possible to treat two problems simultaneously with one drug. You should also encourage endurance exercise over resistance training. Before Bill begins exercising, his blood pressure should be controlled to less than 180/105 mm Hg. While the blood pressure–lowering effects of exercise and antihypertensive drugs are additive, this should not be of concern to individuals with hypertension who exercise. Regular exercise provides many health benefits in addition to lowering blood pressure.

Roughly 24% of the U.S. population has hypertension, according to data collected between 1988 and 1991 for the Third National Health and Nutrition Examination Survey (Burt et al. 1995). In 1972, the National Heart, Lung, and Blood Institute (NHLBI) of the National Institutes of Health established the National High Blood Pressure Education Program (NHBPEP). Since then, the percentage of Americans who are aware that they have high blood pressure (BP) has increased from 51% (1976-1980 survey) to 68.4% (1991-1994 survey), according to the latest summary from the Joint National Committee on Prevention, Detection, Evaluation, and Treatment of High Blood Pressure (National Institutes of Health [NIH] 1997). Although it is beyond the goals of this chapter to discuss the pharmacologic management of hypertension, it is worth pointing out that, despite an improved awareness, this disease is still not being treated as comprehensively as it should be (Mosterd et al. 1999).

Health professionals encourage increasing physical activity as a nonpharmacologic treatment to help manage hypertension (NIH 1997). Unfortunately, although regular exercise helps lower BP, the extent of BP reduction appears to be limited (Gordon et al. 1990; van Baak 1994). Regular exercise does not routinely alleviate the need for drug therapy in the management of hypertension.

Hagberg and Brown (1995) reviewed the literature on exercise and hypertension. No fewer than 47 publications focused on how endurance exercise affects individuals with essential hypertension. These studies varied widely in design. Still, the authors could conclude that exercise training reduced diastolic BP in 78% of the groups that had an initial diastolic BP greater than 90 mm Hg; it reduced systolic BP in 70% of the groups that had an initial systolic BP greater than 140 mm Hg. Reductions in BP averaged roughly 10 mm Hg. Hagberg and Brown (1995) also point out that data are extremely limited about African-American hypertensives, despite the high incidence of hypertension and hypertension-associated morbidity and mortality among this population. At least one clinical study, however, has shown that endurance exercise lowers BP in African-American hypertensives (Kokkinos et al. 1995).

Resistance exercise or weight training is not recommended as the sole mode of exercise for hypertensives. Such exercise has not consistently reduced BP in hypertensive subjects (American College of Sports Medicine 1993). Acutely marked increases in BP are seen during resistance exercise (MacDougall et al. 1992). Hypertension is an important health issue, and readers who are interested in more detail should refer to *Physical Activity and Cardiovascular Health*, a symposium edited by Arthur S. Leon, MD (1997), and to the review by Gordon and colleagues (1990).

Because hypertension is so prevalent in the general population, sports medicine practitioners at all levels are likely to encounter individuals who wish to exercise while taking antihypertensive medications. Indeed, there are more than 150 antihypertensive drugs and/or drug combinations currently on the market. This chapter presents some concerns and recommendations regarding persons who exercise while taking one of the broad range of antihypertensive drugs.

In 1988, Chick, Halperin, and Gacek described the characteristics of the ideal antihypertensive agent for patients who exercise: no myocardial depressive effect during exercise; not arrhythmogenic; no detrimental effects on the exercise-induced redistribution of blood flow to exercising muscles; and no detrimental effects on substrate utilization. Several drugs discussed in this chapter appear to come close to meeting this ideal. Because some have become available only recently, however, their effects on the exercise response are as yet unknown. Table 3.1 summarizes the

Table 3.1   Antihypertensive Agents

Beta-blockers (see chapter 1)	Fosinopril (Monopril)
Diuretics (see chapter 2)	Lisinopril (Prinivil, Zestril)
Alpha-blockers	Moexipril (Univasc)
Doxazosin (Cardura)	Perindopril (Aceon)
Prazosin (Minipress)	Quinapril (Accupril)
Terazosin (Hytrin)	Ramipril (Altace)
Calcium-channel blockers	Spirapril (Renormax)
Benzothiazepines	Trandolapril (Mavik)
Diltiazem (Cardizem)	**Angiotensin II receptor antagonists**
Phenylalkylamines	
Verapamil (Calan, Isoptin)	Candesartan (Atacand)
Dihydropyridines	Eprosartan (Teveten)
Amlodipine (Norvasc)	Losartan (Cozaar)
Felodipine (Plendil)	Telmisartan (Micardis)
Isradipine (DynaCirc)	Valsartan (Diovan)
Nicardipine (Cardene)	**Sympatholytics**
Nifedipine (Procardia)	Clonidine (Catapres)
Nisoldipine (Sular)	Guanabenz (Wytensin)
Angiotensin-converting enzyme (ACE) inhibitors	Guanadrel (Hylorel)
	Methyldopa (Aldomet)
Benazepril (Lotensin)	**Vasodilators**
Captopril (Capoten)	Hydralazine (Apresoline)
Enalapril (Vasotec)	Minoxidil (Loniten)

different categories of drugs (not including beta-blockers and diuretics, discussed already) that are commonly used as antihypertensive agents.

The members of the calcium-channel antagonists, or "calcium blockers," are more diverse than the beta-blocker or alpha-blocker groups. Differences among the calcium-channel blockers involve variations in both chemical structure and subcellular mechanism of action. However, all calcium-channel antagonists lower BP.

For the purposes of this discussion, the agents within the alpha-blocker, angiotensin-converting enzyme (ACE) inhibitor, and angiotensin II antagonist groups are highly similar. Data on exercising while taking angiotensin II receptor blockers, however, are not readily available. Hydralazine, methyldopa, and some members of the sympatholytics group (guanethidine, reserpine) are older drugs that are no longer commonly used to treat hypertension (NIH 1997), and these drugs will not be discussed in this chapter. Because of the large number of available antihypertensive drugs and drug combinations, rather than discuss them individually, it makes sense to survey them as antihypertensive drug categories. And although some of these drugs are used to treat other conditions (e.g., ACE inhibitors are also used in the management of heart failure; calcium-channel blockers are used in the management of ischemic heart disease), the discussion here will focus on their use as antihypertensive agents.

How Exercise Affects the Action of Antihypertensive Drugs

What happens when subjects taking antihypertensive drugs start exercising? What is the impact of regular exercise on the actions of these drugs? Aside from some of the obvious overlapping cardiovascular effects, little is known on this issue. Since exercise stimulates catecholamine secretion, increases cardiac output, and redistributes blood flow, some of the effects of exercise on the actions of these drugs might seem predictable. However, exercise may also affect the pharmacokinetics of these drugs, thus making responses somewhat uncertain. In this section, we will briefly discuss the effects of exercise on the pharmacology and pharmacokinetics of these drugs. The majority of the discussion on metabolic interrelationships between exercise and these drugs occurs later in the chapter.

Effects on Pharmacology

Exercise can affect the cardiovascular actions of antihypertensive agents. In this section, we will look at three special cardiovascular actions: blood pressure, heart rate, and left ventricular hypertrophy.

Cardiovascular Actions: Blood Pressure

It is important to note the differences between the effects of endurance exercise and resistance exercise on BP. Both endurance exercise and resistance exercise increase BP acutely. As a session of endurance exercise progresses, systolic BP rises steadily secondary to the increase in cardiac output. Diastolic BP remains unchanged; it may even decrease in an attempt to facilitate blood flow to skeletal muscles. Endurance exercise at intensities of 40% to 70% $\dot{V}O_2$max appear to lower systolic BP slightly more and lower diastolic BP to the same degree as exercise at higher levels of intensity (Hagberg and Brown 1995). Stationary cycling increases mean BP by 21 to 28 mm Hg in hypertensives even while patients are taking antihypertensive agents such as ACE inhibitors, beta-blockers, or calcium-channel blockers (Agostoni et al. 1993). When hypertensive subjects taking antihypertensive agents from the beta-blocker and diuretic categories were given a treadmill exercise test, systolic pressure during exercise was lower, but diastolic pressure actually increased (Miller et al. 1983).

Long-term, endurance exercise exerts a beneficial lowering of BP, lowering both systolic and diastolic BP about 10 mm Hg in patients with essential hypertension and perhaps even more in patients with secondary causes of hypertension (Jacober and Sowers 1995). An exercise program may begin to ameliorate elevated BP within 3 weeks, but after 3 months further reductions are unlikely (Jacober and Sowers 1995).

While linear, predictable increases in BP are usually seen during a session of sustained aerobic exercise, enormous elevations in BP have been seen in weightlifters. Acute increases in systolic pressures over 400 mm Hg have been documented in subjects not taking antihypertensive drugs (MacDougall et al. 1985, 1992), with brachial artery pressures as high as 480/350 (see figure 3.1) in one bodybuilder during a leg press (MacDougall et al. 1985)! MacDougall and colleagues (1992) later investigated various factors affecting BP during weightlifting.

In general, while the acute effects of exercise oppose the principal pharmacologic action of antihypertensive drugs, the rises in BP occurring during exercise are tempered or lessened by the presence of these antihypertensive agents. Conversely, BP decreases in response to a long-term aerobic exercise program. Details of the responses of white male hypertensives to exercise conditioning have been nicely summarized by Duncan and colleagues (1985; figure 3.2). These issues are important to consider since modification of BP control is the most relevant issue regarding the effects of exercise on the pharmacology of antihypertensive (or hypotensive) agents. Although the increases in BP seen during resistance exercise are extreme, the duration of these elevations in BP are relatively short-lived and, therefore, unlikely to substantially compromise the long-term antihypertensive efficacy of these drugs.

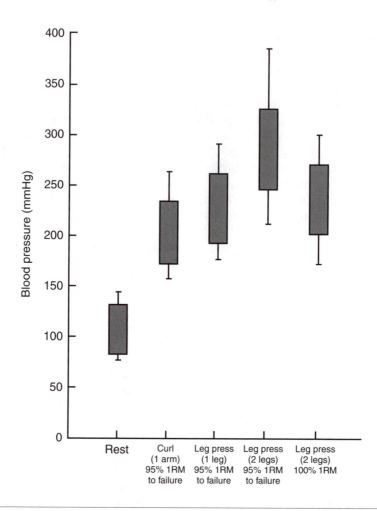

Figure 3.1   Peak systolic and diastolic BPs reached during various exercises at 95% and 100% of all subjects' single maximum lift (1RM). Mean and *SD*, *n* = 5.

Adapted from MacDougall et al. 1985.

Cardiovascular Actions: Heart Rate

Regarding the interaction of exercise and antihypertensive drugs on heart rate (HR), most antihypertensive drugs—aside from beta-blockers, which are discussed in chapter 1—have little effect on resting or exercise HR. Exercising while taking any of the drugs discussed in this chapter will lead to predictable increases in HR, although, in some cases, not to the same degree as would occur in the absence of the drug(s). However, three agents—clonidine, diltiazem, and verapamil—deserve mention, because these drugs can affect HR.

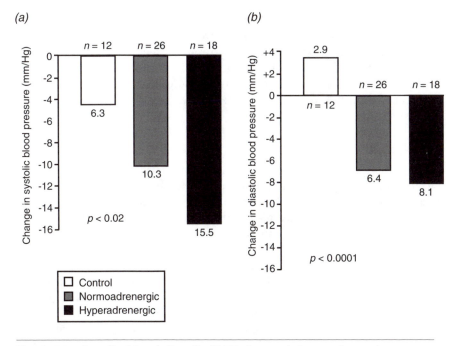

Figure 3.2 Systolic *(a)* and diastolic *(b)* BP changes in hyperadrenergic, normoadrenergic, and control groups following 16 weeks of physical training. Values within bar represent mean changes from baseline. *p* value from one-way analysis of variance.

Adapted from Duncan et al. 1985.

Clonidine is a centrally acting sympatholytic agent. When hypertensive subjects stabilized on clonidine were exercised, HR increased in proportion to exercise intensity, albeit not as much as when the subjects were not receiving the drug (Davies et al. 1989; Lund-Johansen 1974). While individual exercise sessions stimulate catecholamine output acutely, it has been shown that long-term regular exercise leads to a reduction in exercise-induced catecholamine output (Duncan et al. 1985). Thus, if subjects stabilized on clonidine exercise regularly, they may experience an additive drop in either HR or BP due to attenuation in overall sympathetic tone.

Diltiazem and verapamil are calcium-channel blockers that can suppress conduction through the atrioventricular (AV) node; both agents are used in clinical medicine to control ventricular rate in patients with atrial fibrillation. Indeed, these agents are preferred over digitalis because they control ventricular rate during exertion more effectively. In subjects that do not have atrial tachyarrhythmias, their effects on exercise HR are much less pronounced. In hypertensive subjects, verapamil suppressed exercise HR compared to placebo, but much less so than a beta-blocker (Mooy et al. 1987). Dihydropyridine-type calcium channel blockers do not demonstrate the suppressive effects on exercise HR seen with either diltiazem (Palatini et al. 1995) or verapamil (Halperin et al. 1993) in hypertensives. In normotensive volunteers, exercise does not appear to modify the effect of diltiazem or verapamil on HR (Gordon et al. 1986).

Cardiovascular Actions: LVH

The presence of left ventricular hypertrophy (LVH) in patients with long-standing hypertension is a serious risk factor for coronary heart disease (Koren et al. 1991; Levy et al. 1990). Endurance athletes can also develop LVH, although exercise-induced LVH is not associated with the same complications as is hypertension-induced LVH (Kokkinos et al. 1995).

What happens to LVH when hypertensive patients exercise? Kokkinos and colleagues (1995) studied the effects of regular exercise or no exercise in hypertensive African-American males who received a combination of indapamide, verapamil, and enalapril for treatment of their hypertension. The exercise regimen involved cycling on a stationary bicycle for 20 to 60 min at 60% to 80% of predicted maximum HR. After 16 weeks, larger reductions from baseline were seen in interventricular septal thickness, left ventricular mass, and left ventricular mass index than among the nonexercise group (see table 3.2). The effects of exercise appeared to be additive to the LVH-lowering effect of the medications these subjects were receiving, since these three drugs are known to independently reduce LVH (Houston 1989). Nevertheless, it is felt that exercise intensity should be restricted in subjects with preexisting LVH because exercise may further impair coronary vasodilation, thereby increasing the risk of myocardial ischemia and potentially fatal cardiac arrhythmias (Jacober and Sowers 1995).

Since LVH is an independent risk factor for coronary artery disease (Koren et al. 1991; Levy et al. 1990), it is no longer acceptable to simply lower the elevated BP in individuals with hypertension. As a result, it is desirable to prescribe antihypertensive agents that promote a beneficial reduction in LVH (Houston 1989; NIH 1997). Antihypertensive drugs that lower LVH are (Houston 1989)

- ACE inhibitors,
- alpha-receptor antagonists,
- calcium-channel blockers,
- clonidine,
- guanabenz,
- guanfacine,

Table 3.2 Echocardiographic Data on 15 Patients in the Exercise Group and 17 Patients in the No-Exercise Group

Variable	Exercise group (n = 15)		No-exercise group (n = 17)		p value	
	Baseline	16 weeks	Baseline	16 weeks	Unadjusted	Adjusted
Posterior-wall thickness (mm)	13.3 ± 1.5	12.3 ± 1.3	11.9 ± 2.0	11.9 ± 1.9	0.04	0.20
Interventricular septal thickness (mm)	14.9 ± 2.3	14.0 ± 1.7	13.7 ± 2.0	13.7 ± 2.1	0.008	0.03
Left ventricular systolic dimension (mm)	31 ± 5	30 ± 5	35 ± 7	34 ± 6	0.49	0.92
Left ventricular diastolic dimension (mm)	49 ± 5	48 ± 4	51 ± 6	51 ± 6	0.62	0.29
Left ventricular mass (g)	346 ± 95	304 ± 72	323 ± 69	326 ± 83	0.01	0.02
Left-ventricular-mass index*	163 ± 45	143 ± 34	150 ± 27	149 ± 32	0.02	0.04
Ejection fraction (%)	72 ± 11	74 ± 11	64 ± 11	69 ± 12	0.43	0.81
Fractional shortening (%)	37 ± 8	38 ± 9	32 ± 5	36 ± 8	0.18	0.53

*The left-ventricular-mass index is the left ventricular mass divided by the body-surface area.

Plus-minus values are means ± SD. p values are for the comparison of changes from baseline between groups.

Table 3.2 Reprinted, by permission, from P.F. Kokkinos, P. Narayan, J.A. Colleran, A. Pittaras, A. Notargiacomo, D. Reda, and V. Papademetriou, 1995, "Effects of regular exercise on blood pressure and left ventricular hypertrophy in African-American men with severe hypertension," *New England Journal of Medicine* 333: 1462-1467. Copyright © 1995 Massachusetts Medical Society. All rights reserved.

- indapamide,
- labetalol,
- methyldopa, and
- reserpine.

Effects on Pharmacokinetics

Data regarding the effects of exercise on the pharmacokinetics of these drugs are not readily available. However, some generalizations can be offered. The clearance (either renal or hepatic) of flow-limited drugs should decrease acutely during exercise. Captopril (ACE inhibitor), diltiazem (calcium-channel blocker), hydralazine (vasodilator), nifedipine (calcium-channel blocker), and verapamil (calcium-channel blocker) are antihypertensive agents that are known to be flow-limited drugs. Since all of these drugs are relatively short-lived agents, it is possible that sustained endurance exercise might exert a significant effect on the drug's pharmacokinetics. Theoretically, then, exercise might potentiate the actions of these flow-limited drugs. However, because BP rises acutely during exercise, any potentiation of the drug's antihypertensive action owing to delayed clearance would likely be insignificant. Further complicating the issue is the fact that hepatic drug metabolic capacity increases as overall fitness level improves (Boel et al. 1984).

Verapamil is an example of a drug that, when administered orally, is susceptible to extensive elimination as it passes through the liver; its clearance is highly dependent on blood flow to the liver. Since exercise diverts blood flow away from the liver (George 1979), exercise would be expected to delay the removal of verapamil from the circulation, thereby potentiating its duration of action. Van Baak, Mooij, and Schiffers (1992) showed that verapamil serum concentrations increased during submaximal aerobic exercise more than could be accounted for by the exercise-induced decrease in hepatic clearance. They attributed this to a corresponding decrease in verapamil volume of distribution. However, an earlier study using a much longer period of submaximal exercise found no changes in verapamil pharmacokinetics (Mooy et al. 1986). The reader is referred to the text by Somani (1996), which reviews this topic in great detail.

How Antihypertensive Drugs Affect Exercisers

With more than a hundred different antihypertensive drugs on the U.S. market alone, there isn't space in this book to review all the particular effects of each individual drug on responses during exercise. Much more information is available in several good reviews of this topic (see Chick,

Halperin, and Gacek 1988; Lowenthal and Kendrick 1985; Omvik and Lund-Johansen 1990, 1993). In this section, we will discuss, in general terms, the hemodynamic, pulmonary, and metabolic effects of antihypertensive agents. Throughout this section, readers should keep in mind that patients with hypertension often develop LVH (Mosterd et al. 1999) and display diminished exercise capacity (Lim et al. 1996), relative to normotensive subjects.

Hemodynamic Actions

We look first at hemodynamic actions—effects on exercise BP, HR, and cardiac output—among the calcium-channel antagonists, ACE inhibitors, alpha-blockers, and sympatholytics. In general, all antihypertensive agents exert an immediate (Omvik and Lund-Johansen 1990) and a sustained (Omvik and Lund-Johansen 1993) lowering of exercise BP. The effects on exercise HR differ among the agents; some of these issues have been discussed above.

Calcium-Channel Antagonists

Readers should not conclude that all members of the calcium-channel blocker group have similar cardiovascular effects. The dihydropyridines, of which nifedipine is the prototype, are strong vasodilators with little (if any) negative chronotropic (Palatini et al. 1995), dromotropic, or inotropic effects. The dihydropyridines also induce greater peripheral vasodilation than either diltiazem or verapamil. Diltiazem (Roth et al. 1986) and verapamil (Lang et al. 1983) exert strong inhibitory actions on conduction through the calcium-dependent AV nodal tissue; as a result, reflex tachycardia, which is seen with the dihydropyridine subgroup, does not occur (Kindermann 1987). Peripheral resistance (Palatini et al. 1995) and exercise BP (Gambini et al. 1991) are generally lowered more by calcium-channel blockers of the dihydropyridine type. The stronger peripheral vasodilatory actions of the dihydropyridine agents appear to exert detrimental effects on exercise hemodynamics. Nifedipine, but not diltiazem or verapamil, produced a detrimental effect on the oxygen uptake/percent maximum HR ratio in healthy males (Gordon et al. 1986).

Even though they suppress AV node conduction, diltiazem (Cohen-Solal et al. 1993) and verapamil (Mooy et al. 1987; Petri, Arends, and van Baak 1986) exert less of a depressive effect on exercise HR than do beta-blockers. Nifedipine does not affect exercise HR at $\dot{V}O_2$max or during submaximal exercise (Derman, Sims, and Noakes 1992). No differences are seen between diltiazem and nifedipine on cardiac output during exercise in hypertensive patients, even though exercise HR is lower with diltiazem (Yamakado et al. 1985).

ACE Inhibitors

Enalapril had no effect on exercise HR in hypertensive subjects during submaximal (van Baak et al. 1991) or maximal (Leon et al. 1986) exercise, although the drug did decrease exercise BP. In normotensive subjects, captopril decreased systolic, diastolic, and mean exercise BPs, but did not affect exercise HR during a graded exercise test (Fagard et al. 1982; figure 3.3).

Alpha-Blockers

Alpha-blockers reduce exercise diastolic, but not exercise systolic, BP (Thompson et al. 1989). Total peripheral resistance during exercise is reduced, but prazosin had no effect on cardiac output in hypertensive

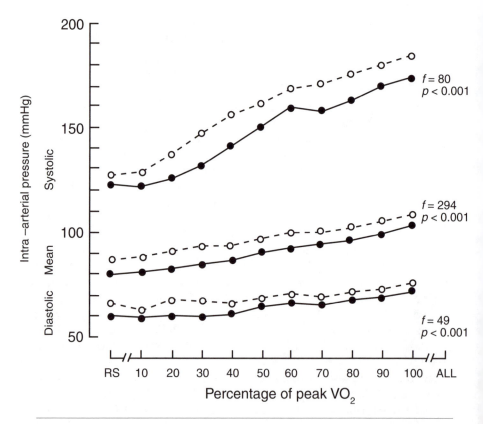

Figure 3.3   Systolic, diastolic, and mean intra-arterial pressure during placebo (○) and during captopril (●) in subjects at rest sitting (RS), during exercise (per 10% of peak $\dot{V}O_2$), and for all data combined (± *SE*). F value refers to effect of captopril.

Adapted from Fagard et al. 1982.

subjects during intermediate and maximal intensity cycling (Mulvihill-Wilson et al. 1983). Alpha-blockers do not decrease cardiac output (Gillin et al. 1989) or ejection fraction (Inouye et al. 1984b), even when administered for 2 months. Ejection fraction increased slightly in hypertensive subjects during bicycle exercise after chronic administration of doxazosin (Gillin et al. 1989).

Doxazosin had no effect on exercise HR at 30% or 50% $\dot{V}O_2$max, but slightly increased it at 75% $\dot{V}O_2$max and increased cardiac output at 50% $\dot{V}O_2$max, compared to placebo, in hypertensive male runners during treadmill exercise (Fahrenbach et al. 1995). Prazosin increases exercise HR acutely (Kenney et al. 1991; Mulvihill-Wilson et al. 1983), but chronic administration had no effect on exercise HR after either dynamic or isometric exercise (Mancia et al. 1980). Among the currently marketed alpha-blockers, prazosin has a half-life of 2 to 4 h, much shorter than that of either terazosin (12 h) or doxazosin (24 h). This factor, along with the lack of a sustained period of drug administration, may explain some of the divergent observations between prazosin and doxazosin on exercise HR (Mulvihill-Wilson et al. 1983). The mechanism for alpha-blockers to increase exercise HR is unclear, since these drugs do not affect skin blood flow (Kenney et al. 1991) or $\dot{V}O_2$ (Fahrenbach et al. 1995; Mulvihill-Wilson et al. 1983).

Sympatholytics

Clonidine, guanabenz, and guanfacine all possess a central sympatholytic action. Exercise increases catecholamine output acutely, but centrally acting sympatholytic agents inhibit the release of norepinephrine (Manhem et al. 1981). Thus, drugs of this type can blunt the sympathetic response to exercise (Maurer et al. 1983; Davies et al. 1989). In general, the sympatholytic effect of clonidine is more pronounced at rest than during exercise (Maurer et al. 1983). Clonidine decreases exercise HR in normotensive subjects (Maurer et al. 1983) and in hypertensive subjects (Davies et al. 1989; Manhem and Hokfelt 1981), although the negative chronotropic effect of beta-blockers is more dramatic than that of clonidine (Virtanen, Janne, and Frick 1982). Guanabenz did not affect exercise HR in hypertensive subjects (Dziedzic et al. 1983), perhaps because only a single dose was studied. While clonidine exerts an inhibitory effect on the sympatho-adrenomedullary system, BP and HR still increase during exercise, though not to the same degree as without clonidine (Davies et al. 1989; Manhem and Hokfelt 1981). Clonidine did not affect cardiac output during exercise (Lund-Johansen 1974). It has been shown to decrease exercise systolic BP in normotensives (Maurer et al. 1983), but to have no effect on exercise systolic BP in individuals with hypertension (Virtanen, Janne, and Frick 1982).

Pulmonary Actions

Little information is available about how the antihypertensive agents affect pulmonary function during exercise. Single doses of diltiazem, nifedipine, and verapamil (Gordon et al. 1986) or short courses of verapamil (Petri, Arends, and van Baak 1986) had no effect on ventilation, CO_2 production, or respiratory exchange ratio in 12 healthy subjects during cycle ergometry. However, nifedipine (Sharma, Pande, and Guleria 1986) and felodipine (Patel and Peers 1988) have been beneficial in exercise-induced bronchoconstriction, whereas inhaled diltiazem has not (Hendeles et al. 1988). Kindermann (1987) reviewed the pulmonary effects of calcium-channel blockers during exercise and concluded that this drug group has no effect on respiratory exchange ratio or minute ventilation during submaximal or maximal exercise.

Metabolic Actions: Oxygen Uptake

Fagard and colleagues (1993) summarized the effects of antihypertensive drugs on oxygen uptake ($\dot{V}O_2$), but most of the data they reviewed involved studies of beta-blockers. Less data exist regarding the effects on $\dot{V}O_2$ for diuretics, ACE inhibitors, calcium-channel antagonists, and other antihypertensive drugs. The following sections summarize what has been reported, organized again by categories of the antihypertensive agents.

ACE Inhibitors and Effects on $\dot{V}O_2$

Twelve weeks of enalapril therapy in patients with hypertension did not alter $\dot{V}O_2$ during treadmill testing (Leon et al. 1986). When compared with other antihypertensive agents in patients with hypertension, only captopril did not adversely affect either $\dot{V}O_2$ or exercise tolerance during graded cycle ergometry (Agostoni et al. 1993; figure 3.4). One month of captopril had no effect on $\dot{V}O_2$ in normotensive athletes (Carré et al. 1992). Angiotensin-converting enzyme inhibitors are routinely used in patients with heart failure (Meyer et al. 1991); however, these data are beyond the scope of this discussion.

For information comparing ACE inhibitors to other types of antihypertensive agents, see figure 3.5.

Alpha-Blockers and Acute Effects on $\dot{V}O_2$

Doxazosin had no effect on $\dot{V}O_2$ at 30%, 50%, or 75% $\dot{V}O_2$max in hypertensive runners during treadmill exercise (Fahrenbach et al. 1995). Prazosin also did not affect $\dot{V}O_2$, either acutely or after chronic administration, in hypertensive subjects during cycling at intermediate or maximal effort (Mulvihill-Wilson et al. 1983).

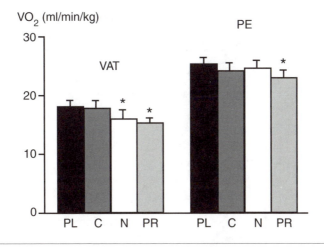

Figure 3.4   Oxygen consumption during administration of three antihypertensive agents and placebo. PL = placebo; C = 50 mg captopril; N = 20 mg nifedipine; PR = 80 mg propranolol; $\dot{V}O_2$ = oxygen consumption; VAT = ventilatory anaerobic threshold; PE = peak exercise. * = $p < 0.01$ vs. placebo.

Adapted from Agostoni et al. 1993.

Sympatholytics and Acute Effects on $\dot{V}O_2$

No data are available about the effects of clonidine and related drugs on $\dot{V}O_2$. Later in the chapter, however, data are provided describing improvements in $\dot{V}O_2$ in response to a training regimen during administration of clonidine.

Calcium-Channel Blockers and Acute Effects on $\dot{V}O_2$

The effects of calcium-channel blockers on $\dot{V}O_2$ are variable. This is likely because these drugs exhibit different pharmacologic profiles, but also because testing subjects within 1 h of ingesting nonsustained-release nifedipine exaggerates its hemodynamic effects. When tests were conducted within 1 h after ingestion of a single dose, nifedipine adversely affected $\dot{V}O_2$ in patients with hypertension (Agostini et al. 1993; see figure 3.5). No detrimental effects were seen in healthy male volunteers when testing was conducted 3 h postingestion (Derman, Sims, and Noakes 1992). In both studies, a 20 mg dose was used, and testing was conducted via cycle ergometry. Cohen-Solal and colleagues (1993) did not observe any effect of diltiazem on $\dot{V}O_2$max in sedentary hypertensives after 6 weeks of continuous administration.

When different calcium-channel blockers (e.g., diltiazem, nifedipine, verapamil) were compared in healthy males, only nifedipine was found to exert detrimental effects on oxygen uptake, but this was

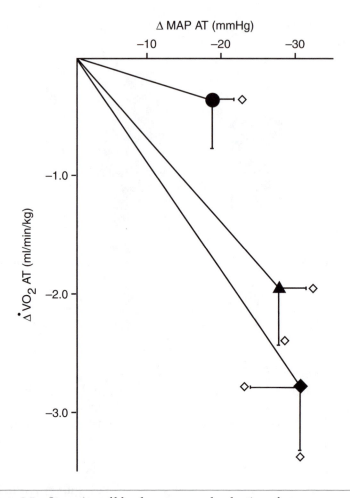

Figure 3.5 Lowering of blood pressure and reduction of oxygen consumption at ventilatory anaerobic threshold (VAT). ● = captopril; ▲ = nifedipine; ◆ = propranolol; ◇ = $p < 0.01$.

Adapted from Agostoni et al. 1993.

observed only during maximal exercise. Although the reduction in $\dot{V}O_2$ was modest, exercise performance was also diminished by nifedipine but not the other two agents (Gordon et al. 1986; table 3.3). Note that a nonsustained-release form of nifedipine was used in this study.

Oxygen Uptake in Summary

Some major points about $\dot{V}O_2$ deserve emphasis. First, researchers have not always observed a clear relationship between the effect of a drug on

Table 3.3 Effect of Acute Calcium Slow-Channel Antagonism on the Absolute and Relative O_2 Consumption for 70% and 85% of the Maximal Heart Rate

	Placebo	Diltiazem	Nifedipine	Verapamil
70% HR max				
HR (beats/min)	139 ± 5	138 ± 5	137 ± 5	137 ± 5
$\dot{V}O_2$ (l/min)	1.857 ± 0.35	1.859 ± 0.298	1.69* ± 0.309	1.766 ± 0.268
%$\dot{V}O_2$max	53.9 ± 6.5	54.5 ± 6.5	50.4** ± 6.6	52.7 ± 6.5
85% HR max				
HR (beats/min)	169 ± 6	168 ± 6	167 ± 6	167 ± 6
$\dot{V}O_2$ (l/min)	2.59 ± 0.364	2.581 ± 0.294	2.459* ± 0.339	2.503 ± 0.26
%$\dot{V}O_2$max	75.3 ± 4.5	75.9 ± 4.6	73.5** ± 4.7	74.7 ± 4.1

*$p < 0.01$ vs. placebo
**$p < 0.05$ vs. placebo
Data presented as the mean ± SD; $n = 12$. HR = heart rate; $\dot{V}O_2$ = oxygen consumption. Values differed significantly ($p < 0.05$) where indicated.

Adapted from Gordon et al. 1986.

$\dot{V}O_2$ and the effect of the same drug on exercise performance. And, regardless of the effects a given drug has on $\dot{V}O_2$, it is the effect on *exercise duration or performance* that matters. Several studies have demonstrated a direct relationship between the effect on $\dot{V}O_2$ and the effect on performance for beta-blockers; a similar relationship was not demonstrated, however, for other antihypertensive drugs. A decline in exercise performance should not be surprising with beta-blockers, considering that they affect many aspects of the exercise response (see chapter 1). On the other hand, some antihypertensive agents have been shown to exert detrimental effects on maximal exercise performance that were not predicted by corresponding changes in $\dot{V}O_2$max (Derman, Sims, and Noakes 1992).

Another important issue to consider in evaluating studies—and their results—of drugs on $\dot{V}O_2$ is the type of subjects and the mode of exercise they participate in. Most subjects rarely perform at peak levels of exercise; it may be more relevant, therefore, to study *submaximal exercise endurance* rather than maximal exercise capacity (Fagard et al. 1993). Regarding the mode of exercise testing, Cohen-Solal and colleagues (1993) proposed that exercise at a constant workload may be a better method of assessing the effects of antihypertensive agents during exercise in subjects with hypertension than a maximal exercise test of relatively short duration.

Metabolic Actions: Energy Substrates

During sustained exercise, both carbohydrates (derived from glycogen) and free fatty acids (FFAs; derived from triglycerides) are used to meet energy needs. Chapter 1 summarized how beta-blockers interfere with utilization of fats for energy by their ability to block epinephrine-mediated activation of lipolysis (Cleroux et al. 1989; Head 1999; Vanhees et al. 1991). Do other categories of antihypertensive agents interfere with energy utilization during exercise?

Verapamil had no effect on parameters of carbohydrate and fat metabolism during progressive cycling to exhaustion in healthy volunteers (Petri, Arends, and van Baak 1986). Free fatty acid concentrations increased during exercise after a single sublingual dose of nifedipine (Raffestin et al. 1985), but this may have been secondary to nifedipine-induced increases in catecholamine output. Kindermann (1987) reviewed data on calcium-channel blockers and concluded that these drugs do not exert any substantial effect on either glucose or lipid metabolism during exercise.

Enalapril had no effect on glucose or glycerol concentrations, but nonesterified fatty acid (NEFA) concentrations were significantly decreased during submaximal exercise in individuals with essential hypertension. A slight decrease in exercise performance was seen, though this was not statistically significant (van Baak et al. 1991).

Doxazosin had no effect on either carbohydrate or lipid metabolism, or on lactate levels during 15 min of cycling at 60% $\dot{V}O_2$max (Cosenzi et al. 1995).

Metabolic Actions: Lactate Concentrations

Only limited data are available on the issue of lactate concentrations. Lactate levels increased in hypertensive individuals receiving enalapril during submaximal exercise. Exercise endurance was slightly impaired, but not to a statistically significant degree (van Baak et al. 1991). Although changes were not statistically significant, blood lactate at rest and during maximal exercise increased in healthy subjects receiving nifedipine; it decreased, however, during administration of either an ACE inhibitor or a beta-blocker (Derman, Sims, and Noakes 1992). In another study, lactate concentrations were higher at all phases of exercise intensity when subjects were tested 90 min after a single dose of nifedipine. In this study, maximum workload during cycle ergometry was also impaired (Chick et al. 1986).

Metabolic Actions: Hormones

As discussed above, the hormonal response to a single exercise session differs from the response to long-term regular exercise (Duncan et al.

1985). Antihypertensive agents might be expected to affect levels of endogenous hormones. It should not be surprising that centrally acting sympatholytic drugs can affect catecholamine output during exercise. Clonidine can decrease epinephrine and norepinephrine output during exercise by roughly 60% (Maurer et al. 1983) (see figure 3.6). Based on the drug's mechanism, one would expect this. Yet guanabenz had no effect on plasma norepinephrine or renin (Dziedzic et al. 1983). The small number of subjects, and the fact that only a single dose was studied, may explain the lack of documented effect of guanabenz. Manhem and Hokfelt (1981) showed that clonidine decreased renin and aldosterone concentrations during 20 min of cycling at 80% $\dot{V}O_2$max. Joffe and colleagues (1986) thoroughly discussed the effects of clonidine on endogenous hormones.

In normotensives, captopril decreases plasma renin activity (PRA) at exercise intensities of 30%, 60%, and 100% $\dot{V}O_2$max (Fagard et al. 1982; figure 3.7). Manhem and colleagues (1981) found that high-dose captopril had no effect on either norepinephrine or epinephrine output in hypertensive subjects during a submaximal cycling test.

The effects of calcium-channel blockers on catecholamine output vary depending on the agent. Nifedipine has been shown to increase norepinephrine output more than verapamil does (Stein et al. 1984). Diltiazem also increases norepinephrine output (Inouye et al. 1984a). Kindermann (1987) reviewed the effects of calcium-channel blockers on

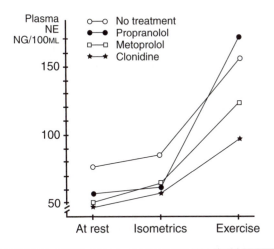

Figure 3.6 Plasma norepinephrine (NE) levels during three different treatments and control.

Adapted from Virtanen, Janne, and Frick 1982.

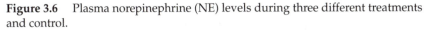

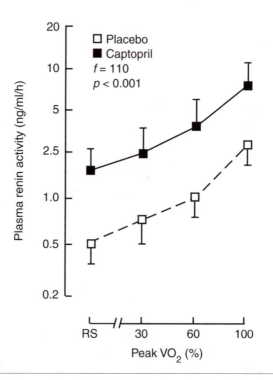

Figure 3.7 Plasma renin activity (PRA) during placebo (□) and captopril (■) in subjects at rest sitting (RS) and at 30, 60, and 100% of peak $\dot{V}O_2$. Values are mean $\pm$ *SE*; $f = 110$ (refers to effect of captopril); $p < 0.001$.

Adapted from Fagard et al. 1982.

the hormonal response to exercise and concluded that there were no significant effects on growth hormone, insulin, or other hormones.

Prazosin acutely increases plasma renin in hypertensive subjects during maximal cycling, but this effect disappears after chronic administration. Conversely, both acute and chronic prazosin increase plasma norepinephrine levels during exercise compared to placebo (Mulvihill-Wilson et al. 1983).

Table 3.4 summarizes how antihypertensive agents affect exercisers and their physiology.

How Antihypertensive Drugs Affect Exercise Performance

Blood pressure and physical activity are intimately related; BP increases acutely during exercise (MacDougall et al. 1985), and, conversely, low

Table 3.4   Effect of Calcium-Channel Blockers and Other Antihypertensive Agents on Exercise Parameters

	$\dot{V}O_2$max	HR	BP	CO	SVR	Training
Calcium-channel blockers						
Nifedipine	NC	I	D	I	D	NC
Verapamil	NR	D	D	NC	D	NR
Diltiazem	NR	D	D	NC	D	NR
Other antihypertensive agents						
Converting enzyme inhibitors	NC	D	NC	D		
Central alpha agonists	D	D	NC	D		
Alpha blockers	NC	D	NC	D		
Diuretics	NC	D	NR	D		

HR = heart rate
BP = blood pressure
CO = cardiac output
SVR = systemic vascular resistance
NC = no significant change
NR = not reported
I = increased
D = decreased

Adapted from Chick, Halperin, and Gacek 1988.

BP can compromise activity levels (Bou-Holaigah et al. 1995). Hypertensive patients often complain of weakness after acute reduction in BP (Agostoni et al. 1993). When studying the effect of BP-modifying drugs on athletic performance, one should consider the population selected and the mode of exercise; these factors can impact the results dramatically. Clinicians should be aware that patients with hypertension exhibit decreases in exercise capacity of as much as 30% compared to age-matched controls (Lim et al. 1996). In untreated hypertensives, cardiac output decreases by 1% to 2% per year (Omvik and Lund-Johansen 1993).

Blood pressure-lowering drugs may substantially affect exercise performance. During aerobic exercise, systolic BP increases while diastolic BP remains unchanged or may even decrease slightly. You should consider these variables when assessing the effects of various medications on the BP response to exercise. Fagard and colleagues (1993) have reviewed the effects of antihypertensive agents on exercise performance. Let's look at how some categories of antihypertensives affect performance.

ACE Inhibitors and Performance

Single doses of cilazapril in healthy males increased ratings of perceived exertion (RPE) during submaximal exercise and decreased the time to exhaustion during maximal exercise (Derman, Sims, and Noakes 1992). In contrast, after 8-12 weeks of cilazapril administration, treadmill exercise duration improved slightly in a study of hypertensive subjects (White et al. 1988). The duration of drug administration and the type of subjects studied may explain why different results were obtained with the same drug. Chronic, 12-week administration of enalapril had no effect on RPE in hypertensive subjects during treadmill testing (Leon et al. 1986). In other studies of hypertensive subjects, enalapril decreased cycling performance by 3% (Vanhees et al. 1991) and decreased submaximal exercise performance by 12% (van Baak et al. 1991), but these observations were not statistically significant. Finally, 1 month of captopril administration had no effect on maximal cycling performance or on isokinetic muscle strength in normotensive athletes (Carré et al. 1992; figure 3.8 and table 3.5).

Calcium-Channel Blockers and Performance

In 1987, Kindermann reviewed data regarding the effects of calcium-channel blockers on exercise performance and concluded that these agents did not affect maximum and endurance performance, endurance time during prolonged submaximal exercise, or heavy submaximal exercise. Since then, other data have been published. In some studies, nonsustained-release dosage forms of nifedipine, because of its rapid and potent peripheral vasodilatory properties, have been shown to impair performance. During maximal exercise, a single 10 mg oral dose of nifedipine decreased exercise duration, decreased maximum workload, decreased lactate threshold, and increased lactate levels in sedentary subjects during cycle ergometry (Derman, Sims, and Noakes 1992). Sustained-release dosage forms of diltiazem (Chrysant and Miller 1994), nifedipine (Halperin et al. 1993), or verapamil (Halperin et al. 1993) did not affect exercise time in other studies. When maximal power was assessed during cycle ergometry, single doses of nifedipine were not found to be ergolytic (Raffestin et al. 1985). However, when performance time was assessed, in a comparison of nifedipine, diltiazem, and verapamil, only nifedipine (nonsustained release) exerted detrimental effects on cycling performance in healthy males. The detrimental effects on performance were of a greater magnitude than could be accounted for by the changes observed in $\dot{V}O_2$, so the authors concluded that some other physiologic alteration explained this ergolytic effect (Gordon et al. 1986). Diltiazem did not affect exer-

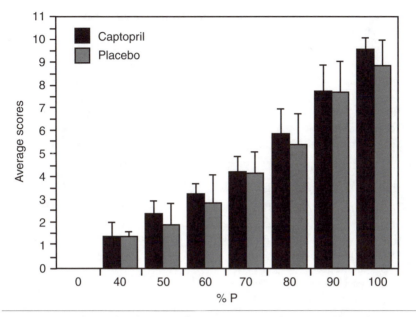

Figure 3.8 Relationship between the average scores (mean ± *SD*) on the Borg scale and the percentage of aerobic power (% P). % P = percentage of maximum power.

Adapted from Carré et al. 1992.

Table 3.5 Effect of Captopril on Isokinetic Quadriceps Muscle Strength

	Q/kg 60 degrees · s⁻¹ Nm	Q/kg 180 degrees · s⁻¹ Nm	FI
Captopril	2.71 ± 0.3	1.85 ± 0.2	0.66 ± 0.11
Placebo	2.74 ± 0.4	1.86 ± 0.3	0.66 ± 0.12
p	NS	NS	NS

Q/kg-strength peak related to body weight in Nm.
FI-fatigability index at 180 degrees · s⁻¹ (mean ± SD).

Adapted from Carré et al. 1992.

cise duration relative to placebo in sedentary hypertensives, as seen in table 3.6 (Cohen-Solal et al. 1993).

A few studies have compared verapamil with beta-blockers in hypertensive subjects. In one, verapamil decreased cycling performance by

Table 3.6   Effects of Placebo, Atenolol, and Diltiazem on Cardiopulmonary Parameters of Exercise Capacity

	Placebo	Atenolol	Diltiazem
Maximal HR (beats · min^{-1})	161 ± 20	130 ± 22[b, c]	149 ± 22
Exercise duration (s)	823 ± 344	839 ± 352	839 ± 355
Ventilatory threshold[a] (ml/min/kg)	16.3 ± 6.7	15.3 ± 6.1	15.8 ± 6.6
Maximal $\dot{V}O_2$ (ml/min/kg)	24.9 ± 7.7	23.2 ± 7.5	23.3 ± 8.7
Maximal O_2 pulse (ml/min/kg/beat · 10^3)	155 ± 38	179 ± 44[c, d]	155 ± 48
$\Delta \dot{V}O_2$/time (ml/min/kg/s · 10^3)	20.0 ± 2.8	19.1 ± 2.7	19.2 ± 2.7

[a] n = 12 for placebo, 13 for atenolol, and 11 for diltiazem
[b] $p < 0.05$ vs. placebo
[c] $p < 0.05$ vs. diltiazem
[d] $p < 0.005$ vs. placebo
Adapted from Cohen-Solal et al. 1993.

7% among hypertensive subjects, but these changes were not statistically significant (Vanhees et al. 1991). In another, verapamil had no effect on cycling exercise endurance despite its effects on exercise HR and exercise BP (Mooy et al. 1987). Likewise, verapamil had no detrimental effect on maximal exercise capacity or RPE in healthy volunteers exercised on a bicycle ergometer to exhaustion (Petri, Arends, and van Baak 1986).

In subjects with atrial fibrillation, a setting where calcium-channel blockers can exert dramatic effects on exercise HR, the effect on performance was varied. In one such study, verapamil improved exercise performance (Lang et al. 1983), whereas in another study diltiazem had no effect on exercise performance (Steinberg et al. 1987), despite the fact that both drugs reduced exercise HR. The mode of exercise testing (e.g., bicycle ergometry and Master's step test in the verapamil study; the Bruce or modified Bruce treadmill protocol in the diltiazem study) may have been responsible for these divergent results. This is plausible, since the two calcium-channel blockers significantly reduced both resting and exercise HRs. Thus, the type of subjects, the type of exercise testing, and the drug in question all can affect the interpretation of the relationship between drug-induced changes on HR and how this impacts on exercise performance.

Alpha-Blockers and Performance

Alpha-blockers do not appear to affect performance during endurance exercise. Prazosin had no detrimental effects on either treadmill or cycle ergometer performance in hypertensive joggers (Thompson et al. 1989). Terazosin had no detrimental effect on exercise performance in hypertensive subjects (Ligueros et al. 1992). Several groups of investigators compared doxazosin with atenolol and found that doxazosin did not impair exercise performance during running (Fahrenbach et al. 1995) or during cycling (Gillin et al. 1989). In yet another comparison (Cosenzi et al. 1995), 15 min of cycling at 60% $\dot{V}O_2$max was not adversely affected by doxazosin.

Summary of Effects of Antihypertensive Agents on Performance

Several reviews have been published summarizing data on the effects of antihypertensive drugs on athletic performance (Chick, Halperin, and Gacek 1988; Fagard et al. 1993). In both reviews, the bulk of the data focused on beta-blockers. For the other categories of antihypertensive agents, much less data are available. Chick and colleagues recommended avoiding beta-blockers and diuretics (Chick, Halperin, and Gacek 1988), precisely the drug categories that are preferred by the medical community for the treatment of hypertension (NIH 1997). Chick and colleagues concluded that any of the other drug categories would be better choices than beta-blockers or diuretics. However, it seems that drugs like clonidine, which directly interfere with the sympathetic response to exercise, should be avoided also. Although not well-studied, the alpha-blocker drug doxazosin might become a worthwhile agent in the hypertensive athlete, since this drug does not affect performance and also does not appear to affect skin blood flow (Kenney et al. 1991) or cardiovascular or thermoregulatory responses to severe exercise in heat (Franke et al. 1993).

Can a Conditioning Effect Be Achieved While Taking Antihypertensive Drugs?

If we are successful in getting more of the sedentary, deconditioned population to start exercising, it would be helpful to know if improvements in cardiovascular fitness can be achieved in patients taking antihypertensive drugs. Unfortunately, the literature provides very little data on this topic for this large group of drugs. However, there is some hope; even though a drug may depress $\dot{V}O_2$ acutely, increases in $\dot{V}O_2$max *in response to a conditioning regimen* can still occur during administration of the same drug. For example, even with the beta-blockers, drugs known to exert multiple negative aspects on the exercise response, a noticeable increase in $\dot{V}O_2$ during a training regimen has been documented during chronic administration of these drugs (Duncan et al. 1990). Some additional information on this topic is summarized below.

When healthy, sedentary subjects participated in an intense (5 times per week at >85% maximum HR), 6-week exercise regimen, researchers found that $\dot{V}O_2$ increased in subjects receiving the calcium-channel blocker nifedipine and in subjects receiving placebo. There were no differences between the placebo and nifedipine groups with regard to degree of improvement (Duffey, Horwitz, and Brammell 1984). In a study of diltiazem, exercise duration increased by 19% in hypertensive subjects receiving placebo, by 22% in subjects receiving diltiazem, and by only 10% in subjects receiving propranolol during a 10-week exercise program (Stewart et al. 1990).

Looking at the sympatholytics category to examine performance and conditioning effects, Davies and colleagues (1989) assessed the effects of an 8-week walking/jogging program on hypertensive subjects receiving transdermal clonidine. Oxygen uptake improved during the 8 weeks despite continuous administration of clonidine (see figures 3.9, 3.10, and 3.11). Transdermal clonidine did not interfere with the ability of the subjects to gradually lengthen their jogging time (Davies et al. 1989).

Sometimes antihypertensive agents are used in combination, and in one study the combination of indapamide, verapamil, and enalapril in African-American hypertensive males did not prevent an increase in peak $\dot{V}O_2$ from occurring during a 32-week exercise program (Kokkinos et al. 1995). This particular study did not measure the effects on exercise performance.

Beyond these data, only questions exist. Research that explores how chronic administration of antihypertensive drugs affects the response to regular exercise is urgently needed.

Avoiding Potential Complications

Beta-blockers interfere with energy utilization and sympathetic regulation of the exercise response. Diuretics can also interfere with exercise performance. Much less is known, however, about other classes of antihypertensive agents when used during exercise. This issue needs urgent investigation considering both the number of drugs used in the treatment of hypertension and the number of hypertensive individuals. Fluid replacement after exercise is always important, but individuals with hypertension should be careful with high sodium- and/or potassium-containing fluids.

NCAA and USOC Status

Other than beta-blockers and diuretics, antihypertensive drugs are not banned for use in competition by the NCAA and USOC. Nevertheless,

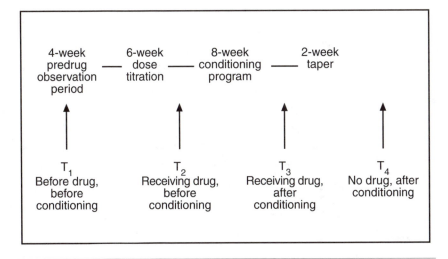

Figure 3.9   Phases of the study.

Adapted from Davies et al. 1989.

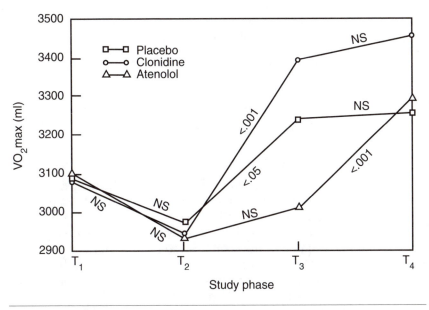

Figure 3.10 $\dot{V}O_2$max with incremental bicycle exercise at four time points of the study. NS = not significant.

Adapted from Davies et al. 1989.

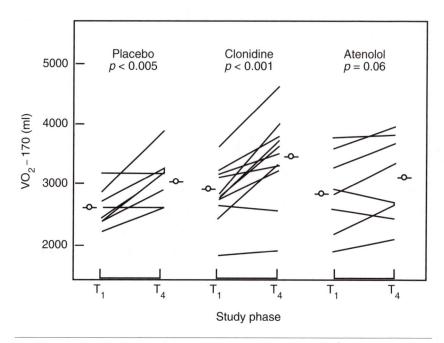

Figure 3.11   Oxygen uptake at a heart rate of 170 beats/min ($\dot{V}O_2$ 170) at baseline (T1) and at the end of the study (T4). There was no active medication at either time point.

Adapted from Davies et al. 1989.

since many antihypertensive agents are marketed *in combination with a diuretic,* these combination products are banned.

Guidelines for Using Antihypertensive Drugs

Since it has been recommended that BP be lowered to at least 180/105 before a hypertensive patient embarks on an exercise program (Jacober and Sowers 1995), individuals with hypertension will likely be receiving drugs when they meet with an exercise counselor. Houston considers beta-blockers one of the least desirable antihypertensive agents for the exercisers. He suggests that these individuals with hypertension should receive calcium-channel blockers or ACE inhibitors (Houston 1992). Physicians and sports medicine personnel should realize that among all types of antihypertensive drugs, calcium-channel blockers and ACE inhibitors appear to impair $\dot{V}O_2$max and performance less than the other types. Doxazosin, since it preserves cardiac output, can be administered once daily, and does not exert ergolytic effects on performance, appears especially attractive in the hypertensive athlete. If the hypertensive individual intends to exercise, particularly if he or she intends to exercise aerobically, it may be best to select agents other than those of the beta-blocker or diuretic categories.

References

Agostoni, P.G., Doria, E., Alimento, M., Riva, S., Muratori, M., and Tamborini, G. 1993. Modification of exercise performance by sharp reduction of blood pressure. *Chest* 104:1755-1758.
American College of Sports Medicine. 1993. Position stand. Physical activity, physical fitness, and hypertension. *Med Sci Sports Exerc* 25(10):i-x.
Boel, J., Andersen, L.B., Rasmussen, B., Hansen, S.H., and Dossing, M. 1984. Hepatic drug metabolism and physical fitness. *Clin Pharmacol Ther* 36:121-126.
Bou-Holaigah, I., Rowe, P.C., Kan, J., and Calkins, H. 1995. The relationship between neurally mediated hypotension and the chronic fatigue syndrome. *JAMA* 274:961-967.
Burt, V.L., Whelton, P., Roccella, E.J., Brown, C., Cutler, J.A., Higgins, M., Horan, M.J., and Labarthe, D. 1995. Prevalence of hypertension in the U.S. adult population: Results from the Third National Health and Nutrition Examination Survey, 1988-1991. *Hypertension* 25:305-313.
Carré, F., Handschuh, R., Beillot, J., Dassonville, J., Rochcongar, P., Guivarc'h, P.H., and Lessard, Y. 1992. Effects of captopril chronic intake on the aerobic performance and muscle strength of normotensive trained subjects. *Int J Sports Med* 13:308-312.
Chick, T.W., Halperin, A.K., and Gacek, E.M. 1988. The effect of antihypertensive medications on exercise performance: A review. *Med Sci Sports Exerc* 20:447-454.
Chick, T.W., Halperin, A.K., Jackson, J.E., and Van As, A. 1986. The effect of nifedipine on cardiopulmonary responses during exercise in normal subjects. *Chest* 89:641-646.
Chrysant, S.G., and Miller, E. 1994. Effects of atenolol and diltiazem-SR on exercise and pressure load in hypertensive patients. *Clin Cardiol* 17:670-674.
Cleroux, J., Van Nguyen, P., Taylor, A.W., and Leenen, F.H.H. 1989. Effects of beta-1 plus beta-2 blockade on exercise endurance and muscle metabolism in humans. *J Appl Physiol* 66:548-554.
Cohen-Solal, A., Baleynaud, S., Laperche, T., Sebag, C., and Gourgon, R. 1993. Cardiopulmonary response during exercise of a beta-1-selective beta-blocker (atenolol) and a calcium-channel blocker (diltiazem) in untrained subjects with hypertension. *J Cardiovasc Pharmacol* 22:33-38.
Cosenzi, A., Sacerdote, A., Bocin, E., Molino, R., Mangiarotti, M., and Bellini, G. 1995. Metabolic effects of atenolol and doxazosin in healthy volunteers during prolonged physical exercise. *J Cardiovasc Pharmacol* 25:142-146.
Davies, S.F., Graif, J.L., Husebye, D.G., Maddy, M.M., McArthur, C.D., Path, M.J., O'Connell, M.B., Iber, C., and Davidman, M. 1989. Comparative effects of transdermal clonidine and oral atenolol on acute exercise performance and response to aerobic conditioning in subjects with hypertension. *Arch Intern Med* 149:1551-1556.

Derman, W.E., Sims, R., and Noakes, T.D. 1992. The effects of antihypertensive medication on the physiological response to maximal exercise testing. *J Cardiovasc Pharmacol* 19(suppl 5):S122-S127.

Duffey, D.J., Horwitz, L.D., and Brammell, H.L. 1984. Nifedipine and the conditioning response. *Am J Cardiol* 53:908-911.

Duncan, J.J., Farr, J.E., Upton, S.J., Hagan, R.D., Oglesby, M.E., and Blair, S.N. 1985. The effects of aerobic exercise on plasma catecholamines and blood pressure in patients with mild essential hypertension. *JAMA* 254:2609-2613.

Duncan, J.J., Vaandrager, H., Farr, J.E., Kohl, H.W., and Gordon, N.F. 1990. Effect of intrinsic sympathomimetic activity on the ability of hypertensive patients to derive a cardiorespiratory training effect during chronic beta-blockage. *Am J Hypertens* 3:302-306.

Dziedzic, S.W., Elijovich, F., Felton, K., Yeager, K., and Krakoff, L.R. 1983. Effect of guanabenz on blood pressure responses to posture and exercise. *Clin Pharmacol Ther* 33:151-155.

Fagard, R., Lijnen, P., Vanhees, L., and Amery, A. 1982. Hemodynamic response to converting enzyme inhibition at rest and exercise in humans. *J Appl Physiol: Respirat Environ Exercise Physiol* 53:576-581.

Fagard, R., Staessen, J., Thijs, L., and Amery, A. 1993. Influence of antihypertensive drugs on exercise capacity. *Drugs* 46(suppl 2):32-36.

Fahrenbach, M.C., Yurgalevitch, S.M., Zmuda, J.M., and Thompson, P.D. 1995. Effect of doxazosin or atenolol on exercise performance in physically active, hypertensive men. *Am J Cardiol* 75:258-263.

Franke, W.D., Hickey, M.S., Ward, C.W., and Davy, K.P. 1993. Effects of alpha-1-receptor blockade on the cardiovascular and thermoregulatory responses to severe exercise in the heat. *J Sports Med Phys Fitness* 33:146-151.

Gambini, G., Valori, C., Bianchi, L., and Bozza, M. 1991. Acute and short-term effects of nitrendipine and diltiazem at rest and during exercise in hypertensive patients. *Clin Ther* 13:680-686.

George, C.F. 1979. Drug kinetics and hepatic blood flow. *Clin Pharmacokinet* 4:433-448.

Gillin, A.G., Fletcher, P.J., Horvath, J.S., Hutton, B.F., Bautovich, G.J., and Tiller, D.J. 1989. Comparison of doxazosin and atenolol in mild hypertension, and effects on exercise capacity, hemodynamics and left ventricular function. *Am J Cardiol* 63:950-954.

Gordon, N.F., Scott, C.B., Wilkinson, W.J., Duncan, J.J., and Blair, S.N. 1990. Exercise and mild essential hypertension. Recommendations for adults. *Sports Med* 10:390-404.

Gordon, N.F., van Rensburg, J.P., Kawalsky, D.L., Russell, H.M., Celliers, C.P., and Myburgh, D.P. 1986. Effect of acute calcium slow-channel antagonism on the cardiorespiratory response to graded exercise testing. *Int J Sports Med* 7:254-258.

Hagberg, J.M., and Brown, M.D. 1995. Does exercise training play a role in the treatment of essential hypertension? *J Cardiovasc Risk* 2:296-302.

Halperin, A.K., Icenogle, M.V., Kapsner, C.O., Chick, T.W., Roehnert, J., and Murata, G.H. 1993. A comparison of the effect of nifedipine and verapamil on exercise performance in patients with mild to moderate hypertension. *Am J Hypertens* 6:1025-1032.

Head, A. 1999. Exercise metabolism and beta-blocker therapy. *Sports Med* 27:81-96.

Hendeles, L., Hill, M., Harman, E., Moore, P., and Pieper, J. 1988. Dose-response of inhaled diltiazem on airway reactivity to methacholine and exercise in subjects with mild asthma. *Clin Pharmacol Ther* 43:387-392.

Houston, M.C. 1989. New insights and new approaches for the treatment of essential hypertension: Selection of therapy based on coronary heart disease risk factor analysis, hemodynamic profiles, quality of life, and subsets of hypertension. *Am Heart J* 117:911-951.

Houston, M.C. 1992. Exercise and hypertension. Maximizing the benefits in patients receiving drug therapy. *Postgrad Med* 92:139-144, 150.

Inouye, I.K., Massie, B.M., Benowitz, N., Simpson, P., and Loge, D. 1984a. Antihypertensive therapy with diltiazem and comparison with hydrochlorothiazide. *Am J Cardiol* 53:1588-1592.

Inouye, I., Massie, B., Benowitz, N., Simpson, P., Loge, D., and Topic, N. 1984b. Monotherapy in mild to moderate hypertension: Comparison of hydrochlorothiazide, propranolol and prazosin. *Am J Cardiol* 53:24A-28A.

Jacober, S.J., and Sowers, J.R. 1995. Exercise and hypertension. *JAMA* 273:1965.

Joffe, B.I., Haitas, B., Edelstein, D., Panz, V., Lamprey, J.M., Baker, S.G., and Seftel, H.C. 1986. Clonidine and the hormonal responses to graded exercise in healthy subjects. *Horm Res* 23:136-141.

Kenney, W.L., Tankersley, C.G., Newswanger, D.L., and Puhl, S.M. 1991. Alpha-1-adrenergic blockade does not alter control of skin blood flow during exercise. *Am J Physiol (Heart Circ Physiol)* 260:H855-H861.

Kindermann, W. 1987. Calcium antagonists and exercise performance. *Sports Med* 4:177-193.

Kokkinos, P.F., Narayan, P., Colleran, J.A., Pittaras, A., Notargiacomo, A., Reda, D., and Papademetriou, V. 1995. Effects of regular exercise on blood pressure and left ventricular hypertrophy in African-American men with severe hypertension. *N Engl J Med* 333:1462-1467.

Koren, M.J., Devereux, R.B., Casale, P.N., Savage, D.D., and Laragh, J.H. 1991. Relation of left ventricular mass and geometry to morbidity and mortality in uncomplicated essential hypertension. *Ann Intern Med* 114:345-352.

Lang, R., Klein, H.O., Weiss, E., David, D., Sareli, P., Levy, A., Guerrero, J., Di Segni, E., and Kaplinsky, E. 1983. Superiority of oral verapamil therapy to digoxin in treatment of chronic atrial fibrillation. *Chest* 83:491-499.

Leon, A.S., ed. 1997. *Physical activity and cardiovascular health: A national consensus.* Champaign, IL: Human Kinetics.

Leon, A.S., McNally, C., Casal, D., Grimm, R., Crow, R., Bell, C., and Hunninghake, D.B. 1986. Enalapril alone and in combination with hydrochlorothiazide in the treatment of hypertension: Effect on treadmill exercise performance. *J Cardiopulmonary Rehabil* 6:251-256.

Levy, D., Garrison, R.J., Savage, D.D., Kannel, W.B., and Castelli, W.P. 1990. Prognostic implications of echocardiographically determined left ventricular mass in the Framingham Heart Study. *N Engl J Med* 322:1561-1566.

Ligueros, M., Unwin, R., Wilkins, M.R., Humphreys, J., Coles, S.J., and Cleland, J. 1992. A comparison of the effects of the selective peripheral alpha 1-blocker terazosin with selective beta 1-blocker atenolol on blood pressure, exercise performance and the lipid profile in mild-to-moderate essential hypertension. *Clin Auton Res* 2:373-381.

Lim, P.O., MacFadyen, R.J., Clarkson, P.B.M., and MacDonald, T.M. 1996. Impaired exercise tolerance in hypertensive patients. *Ann Intern Med* 124(1 pt 1):41-55.

Lowenthal, D.T., and Kendrick, Z.V. 1985. Drug-exercise interactions. *Ann Rev Pharmacol Toxicol* 25:275-305.

Lund-Johansen, P. 1974. Hemodynamic changes at rest and during exercise in long-term clonidine therapy of essential hypertension. *Acta Med Scand* 195:111-115.

MacDougall, J.D., McKelvie, R.S., Moroz, D.E., Sale, D.G., McCartney, N., and Buick, F. 1992. Factors affecting blood pressure during heavy weight lifting and static contractions. *J Appl Physiol* 73:1590-1597.

MacDougall, J.D., Tuxen, D., Sale, D.G., Moroz, J.R., and Sutton, J.R. 1985. Arterial blood pressure response to heavy resistance exercise. *J Appl Physiol* 58:785-790.

Mancia, G., Ferrari, A., Gregorini, L., Ferrari, C., Bianchini, C., Terzoli, L., Leonetti, G., and Zanchetti, A. 1980. Effects of prazosin on autonomic control of circulation in essential hypertension. *Hypertension* 2:700-707.

Manhem, P., Bramnert, M., Hulthen, U.L., and Hokfelt, B. 1981. The effect of captopril on catecholamines, renin activity, angiotensin II and aldosterone in plasma during physical exercise in hypertensive patients. *Eur J Clin Invest* 11:389-395.

Manhem, P., and Hokfelt, B. 1981. Prolonged clonidine treatment: Catecholamines, renin activity and aldosterone following exercise in hypertensives. *Acta Med Scand* 209:253-260.

Maurer, W., Hausen, M., Kramer, B., and Kubler, W. 1983. Effect of the centrally acting agent clonidine on circulating catecholamines at rest and during exercise. Comparison with the effects of beta-blocking agents. *Chest* 83(2 suppl):366-369.

Meyer, T.E., Casadei, B., Coats, A.J.S., Davey, P.P., Adamopoulos, S., Radaelli, A., and Conway, J. 1991. Angiotensin-converting enzyme inhibition and physical training in heart failure. *J Intern Med* 230:407-413.

Miller, A.J., Kaplan, B.M., Upton, M.T., Grais, M., and Abrams, D.L. 1983. Treadmill exercise testing in hypertensive patients treated with hydrochlorothiazide and beta-blocking drugs. *JAMA* 250:67-70.

Mooy, J., Arends, B., Kemenade, J.V., Boehm, R., Rahn, K.H., and van Baak, M. 1986. Influence of prolonged submaximal exercise on the pharmacokinetics of verapamil in humans. *J Cardiovasc Pharmacol* 8:940-942.

Mooy, J., van Baak, M., Bohm, R., Does, R., Petri, H., van Kemenade, J., and Rahn, K.H. 1987. The effects of verapamil and propranolol on exercise tolerance in hypertensive patients. *Clin Pharmacol Ther* 41:490-495.

Mosterd, A., D'Agostino, R.B., Silbershatz, H., Sytkowski, P.A., Kannel, W.B., Grobbee, D.E., and Levy, D. 1999. Trends in the prevalence of hypertension, antihypertensive therapy, and left ventricular hypertrophy from 1950 to 1989. *N Engl J Med* 340:1221-1227.

Mulvihill-Wilson, J., Gaffney, F.A., Pettinger, W.A., Blomqvist, C.G., Anderson, S., and Graham, R.M. 1983. Hemodynamic and neuroendocrine responses to acute and chronic alpha-adrenergic blockade with prazosin and phenoxybenzamine. *Circulation* 67:383-393.

National Institutes of Health. 1997. *The sixth report of the Joint National Committee on the Prevention, Detection, Evaluation, and Treatment of High Blood Pressure.* U.S. Department of Health and Human Services, NIH Publication no. 98-4080, November.

Omvik, P., and Lund-Johansen, P. 1990. The initial hemodynamic response to newer antihypertensive agents at rest and during exercise: Review of visacor, doxazosin, nisoldipine, tiapamil, perindoprilat, pinacidil, dilevalol, and carvedilol. *Cardiovasc Drugs Ther* 4:1135-1143.

Omvik, P., and Lund-Johansen, P. 1993. Long-term hemodynamic effects at rest and during exercise of newer antihypertensive agents and salt restriction in essential hypertension: Review of epanolol, doxazosin, amlodipine, felodipine, diltiazem, lisinopril, dilevalol, carvedilol, and ketanserin. *Cardiovasc Drugs Ther* 7:193-206.

Palatini, P., Casiglia, E., Graniero, G.R., Dorigatti, F., Lotoro, F., Vriz, O., and Pessina, A.C. 1995. Diltiazem vs. nicardipine on ambulatory and exercise blood pressure and on peripheral hemodynamics. *Int J Clin Pharmacol Ther* 33:38-42.

Patel, K.R., and Peers, E. 1988. Felodipine, a new calcium antagonist, modifies exercise-induced asthma. *Am Rev Resp Dis* 138:54-56.

Petri, H., Arends, B.G., and van Baak, M.A. 1986. The effect of verapamil on cardiovascular and metabolic responses to exercise. *Eur J Appl Physiol* 55:499-502.

Raffestin, B., Denjean, A., Legrand, A., Derrieux, C., Boillot, J., Comoy, E., Martre, H., and Lockhart, A. 1985. Effects of nifedipine on responses to exercise in normal subjects. *J Appl Physiol* 58:702-709.

Roth, A., Harrison, E., Mitani, G., Cohen, J., Rahimtoola, S.H., and Elkayam, U. 1986. Efficacy and safety of medium- and high-dose diltiazem alone and in combination with digoxin for control of heart rate at rest and during exercise in patients with chronic atrial fibrillation. *Circulation* 73:316-324.

Sharma, S.K., Pande, J.N., and Guleria, J.S. 1986. The effect of nifedipine on exercise-induced asthma. *J Asthma* 23:15-17.

Somani, S.M., ed. 1996. *Pharmacology in exercise and sports.* Boca Raton, FL: CRC Press.

Stein, D.T., Lowenthal, D.T., Porter, R.S., Falkner, B., Bravo, E.L., and Hare, T.W. 1984. Effects of nifedipine and verapamil on isometric and dynamic exercise in normal subjects. *Am J Cardiol* 54:386-389.

Steinberg, J.S., Katz, R.J., Bren, G.B., Buff, L.A., and Varghese, P.J. 1987. Efficacy of oral diltiazem to control ventricular response in chronic atrial fibrillation at rest and during exercise. *J Am Coll Cardiol* 9:405-411.

Stewart, K.J., Effron, M.B., Valenti, S.A., and Kelemen, M.H. 1990. Effects of diltiazem or propranolol during exercise training of hypertensive men. *Med Sci Sports Exerc* 22:171-177.

Thompson, P.D., Cullinane, E.M., Nugent, A.M., Sady, M.A., and Sady, S.P. 1989. Effect of atenolol or prazosin on maximal exercise performance in hypertensive joggers. *Am J Med* 86(1B):104-109.

van Baak, M.A. 1994. Hypertension, beta-adrenoceptor blocking agents and exercise. *Int J Sports Med* 15:112-115.

van Baak, M.A., Mooij, J.M., Wijnen, J.A., and Tan, F.S. 1991. Submaximal endurance exercise performance during enalapril treatment in patients with essential hypertension. *Clin Pharmacol Ther* 50:221-227.

van Baak, M.A., Mooij, J.M.V., and Schiffers, P.M.H. 1992. Exercise and the pharmacokinetics of propranolol, verapamil, and atenolol. *Eur J Clin Pharmacol* 43:547-550.

Vanhees, L., Fagard, R., Lijnen, P., and Amery, A. 1991. Effect of antihypertensive medication on endurance exercise capacity in hypertensive sportsmen. *J Hypertens* 9:1063-1068.

Virtanen, K., Janne, J., and Frick, M.H. 1982. Response of blood pressure and plasma norepinephrine to propranolol, metoprolol and clonidine during isometric and dynamic exercise in hypertensive patients. *Eur J Clin Pharmacol* 21:275-279.

White, W.B., McCabe, E.J., Hager, W.D., and Schulman, P. 1988. The effects of the long-acting angiotensin-converting enzyme inhibitor cilazapril on casual, exercise, and ambulatory blood pressure. *Clin Pharmacol Ther* 44:173-178.

Yamakado, T., Oonishi, N., Nakano, T., and Takezawa, H. 1985. Effects of nifedipine and diltiazem on hemodynamic responses at rest and during exercise in hypertensive patients. *Jpn Circ J* 49:415-421.

4
CHAPTER

Sympathomimetics

CASE STUDY

■ *CASE*   Wayne is close to realizing his dream of being a professional player in the National Hockey League (NHL). He already has been chosen as a member of the U.S. Olympic hockey team with his best friend, Mike. Randomly selected for drug testing at the Salt Lake City Games, Mike subsequently is informed that he tested positive for pseudoephedrine, a banned substance. Both he and Wayne are bewildered: they have routinely used pseudoephedrine (Sudafed) before other hockey games and not been told this is illegal. Is pseudoephedrine a banned substance? Does it possess ergogenic properties?

■ *COMMENT*   Pseudoephedrine is allowed in the NHL and in other game situations, but since it is a sympathomimetic (i.e., an amphetamine-like) drug and falls within the category of substances classified as "stimulants," it is banned for use during Olympic competition. Even at recommended doses, however, it does not appear to possess ergogenic properties.

$\mathbf{F}$rom 1993 through 1996, stimulants accounted for roughly 60-65% of positive drug test results from 25 International Olympic Committee (IOC) laboratories (Mottram 1999). These statistics are difficult to interpret, considering that these labs analyze roughly 80 specimens per week, a figure that contrasts sharply with the millions of athletes who participate in sports. In the January 26, 1998 issue, *Sports Illustrated* reported that 20% of players in the NHL routinely use pseudoephedrine (PSE) to increase their energy. Companies market many drugs of this type, though they are not intended to be used as psychostimulants. Rather, these drugs are generally used as decongestants and are given orally or via nasal inhalation. Phenylpropanolamine (PPA) is also used to suppress appetite; it is the active ingredient in over-the-counter (OTC) diet products like Acutrim and Dexatrim. The list of sympathomimetics includes

- ephedrine,
- epinephrine,
- naphazoline (Privine, Vasocon),
- oxymetazoline (Afrin),
- phenylephrine (Neo-Synephrine),
- phenylpropanolamine (Acutrim, Dexatrim),
- pseudoephedrine (Sudafed),
- tetrahydrozoline (Tyzine, Visine),
- xylometazoline (Otrivin),
- beta-agonists (see chapter 5), and
- psychostimulants (see chapter 15).

In the hospital setting, sympathomimetic drugs are given intravenously to increase systemic blood pressure (BP) or stimulate heart rate (HR), but these pharmacologic effects can also occur when sympathomimetic agents are ingested orally. Technically, beta-agonist bronchodilators and psychostimulants of the amphetamine type are also sympathomimetics, but these drugs will be discussed in other chapters.

It is uncertain how many people use sympathomimetic decongestants since many products are sold without a prescription. In 1997 the FDA announced it would curb sale of nonprescription diet supplements containing ephedrine alkaloids in an attempt to prevent "basement chemists" from obtaining large quantities of precursor chemicals used in the manufacture of methamphetamine (Methamphetamine Control Act of 1997). Then, in August 1999, a report from the General Accounting Office (GAO) announced that the FDA did not have the evidence necessary to put restrictions on ephedra-containing products.

Ephedra, also known as ma huang, epitonin, and *Sida cordifolia,* is an alkaloid found naturally in some plants. The active principle in ephedra is ephedrine. Ephedrine, the drug, is found only in prescription drug products; however, some herbal products contain the alkaloid ephedra.

One should not underestimate the effects of ephedra; just because an herbal product is labeled "natural" does not mean that serious side effects will not occur. Since 1994 the FDA has received and investigated more than 800 reports of adverse events associated with the use of more than 100 different ephedrine-containing dietary supplement products (Nightingale 1997). Side effects to ephedrine can include tremor, increased BP, cardiac arrhythmia, psychosis, seizure, myocardial infarction, and even death. Even if none of these adverse effects are experienced, the athlete still risks disqualification owing to the fact that products containing ephedrine are classified as stimulants and thus are banned substances.

The selected sympathomimetic agents listed at the beginning of the chapter do not include drugs that are used only in hospitalized individuals (e.g., norepinephrine, dobutamine, dopamine), nor are these substances reviewed in this chapter. Instead, the focus in this chapter is on ephedrine, pseudoephedrine, and phenylpropanolamine, the agents that are administered systemically and that have been involved in what limited research has been conducted on sympathomimetics in sports.

Many of the concepts that pertain to these three drugs are relevant as well to the other drugs listed at the beginning of the chapter. Phenylpropanolamine and phenylephrine are potent sympathomimetics; phenylephrine is used as a topical vasoconstrictor in eye and nose drops. Sympathomimetics found most commonly as decongestants in cough and cold preparations are pseudoephedrine and phenylpropanolamine. Naphazoline, oxymetazoline, tetrahydrozoline, and xylometazoline are used only as topical vasoconstrictors in the eye and/or nose.

Ephedrine is an agonist at both alpha- and beta-receptors. In addition, it stimulates the release of norepinephrine from storage sites in sympathetic neurons. Pseudoephedrine is a less potent isomer of ephedrine. Some researchers have determined that 120 mg of pseudoephedrine is equivalent to 48 mg of ephedrine (Gillies et al. 1996), but potency relationships between these two drugs depend on the pharmacologic parameter being assessed. Drew and colleagues (1978) determined that, based on BP response, 60 mg of ephedrine was roughly equivalent to 210 mg pseudoephedrine, but when bronchodilation (i.e., FEV-1 [forced expiratory volume in 1 s]) was assessed, 60 mg of ephedrine was more than twice as potent as 210 mg of pseudoephedrine.

How Exercise Affects the Action of Sympathomimetics

We look next at the effects exercise has on the action of sympathomimetics that the exerciser is taking. Relatively few studies have been made of how exercise affects either the pharmacokinetics or pharmacology of these drugs.

Effects on Pharmacology

While exercise does not appear to alter the pharmacologic action of these drugs, it is worth noting that the pressor effects of these sympathomimetics may be additive with the pressor effects of resistance exercise (see later discussion). For pseudoephedrine, there is a poor correlation between serum concentrations and either cardiovascular or subjective responses (Bye et al. 1975). Although serum drug concentrations were not measured, Swain and colleagues could not demonstrate any dose-response relationship regarding the effects of either phenylpropanolamine or pseudoephedrine on HR or BP in elite cyclists during cycle ergometry testing. More importantly, the pressor effects of these drugs did not appear to augment the cardiovascular response of subjects to exercise while receiving placebo (Swain et al. 1997).

Effects on Pharmacokinetics

For ephedrine, 2 h of exercise at 50% $\dot{V}O_2$max had no effect on the urinary excretion after intranasal administration (6 drops every 2 h for 4 doses), although there was an inverse correlation between urinary pH and the amount of ephedrine in the urine. Ephedrine was detected in all urine samples that were collected hourly over 10 h; all 8 volunteers had at least one urine sample with an ephedrine concentration >5 mcg/ml (Lefebvre et al. 1992).

For pseudoephedrine, urine samples obtained 180 min after oral ingestion of a 120 mg dose were positive in 8 of 10 male cyclists. Sixty minutes after the end of a 1 h time trial and 240 min after ingestion, pseudoephedrine was detected in urine samples from all 10 cyclists. Urine pH was lower in the second sample, again suggesting that the urine pH influenced urinary clearance of pseudoephedrine (Gillies et al. 1996).

Swain and colleagues (1997) measured urine concentrations in elite cyclists after ingestion of oral doses of phenylpropanolamine and pseudoephedrine. Although the effects of exercise on the pharmacokinetics of these drugs were not measured, relatively modest doses of each drug were found to produce urine concentrations that exceeded the IOC's upper limit of 10 mcg/ml.

How Sympathomimetics Affect Exercisers

All sympathomimetics carry standard warnings about use in individuals with hypertension or diabetes mellitus. These precautions are derived largely from the observed effects of more potent agents, such as norepinephrine and epinephrine (Bright, Sandage, and Fletcher 1981). Further, these recommendations are based largely on data derived from nonexercising subjects. Limited data have been generated on the effects of these drugs during exercise.

Cardiovascular Actions

Sympathomimetics exert variable effects on HR during exercise. Pseudoephedrine at 120 mg had no significant effect on resting HR, the time to reach target HR, or the time required to recover to baseline HR in healthy males during treadmill exercise. However, premature ventricular contractions (PVCs) were noted in 2 of the 6 subjects (Bright, Sandage, and Fletcher 1981). In another treadmill-exercise challenge, a single 60 mg dose of pseudoephedrine increased exercise HR in female athletes (Clemons and Crosby 1993). A single 40 mg dose of ephedrine did not affect exercise HR during cycle ergometry in healthy students (DeMeersman, Getty, and Schaefer 1987). When male cyclists were given two different doses of phenylpropanolamine and pseudoephedrine during cycle ergometry, exercise HR did not differ from that resulting from administration of placebo (Swain et al. 1997). It is possible that the beta-agonist effects of these drugs on exercise HR are overshadowed by the powerful chronotropic effects of endogenous catecholamines when measurements are taken during maximal exercise.

Phenylpropanolamine is a potent sympathomimetic! Cerebral hemorrhages have occurred after ingestion of doses above 100 mg. Doses just slightly higher than the recommended dose of 25 mg can increase BP substantially. Oral doses of 37.5 mg increased supine systolic BP by an average of 18.5 mm Hg (range 8-43) in normotensive volunteers (Pentel, Aaron, and Paya 1985). BP increased to an average of 173/103 mm Hg in normotensive volunteers after they had ingested 150 mg phenylpropanolamine without caffeine, and significant increases in BP occurred when 75 mg doses were administered with 400 mg of caffeine (Lake et al. 1989). The pressor effects of phenylpropanolamine are additive to increases seen during handgrip exercise (Pentel and Eisen 1988); the same is not true during bicycle-ergometer testing (Davies et al. 1989; Swain et al. 1997). Ephedrine (40 mg) did not affect exercise BP (DeMeersman, Getty, and Schaefer 1987). Pseudoephedrine in doses of 1 mg/kg increased systolic BP during cycling, but doses of 2 mg/kg did not (Swain et al. 1997). Pseudoephedrine after single doses of 60 to 120 mg revealed no effect on exercise BP during treadmill testing in either men (Bright, Sandage, and Fletcher 1981) or women (Clemons and Crosby 1993). Again, the difference is probably due to the dominating effects on the cardiovascular system from acute, exercise-induced increases in circulating catecholamines, which likely masked any pharmacologic effect from the drugs.

Pulmonary Actions

Studies of healthy volunteers and elite athletes reveal that oral doses of ephedrine (DeMeersman, Getty, and Schaefer 1987; Sidney and Lefcoe 1977), pseudoephedrine (Clemons and Crosby 1993; Swain et al. 1997), and phenylpropanolamine (Swain et al. 1997) do not affect oxygen uptake ($\dot{V}O_2$). In a clinical study, the effects of IV ephedrine at 0.1 mg/kg were studied in healthy male volunteers. Within minutes after the subjects were injected, both their $\dot{V}O_2$ and cardiac index (CI) increased; the $\dot{V}O_2$/CI ratio, however, did not change. The authors concluded that ephedrine increases oxygen demand and supply in a similar magnitude (Radstrom et al. 1995).

Metabolic Actions

To study metabolic actions, researchers worked with healthy males and subjected them to treadmill exercise. After single doses (in the 60-120 mg range) of pseudoephedrine, the subjects' postexercise blood glucose or insulin levels did not show effects from the drug (Bright, Sandage, and Fletcher 1981). A criticism of this older study might be that the bout of exercise was too brief; exercise was terminated when each subject reached 85% of their predicted maximal exercise HR. While the actual duration of exercise was not stated, it is possible that had researchers used a longer period of exercise, the drug might have produced different results. Pseudoephedrine has beta-agonist properties. Beta-stimulation by endogenous epinephrine is an important step in the control of glucose uptake and glycogen breakdown in skeletal muscle during exercise (Hargreaves 1995). Glucose utilization by skeletal muscle is affected by both exercise intensity and duration (Hargreaves 1995).

Two groups of investigators assessed the effects of sympathomimetics on lactate levels during aerobic exercise. The researchers found that the "anaerobic threshold" occurred at identical levels of exercise intensity when ephedrine at 40 mg was compared with placebo's effects (DeMeersman, Getty, and Schaefer 1987). Postexercise lactate levels were not affected by pseudoephedrine 120 mg in cyclists subjected to a 1 h cycling time trial (Gillies et al. 1996).

In conclusion, although data are limited, at typical doses the sympathomimetics discussed in this chapter appear to have no effects on exercise metabolism.

How Sympathomimetics Affect Exercise Performance

The effects of common OTC sympathomimetics have not been studied much in athletes and other physically active individuals. Sidney and Lefcoe (1977) studied 40 different exercise performance and physiological variables in healthy males after the subjects had been administered a single, oral dose of ephedrine 24 mg. They did not see beneficial effects on muscle strength, endurance, power, reaction time, hand-eye coordination, anaerobic capacity and speed, or ratings of perceived exertion (RPE) in their study's subjects during maximal and submaximal exercise. Several less comprehensive studies have also been conducted on OTC sympathomimetics. Single doses of ephedrine (DeMeersman, Getty, and Schaefer 1987), pseudoephedrine (Swain et al. 1997), or phenylpropanolamine (Swain et al. 1997) did not affect RPE during cycle ergometry. Ratings of perceived exertion during treadmill exercise did not improve with a single 60 mg dose of pseudoephedrine (Clemons and Crosby 1993). Time to exhaustion during cycle ergometry was not improved in elite cyclists by either phenylpropanolamine or pseudoephedrine (Swain et al. 1997); nor did a single 120 mg dose of pseudoephedrine improve quadriceps strength or the cycling-time trial performance in male cyclists (Gillies et al. 1996). In conclusion, there appears to be no evidence of an ergogenic effect from OTC sympathomimetics.

Avoiding Potential Complications

Blood pressure as high as 480/350 has been recorded in the brachial artery of a bodybuilder during a double-leg press (MacDougall et al. 1985). Because phenylpropanolamine has been shown to augment exercise-induced increases in systolic BP during handgrip exercise, it is possible that weightlifters who concomitantly use phenylpropanolamine, particularly in higher-than-recommended doses, may experience serious vascular events. Even without the added effect of weightlifting, phenylpropanolamine has been associated with intracerebral hemorrhage.

Even though the drugs discussed in this chapter do not seem to be as potent as endogenous norepinephrine, researchers have observed PVCs in healthy males during submaximal exercise after their ingestion of pseudoephedrine 120 mg (Bright, Sandage, and Fletcher 1981).

NCAA and USOC Status

The verdict on sympathomimetics seems to be mixed. The USOC and the IOC prohibit use of sympathomimetics during competition, but the NCAA and the NHL do not. Unfortunately, the list of drugs banned by the IOC has been compiled in the absence of firm scientific data demonstrating ergogenic effects for all the agents on the list, particularly the sympathomimetics (Gillies et al. 1996). For ephedrine, urine concentrations of >5 mcg/ml are grounds for disqualification in cycling competition. Athletic trainers and athletes alike should realize that this threshold can be exceeded simply with a few doses of a nasal spray several hours before urine sampling (Lefebvre et al. 1992)! Currently, the urinary threshold for phenylpropanolamine and pseudoephedrine is set at 10 mcg/ml by the IOC (Mottram 1999), but these limits are easily exceeded by modest oral doses of either drug (Swain et al. 1997).

■ *Two Olympic Examples*

At the 1972 Olympics in Munich, Germany, 16-year-old swimmer Rick Demont had to relinquish his gold medal when ephedrine was detected in a postrace urine sample. He had used the drug product Marax, which contains ephedrine, hydroxyzine, and theophylline, for asthma. On 1 August 1998, Nigerian basketball player Julius Nwosu was suspended for two months when he tested positive for ephedrine at the World Basketball Championships in Athens, Greece. According to the International Basketball Federation, an "abnormally high level" of ephedrine was found in his system. Nwosu blamed the positive test on a vitamin supplement (AP, 2 August 1998). These two cases are highly unfortunate, considering the unsubstantiated ergogenic effects of ephedrine in normal therapeutic doses.

Guidelines for Athletic Trainers

Some guidelines on the use of sympathomimetics during competition or exercising clearly would be helpful. At least 750,000 retail outlets in the United States are licensed to sell OTC drugs, and because more than 100 ephedrine-containing dietary supplement products are available, sports medicine specialists are likely to be called on to advise active individuals about using these substances. The following pointers should be kept in mind:

- Despite the fact that these pharmaceuticals and nutraceuticals do not possess dramatic ergogenic actions, they are banned by the IOC. It is important to realize that athletic organizations vary in their views of these drugs.
- Remind athletes that even when a drug is administered as a nose drop or nasal spray, it can still be detected in a urine sample in quantities high enough for disqualification.
- Counsel athletes about herbal supplements (i.e., nutraceuticals). Any supplement that contains the alkaloid ephedra may produce urine concentrations of ephedrine high enough for detection and disqualification. Since dietary supplements are not regulated for quality control the same way traditional pharmaceuticals are, the amount of active ingredient in ephedra-containing herbal products can vary tremendously. Even though these products produce a heightened state of arousal, there is no evidence that the sympathomimetics discussed in this chapter provide any ergogenic actions.
- Inform athletes that many OTC cough and cold products contain a sympathomimetic drug as the decongestant component. Again, these products may also produce unacceptable urine concentrations of a banned substance.

Guidelines for Physicians

Sports medicine professionals have several issues to communicate with patients and clients concerning sympathomimetics. These range from prescribed medications to herbal supplements and OTC remedies.

- Because herbal supplements are thought to be a more "natural" form of therapy, individuals often are less concerned about these agents compared to traditional drug therapy. Remind your patients that herbal products containing ephedra can produce cardiovascular effects just as powerful as the pure drug ephedrine.
- Phenylpropanolamine is another drug that people often underestimate. It is ubiquitous in cough and cold preparations, and at low doses it is a safe agent. In higher doses (e.g., > 100 mg/dose), however, it can cause dramatic cardiovascular effects. Although all athletes, weightlifters, and bodybuilders should be discouraged from using drugs to potentiate athletic performance, they should also be reminded that sympathomimetics in general are not ergogenic and that using higher doses of phenylpropanolamine in an attempt to achieve an ergogenic effect can lead to serious cardiovascular complications.

- Keep in mind that different athletic governing bodies have different restrictions regarding sympathomimetics; since these drugs are found in so many OTC cough and cold products, many athletes risk disqualification even using something that seems harmless.

References

Bright, T.P., Sandage Jr., B.W., and Fletcher, H.P. 1981. Selected cardiac and metabolic responses to pseudoephedrine with exercise. *J Clin Pharmacol* 21(11-12 pt 1):488-492.

Bye, C., Hill, H.M., Hughes, D.T.D., and Peck, A.W. 1975. A comparison of plasma levels of L(+)pseudoephedrine following different formulations, and their relation to cardiovascular and subjective effects in man. *Eur J Clin Pharmacol* 8:47-53.

Clemons, J.M., and Crosby, S.L. 1993. Cardiopulmonary and subjective effects of a 60 mg dose of pseudoephedrine on graded treadmill exercise. *J Sports Med Phys Fitness* 33:405-412.

Davies, S.F., McArthur, C.D., Husebye, D.G., Maddy, M.M., O'Connell, M.B., and Pentel, P.R. 1989. The effect of phenylpropanolamine on blood pressure during upright bicycle exercise in normal subjects. *Int J Obes* 13:505-510.

DeMeersman, R., Getty, D., and Schaefer, D.C. 1987. Sympathomimetics and exercise enhancement: All in the mind? *Pharmacol Biochem Behav* 28:361-365.

Drew, C.D., Knight, G.T., Hughes, D.T., and Bush, M. 1978. Comparison of the effect of D-(-)-ephedrine and L-(+)-pseudoephedrine on the cardiovascular and respiratory systems in man. *Br J Clin Pharmacol* 6:221-225.

Gillies, H., Derman, W.E., Noakes, T.D., Smith, P., Evans, A., and Gabriels, G. 1996. Pseudoephedrine is without ergogenic effects during prolonged exercise. *J Appl Physiol* 81:2611-2617.

Hargreaves, M. 1995. Skeletal muscle carbohydrate metabolism during exercise. In *Exercise metabolism*, edited by M. Hargreaves. Champaign, IL: Human Kinetics.

Lake, C.R., Zaloga, G., Bray, J., Rosenberg, D., and Chernow, B. 1989. Transient hypertension after two phenylpropanolamine diet aids and the effects of caffeine: A placebo-controlled follow-up study. *Am J Med* 86:427-432.

Lefebvre, R.A., Surmont, F., Bouckaert, J., and Moerman, E. 1992. Urinary excretion of ephedrine after nasal application in healthy volunteers. *J Pharm Pharmacol* 44:672-675.

MacDougall, J.D., Tuxen, D., Sale, D.G., Moroz, J.R., and Sutton, J.R. 1985. Arterial blood pressure response to heavy resistance exercise. *J Appl Physiol* 58:785-790.

Mottram, D.R. 1999. Banned drugs in sport: Does the International Olympic Committee (IOC) list need updating? *Sports Med* 27:1-10.

Nightingale, S.L. 1997. New safety measures are proposed for dietary supplements containing ephedrine alkaloids. *JAMA* 278:15.

Pentel, P.R., Aaron, C., and Paya, C. 1985. Therapeutic doses of phenylpropanolamine increase supine systolic blood pressure. *Int J Obes* 9:115-119.

Pentel, P.R., and Eisen, T. 1988. Effects of phenylpropanolamine and isometric exercise on blood pressure. *Int J Obes* 12:199-204.

Radstrom, M., Bengtsson, J., Ederberg, S., Bengtsson, A., Loswick, A.C., and Bengtson, J.P. 1995. Effects of ephedrine on oxygen consumption and cardiac output. *Acta Anaesthesiol Scand* 39:1084-1087.

Sidney, K.H., and Lefcoe, N.M. 1977. The effects of ephedrine on the physiological and psychological responses to submaximal and maximal exercise in man. *Med Sci Sports* 9:95-99.

Swain, R.A., Harsha, D.M., Baenziger, J., and Saywell Jr., R.M. 1997. Do pseudoephedrine or phenylpropanolamine improve maximum oxygen uptake and time to exhaustion? *Clin J Sport Med* 7:168-173.

5

CHAPTER

Bronchodilators and Respiratory Anti-Inflammatory Agents

CASE STUDY

■ *CASE*   Tom is a cross-country skier who is training for the Winter Olympics. Living in Minnesota, he endures prolonged periods in the cold, dry air. He has been experiencing shortness of breath and coughing for several hours after he completes his workout. A physician has already diagnosed him with exercise-induced bronchoconstriction and has prescribed a metered-dose inhaler containing albuterol for use prior to exercising. What effect will this drug have on his training regimen and his overall performance? Tom worries that albuterol, a sympathomimetic, is a banned drug and that taking it will disqualify him from the upcoming U.S. Olympic team trials. Are there effective alternative drugs he could use?

■ *COMMENT*   Albuterol is a widely prescribed bronchodilator of the class of drugs known as beta-2 agonists. Safe when used as prescribed, overuse of this type of drug can lead to tolerance. Even though albuterol is a sympathomimetic and therefore has adrenergic-like properties, it hardly should be considered an ergogenic agent. Although it is banned for use during competition when *taken systemically*, its use is acceptable when administered via an inhaler. A variety of other drug categories are potential alternatives to albuterol for Tom, but none appears to be as effective, for reasons discussed in this chapter.

$\mathbf{A}$ marathon runner exchanges the equivalent of an estimated 2 months of ventilatory volume during a 2.5 h race (Pierson et al. 1986)! This amount of ventilation can lead not only to an increased drying of respiratory airways but also to a higher intake of pollutants and allergens. In some people, in fact, exercise can even precipitate bronchospasm and anaphylaxis (Montgomery and Deuster 1993). Another type of allergic reaction, such as urticaria, has been associated with temperature extremes, sun exposure, or water exposure (Briner 1993). Some elite athletes can develop exercise-induced hypoxemia, independently of bronchoconstriction (Prefaut, Anselme-Poujol, and Caillaud 1997).

Even apparently healthy athletes sometimes require the use of bronchodilators or respiratory anti-inflammatory drugs. Notable examples are the Olympians Jackie Joyner-Kersee, Amy Van Dyken, and Tom Dolan, all of whom are asthmatic. So it is unfortunate that some highly effective bronchodilators—specifically, the beta-2-receptor agonists—are categorized as banned substances, since evidence of their ergogenic potential is equivocal. However, if exercise-induced decreases in pulmonary function impair athletic performance, a drug that prevents or reverses these detrimental effects on lung function could be construed as being ergogenic. This chapter discusses pulmonary drugs: specifically, bronchodilators, respiratory anti-inflammatory agents, and type-1 histamine receptor antagonists.

Exercise-Induced Bronchoconstriction

About 12 million Americans, roughly 5% of the population, have asthma. Some clinicians report that exercise-induced bronchoconstriction (EIB) occurs in 40% to 90% of these patients with asthma (McFadden and Gilbert 1994), but nearly all people with asthma have respiratory symptoms at least occasionally when exercising vigorously in cold, dry air (Hansen-Flaschen and Schotland 1998).

Generally, it is thought that 10-15% of Olympic athletes have asthma (Storms 1999). Prior to the 1984 Olympic Games in Los Angeles, the USOC screened 597 U.S. Olympic athletes for EIB. Sixty-seven (roughly 11%) were identified as having EIB, including some who were unaware of the cause of their breathlessness after strenuous exercise (Kobayashi and Mellion 1991). Fourteen percent of Finnish athletes (speed and power athletes, distance runners, and swimmers) were found to have current asthmatic symptoms and increased bronchial responsiveness, with the highest incidence occurring in swimmers (Helenius et al. 1998). In another Finnish study (Helenius, Tikkanen, and Haahtela 1998), when a decrease in FEV-1 (forced expiratory volume in 1 s) of 6.5% or more was used as the definition of EIB, a full 26% of elite runners were identified as having EIB. A free running test was used to screen male high school varsity football players, and 9% were found to exhibit significant EIB (Kukafka et al. 1998). A prevalence of 35% was found in 124 professionally coached figure skaters; this rate is higher than from other studies and was thought to be related to the intensity of the exercise and the fact that exercise occurred in cold air (Mannix et al. 1996). More striking still, among cross-country skiers, the incidence of asthma or asthma symptoms is reported to be as high as 80% (Larsson et al. 1993).

Exercise-induced bronchoconstriction is a result of the loss of heat or water (or both) from the respiratory tract. It occurs more readily when the air is cold and dry (Helenius, Tikkanen, and Haahtela 1998), but a history of atopy is also a significant risk factor (Helenius et al. 1998). Airway caliber is essentially unchanged in susceptible individuals during vigorous exercise. When exercise stops, tests of pulmonary airflow, such as FEV-1, show an immediate decline during the next 5 to 10 min, with as much as a 50% decrease compared with baseline. Expiratory airflow gradually returns to preexercise measurements during the following 20 to 90 min (Hansen-Flaschen and Schotland 1998).

This syndrome is commonly called "exercise-induced asthma," but this label is somewhat misleading since asthma is a disease and exercise does not cause individuals to have asthma. *Exercise-induced bronchoconstriction* is a more accurate (and currently preferred) phrase. You may also encounter the following other names to describe the condition:

- Exercise-induced bronchospasm
- Hyperpnea-induced asthma
- Postexercise bronchoconstriction
- Thermally induced asthma

Throughout this chapter, the phrase *exercise-induced bronchoconstriction*, abbreviated EIB, will be used. It is beyond the scope of this book, however, to review the clinical management of disease states. Exercise-induced bronchoconstriction (Bundgaard 1985; Kobayashi and Mellion 1991; McFadden and Gilbert 1994; Morton and Fitch 1992; Storms 1999; Tan and Spector 1998) and exercise-induced allergic reactions (Briner 1993) have been thoroughly reviewed, and readers may turn to these discussions for more in-depth information.

Introduction to Respiratory Drugs

We group the relevant drugs for this discussion into *bronchodilators* and *respiratory anti-inflammatory agents* (see table 5.1). Inhaled beta-adrener-

Table 5.1   Respiratory Drugs

Bronchodilators

Pure beta-receptor agonists

Albuterol (Proventil, Ventolin)[a]

Bitolterol (Tornalate)[a]

Isoproterenol (Isuprel)[a]

Metaproterenol (Alupent)[a]

Pirbuterol (Maxair)[a]

Salmeterol (Serevent)[a]

Terbutaline (Brethair, Brethine, Bricanyl)[a]

Other drugs with beta-receptor agonist properties

Ephedrine[a]

Epinephrine (Bronkaid, Primatene)[b]

Methylxanthines

Caffeine[b]

Theophylline (Slo-bid, TheoDur, others)[a]

Antimuscarinic anticholinergics

Glycopyrrolate (Robinul)[a]

Ipratropium (Atrovent)[a]

Respiratory anti-inflammatory agents

Inhaled corticosteroids

Beclomethasone (Vanceril)[a]

Budesonide (Pulmicort)[a]

Dexamethasone (Decadron)[a]

Flunisolide (Aerobid)[a]

Fluticasone (Flovent)[a]

Triamcinolone (Azmacort)[a]

Mast cell stablizers

Cromolyn (Intal)[b]

Nedocromil (Tilade)[a]

Leukotriene receptor antagonists

Montelukast (Singulair)[a]

Pranlukast (Ultair)[a]

Zafirlukast (Accolate)[a]

5-lipoxygenase inhibitor

Zileuton (Zyflo)[a]

Histamine type-1 receptor antagonists (i.e., antihistamines)

Astemizole (Hismanal)[a]

Azatadine (Optimine)[a]

Azelastine (Asteline NS)[a]

Brompheniramine (Dimetane)[b]

Cetirizine (Zyrtec)[a]

Chlorpheniramine (Chlor-Trimeton)[b]

Clemastine (Tavist)[a]

Cyproheptadine (Periactin)[a]

Dexchlorpheniramine (Polaramine)[a]

Diphenhydramine (Benadryl)

Fexofenadine (Allegra)[a]

Hydroxyzine (Atarax, Vistaril)[a]

Loratadine (Claritin)[a]

Promethazine (Phenergan)[a]

Trimeprazine (Temaril)[a]

Tripelennamine (Pbz)[a]

Triprolidine (Myidyl)[a]

[a] = by prescription only
[b] = available over the counter and by prescription

120

gic agonists and inhaled corticosteroids are used in the treatment of EIB. Antihistamines (i.e., antagonists of type-1 histamine receptors) and corticosteroids are useful for other allergic reactions that can be precipitated by exercise, such as cholinergic urticaria or exercise-induced anaphylaxis.

Although ephedrine is not routinely used as a bronchodilator, it is included in the table since it does have beta-agonist properties. Phenylpropanolamine (Acutrim, Dexatrim) and pseudoephedrine (Sudafed) are mild beta-receptor agonists but do not exhibit bronchodilator properties and will not be discussed here (see chapter 4 for a discussion of all three of these agents as sympathomimetics).

Despite the many corticosteroid and antihistamine preparations on the market, the individual drugs within these classes in general are more similar than different. It is appropriate, therefore, to discuss the drugs in these two groups categorically. Nevertheless, there are some subtle differences among the antihistamines with regard to anticholinergic and sedative side effects, and these will be distinguished where appropriate.

Beta-Receptor Agonists

Beta-agonists, which stimulate the beta-receptors, are the pharmacologic opposite of beta-blockers. Adrenergic stimulation within the bronchial tree is mediated through the beta-2 receptors. Agonism at these beta-receptors leads to relaxation of the bronchiolar smooth muscle. In susceptible athletes, beta-agonists can prevent EIB, which, if it were to develop, could impair aerobic performance.

Isoproterenol was one of the first beta-agonist drugs to be produced, but many other agents have since been developed. These newer, improved drugs have greater specificity for beta-2 receptors (pulmonary tissue) than for beta-1 receptors (cardiac tissue), and they have a longer duration of action than does isoproterenol. Beta-agonists are the most potent of all the bronchodilators in table 5.2 (Godfrey and Konig 1975; McFadden and Gilbert 1994). Because of their potency and their rapid onset of action, beta-agonists are the preferred therapy for prevention of EIB (McFadden and Gilbert 1994). Albuterol (i.e., salbutamol outside the United States), one of the most widely prescribed drugs for asthma, is the most popular beta-receptor agonist.

Because beta-agonists are adrenergic stimulants, one might conclude that their effects on exercise physiology are similar to those of the classic sympathomimetics (e.g., epinephrine, ephedrine, phenylpropanolamine, etc.). It is important to remember, however, that beta-agonists, particularly the beta-2 selective agents, are highly specific drugs. Albuterol, the prototype, does not share the alpha-stimulating

Table 5.2 Effects of Common Anti-Asthma Medications on Exercise-Induced Bronchoconstriction

Agent	Dose (puffs)	Timing before exercise (min)	Effectiveness[a]	Duration of protection (hrs)[b]
Beta-2 aerosols				
Salmeterol	2	10–15	+++	10–12
Albuterol	2	10–15	+++	2.0–2.5
Terbutaline	2	10–15	+++	2.0–2.5
Cromolyn sodium	2	10–15	++	1.5–2.0
Nedocromil sodium	2	10–15	++	1.5–2.0
Methylxanthines	N/A	30–60	+/–	?
Anticholinergics	2	30–60	+/–	?

[a] = Effectiveness is rated as follows: +++, ablation or substantial reduction in the obstructive response at the midpoint of the stimulus-response curve; ++, marked reduction in the obstructive response; and +/–, questionable efficacy.
[b] = A question mark indicates that the duration of the effect is difficult to ascertain because of the variability of protection.
N/A = not applicable

properties of epinephrine—or even the beta-1-stimulating properties of isoproterenol and epinephrine. Further, albuterol does not have any of the central nervous system (CNS) or psychological actions that amphetamine and cocaine possess. When beta-agonists are inhaled—the most popular mode of administration for these drugs in the treatment of asthma—their systemic effects are almost entirely avoided. Readers should not confuse beta-blockers (see chapter 1) that have intrinsic sympathomimetic activity (ISA) with beta-agonists. Though beta-blockers with ISA do exert mild agonistic actions, they have far less ability to stimulate beta-receptors than do the pure beta-agonists.

Theophylline

Methylxanthines (e.g., caffeine and theophylline) are very old drugs. Although caffeine does produce clinically significant bronchodilation, it is used more for its psychologic and metabolic effects than for its pulmonary effects (and will be discussed later in chapter 13). Theophylline, however, has been a mainstay in the treatment of asthma and pulmonary disease for decades. Despite a wealth of research, the mechanism of action for this drug is still unclear, and its utility in the treatment of asthma has recently been questioned. Nevertheless, theophylline is widely prescribed, and many individuals, athletes and nonathletes, may be taking it while exercising. Unlike the beta-agonists, theophylline cannot be given via inhalation.

Antimuscarinic Anticholinergics

Many antimuscarinic anticholinergic drugs are commercially available, but only ipratropium is routinely used in the treatment of pulmonary disease. Glycopyrrolate is sometimes used for its pulmonary effects, but ipratropium is by far the more important of the two for this discussion. Drugs of this type relax bronchiolar smooth muscle by antagonism at cholinergic receptors in the lung, but bronchodilators that work by this mechanism are inferior to the beta-agonists in potency.

Inhaled Corticosteroids

It sometimes seems there are more dosage forms of corticosteroids (i.e., glucocorticoids) than one can keep track of. No fewer than six different compounds are available for administration via oral inhalation. This route of administration is preferred in the treatment of persistent or chronic asthma to minimize the serious adverse effects that occur with long-term systemic corticosteroid use. As the pathophysiology of asthma has become clearer to us, sports medicine specialists have assigned inhaled corticosteroids a greater role in the management of this condition.

Mast Cell Stabilizers

When cromolyn was approved in 1973 for use in the United States, it represented an entirely new approach to the treatment of histamine-mediated allergic conditions. Unlike conventional antihistamines (i.e., type-1 histamine receptor antagonists), cromolyn and nedocromil stabilize mast cells, preventing these cells from releasing histamine, one of the many steps that occur in the allergic response. These drugs are extremely safe—cromolyn is now marketed in the United States in a nonprescription, intranasal form for the treatment of allergic rhinitis—but not very potent. For pulmonary disorders, they are administered by inhalation.

Leukotriene Modifiers

The newest group of respiratory anti-inflammatory agents, leukotriene modifiers affect leukotriene physiology. With its FDA approval in September 1996, zafirlukast became the first leukotriene receptor antagonist available for use in the United States. Approval of zileuton, the first 5-lipoxygenase inhibitor, soon followed in December 1996. More recently (1998), other leukotriene receptor antagonists (e.g., montelukast, pranlukast) have been approved. Leukotrienes are endogenous compounds derived from the ubiquitous-membrane, parent-molecule arachidonic acid. Inhalation of exogenous leukotriene D4 can increase airway responsiveness (Smith et al. 1985).

Leukotriene-modifier drugs are used only for maintenance therapy of chronic asthma; they should not be used to treat an acute asthmatic attack. While montelukast taken daily has been shown to effectively modulate EIB (see figure 5.1; Bronsky et al. 1997; Leff et al. 1998), some clinicians consider the leukotriene modifiers clearly inferior to beta-2 receptor agonists in managing this condition (Hendeles and Marshik 1996). Still, this new class of drugs might become important in managing EIB, because it is unlikely that leukotriene modifiers will ever be banned from use during athletic competition, a notable drawback for both beta-agonists and corticosteroids. See O'Byrne, Israle, and Drazen (1997) for a further review of the antileukotriene drugs.

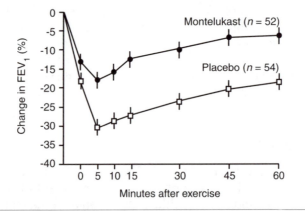

Figure 5.1 Mean (± *SEM*) changes in FEV-1 after exercise challenge after 12 weeks of treatment with montelukast or placebo. Treatment with montelukast was associated with a significant ($p = 0.002$) reduction in EIB.

Type-1 Histamine Receptor Antagonists (Antihistamines)

The many different antihistamines marketed these days are more useful for treating conditions such as exercise-induced cholinergic urticaria than for EIB (Silvers 1992). Drugs of this class interfere with binding of released histamine to type-1 histamine receptors. But it is their side effects, notably drowsiness (or lack thereof) and degree of anticholinergic action, that are the more important issues for this discussion. Hydroxyzine, an antihistamine with potent anticholinergic properties, for example, helps in treating cholinergic urticaria (Briner 1993), whereas terfenadine (removed from the U.S. market in February 1998), an antihistamine with negligible anticholinergic properties, does not (Duffull and Begg 1992).

McFadden and Gilbert (1994) have attempted to rank, according to potency, the various drugs that can be used in EIB, and this article is a good source for additional information (also see table 5.2).

How Exercise Affects the Action of Bronchodilators and Respiratory Anti-Inflammatory Agents

Limited data are available regarding the effects of exercise on either the pharmacology or the pharmacokinetics of these drugs. For the leukotriene modifiers, this issue has yet to be studied.

Effects on Pharmacology

Theoretically, exercise-induced increases in minute ventilation could increase the exposure to allergens, which might challenge the effectiveness of type-1 histamine receptor antagonists in atopic individuals (Montgomery and Deuster 1993). Exercise produces substantial increases in histamine serum concentrations, and cutaneous mast cell degranulation has been noted (Silvers 1992). Susceptible individuals might develop cholinergic urticaria or even exercise-induced anaphylaxis. Thus, in some cases, exercise may compromise the therapeutic effectiveness of type-1 histamine receptor antagonists.

Another issue to consider is that exercise dramatically raises circulating levels of catecholamines. In the case of epinephrine, bronchodilation is enhanced via beta-stimulation. Exercise-induced bronchodilation has been documented in elite athletes, and this effect is additive to the bronchodilatory action of albuterol (Todaro 1996). Further, aerobic training significantly increases exercise-induced bronchodilation in elite athletes (Haas et al. 1987), and it improves ventilatory function in sedentary older individuals (Yerg et al. 1985). Thus, exercise may augment the actions of bronchodilators, but also challenge the effectiveness of antihistamines.

Effects on Pharmacokinetics

Exercise has both acute and long-term effects on the pharmacokinetics of drugs, but unfortunately only limited data are available about these effects on respiratory agents. Theophylline is probably the most extensively studied member of this group, probably because acute toxicity from theophylline is more serious than from any of the other respiratory agents discussed in this chapter. Even without considering the effects of exercise, theophylline is a drug that requires specialized dosing for each individual.

We'll first consider the acute effects of exercise. Note that aerobic exercise diverts blood flow away from the liver and kidneys. This phenomenon interferes with the clearance of flow-limited drugs, but it enhances the clearance of capacity-limited drugs. Caffeine, dexamethasone, diphenhydramine, terbutaline, and theophylline are all examples of respiratory agents that are flow-limited (i.e., those that demonstrate a decrease in clearance during exercise). Several other corticosteroids (not discussed in this chapter) are also flow-limited (see Somani et al. 1990).

The duration of exercise relative to the elimination half-life of the drug determines whether it has a significant effect on a drug's pharmacokinetics. The elimination half-life of theophylline in most adults, for example, averages 4–6 h. According to one study (Schlaeffer et al. 1984), although light to moderate exercise significantly decreased theophylline clearance acutely in normal volunteers, most individuals typically exercise for 60 min or less, so that the acute effects of exercise on theophylline pharmacokinetics would be of little clinical significance. However, for an athlete competing in the Iron Man triathlon, for example, an event that can last 8 h or more, it is quite likely that the activity would prolong theophylline's duration of action. Even in this setting, however, it is unlikely that the acute effects of exercise on theophylline pharmacokinetics would be cause for concern. And it is unlikely that episodic exercise would be problematic in individuals stabilized on theophylline.

Turning to the effects of chronic exercise (i.e., deconditioned vs. conditioned subjects), no data are available about the effects of conditioning on the pharmacokinetics of most of the drugs discussed in this chapter. Since some of these drugs are administered episodically and by inhalation, this issue is likely of minor significance. But for theophylline, a drug that is (a) administered systemically, (b) administered daily, and

(c) potentially toxic, the fitness level of the subject may affect the drug's metabolic rate. Unfortunately, this issue has not been adequately studied, and caution is in order.

How Respiratory Agents Affect Exercisers

This section examines the cardiovascular, pulmonary, and metabolic effects of the respiratory agents during exercise. Table 5.3 first summarizes some physiological effects mediated by beta-2 receptors.

Cardiovascular Actions

We look first at beta-agonists, in passing at bronchodilators, and a bit more at anti-inflammatory agents.

Since *beta-agonists* possess sympathomimetic properties, they might affect exercise HR and, thereby, influence the monitoring of exercise intensity. However, beta-receptors in the heart are predominantly of the beta-1 subtype, and selective beta-2 agonists have little direct effect on HR when administered via inhalation. Studies have shown that albuterol has little effect on maximum exercise HR in elite athletes with (Ienna and McKenzie 1997) and without (Meeuwisse et al. 1992) a history of asthma. Fleck and colleagues (1993), however, did demonstrate that inhaled albuterol at twice the recommended dose (i.e., 360 mcg) increased exercise HR; but this was observed only at intermediate levels of exercise intensity (Fleck et al. 1993). Another study of inhaled albuterol at 360 mcg (in elite cyclists) found no effect on peak exercise HR (Lemmer et al. 1995).

What explains the phenomenon that beta-2 agonists do not augment exercise-induced tachycardia? To start, a drug can simultaneously

Table 5.3   Physiologic Effects Mediated by Beta-2 Receptors

Site	Action
Vascular smooth muscle	Relaxation
Bronchiolar smooth muscle	Relaxation
GI tract smooth muscle	Relaxation
GU tract smooth muscle	Relaxation
Skeletal muscle	Glycogenolysis, K+ uptake, lipolysis
Liver	Glycogenolysis, gluconeogenesis

operate as an agonist and an antagonist at a given receptor. Sorensen, Jensen, and Faergeman (1991) postulated that at lower levels of exercise, HR increases in response to norepinephrine acting via beta-1 receptors, but that at extreme levels of exercise the heart responds to epinephrine acting mainly via beta-2 receptors. Epinephrine is both a beta-1 and beta-2 agonist; however, in the presence of a beta-2 drug, epinephrine cannot bind to the beta-2 receptor. Although the beta-2 agonist is itself a stimulant at that receptor, the drug is a less potent agonist than is endogenous epinephrine. By occupying the receptor, the drug interferes with epinephrine's ability to fully stimulate the receptor. Unlike beta-blockers (see chapter 1), which predictably depress both resting and exercise HR, oral beta-agonists may make it difficult for the athletic trainer to predict the target HR in subjects. Fortunately, beta-agonists are mostly administered by inhalation, making their effects on HR negligible; systemic bioavailability of the drug is limited when administered by this route.

Among the *bronchodilators*, theophylline stimulates resting HR and can produce a mild diuresis, but has negligible effects on exercise HR.

As for the respiratory *anti-inflammatory agents*, we can start with the antihistamines. Since resting HR is mainly under the control of the parasympathetic nervous system (e.g., vagal innervation of the SA node), drugs with antimuscarinic anticholinergic activity can increase resting HR. Because of this, one might assume that drugs with this property also would increase exercise HR. To the contrary, diphenhydramine, an antihistamine with anticholinergic properties, had no effect on exercise HR in the 12 volunteers who were exercised to exhaustion in a study (Montgomery and Deuster 1992). It should be noted, however, that results were assessed 2 h postdose in this study; and with diphenhydramine some clinical effects are not maximal until 6 to 9 h postdose.

Pulmonary Actions and Oxygen Uptake

We begin with beta-agonists and their effects on the pulmonary system. Some scientists believe that exercise increases either the number or sensitivity of beta-receptors. Bronchodilation after maximal effort has been documented in elite athletes with asthma; single doses of inhaled albuterol augmented this response to exercise (Todaro 1996). However, continuous use may diminish the effectiveness of beta-2 agonists. Seven days of inhaled albuterol *worsened* baseline and postexercise FEV-1 in subjects with EIB (Inman and O'Byrne 1996), and daily therapy with the long-acting salmeterol for 1 month was associated with a *decrease* in its duration of action (Nelson et al. 1998). In this latter study, the effective decrease was explained by a change in the pharmacokinetics of salmeterol and not by a change in beta-receptors or pulmonary function. A single dose of inhaled albuterol 15 min prior to exercise *improved* peak flow rate, but still it did not modify minute ventilation in asthmatic athletes (Ienna and McKenzie 1997). Many studies have shown that albuterol exerted significant bronchodilation yet had no beneficial effect on performance (Fleck et al. 1993; Lemmer et al. 1995; Meeuwisse et al. 1992). Taken together, these findings put into perspective the variable nature of the pulmonary response to exercise and to bronchodilators.

As for oxygen uptake ($\dot{V}O_2$) with beta-agonists, single doses of albuterol, administered via inhalation, did not influence $\dot{V}O_2$ at various exercise intensities in athletes with asthma (Freeman, Packe, and Cayton 1989; Ienna and McKenzie 1997) and subjects without asthma (Bedi, Gong, and Horvath 1988; Fleck et al. 1993; Meeuwisse et al. 1992; Sandsund et al. 1998). Intravenous administration of albuterol also had no effect on $\dot{V}O_2$ in nonasthmatics (Violante et al. 1989). The lack of effect on $\dot{V}O_2$ offers another explanation of why beta-agonists do not affect exercise HR.

Regarding the effect of methylxanthines, theophylline is more potent than caffeine both as a bronchodilator and as a CNS stimulant. Caffeine prevented EIB at doses of 7 mg/kg, but not at doses of 3.5 mg/kg (Kivity et al. 1990). For theophylline, doses of roughly 3 mg/kg are superior to placebo, and doses of roughly 5 mg/kg provide even more protection (Magnussen, Reuss, and Jorres 1988). Theophylline can also stimulate respiration centrally by enhancing sensitivity of the medulla to CO_2.

As for $\dot{V}O_2$, theophylline at serum concentrations of 10 to 20 mcg/ml had no effect on $\dot{V}O_2$max in nonasthmatic athletes (Morton, Scott, and Fitch 1989).

Ipratropium is another bronchodilator, and researchers have found that nebulized ipratropium has no effect on cardiac, pulmonary, hemo-dynamic, or subjective parameters during exercise in both asthmatics and nonasthmatics (Freeman, Javaid, and Cayton 1992).

Single, inhaled doses of nedocromil, a mast cell stabilizer, had no effect on pulmonary function tests during exercise (Prefaut, Anselme-Poujol, and Caillaud 1997). The same study found that a single, inhaled dose of nedocromil also had no effect on $\dot{V}O_2$max in master athletes (Prefaut, Anselme-Poujol, and Caillaud 1997).

Anti-inflammatory agents, including inhaled corticosteroids, are another category of respiratory drugs, worthy of separate mention for their effects on pulmonary function. The cardiovascular, metabolic, and pulmonary effects of inhaled corticosteroids during exercise do not appear to be significant. Although corticosteroids can cause hyperglyce-mia, these effects are usually not seen after oral inhalation. The effects of the leukotriene modifiers on these parameters are essentially unknown. A study of montelukast that revealed a significant protective effect on bronchoconstriction (as measured by FEV-1) did not assess other physi-ologic parameters (Leff et al. 1998). For more information, Montgomery and Deuster (1993) have reviewed the limited data on type-1 histamine antagonists.

Metabolic Actions

With the beta-agonist agents, the route of administration also influences the degree of their metabolic effects. Although these effects have already been discussed more thoroughly in chapter 4 on the sympathomimetics, one should not extrapolate findings seen with classic sympathomimetics to the beta-2 agonists.

Four separate groups of investigators measured exercise lactate concentrations to assess the metabolic effect of inhaled beta-2 agonists. Blood lactate increases either when there is a greater reliance on carbohydrate as an energy substrate or when oxygen delivery does not meet demand, both occurrences indicating anaerobic metabolism. In one study, lactate concentrations increased during beta-agonist therapy (compared to placebo) but only at one of seven different workloads (Fleck et al. 1993). In another study, exercise-induced lactate concentrations rose with albuterol, but not with the long-acting agent salmeterol (Robertson et al. 1994). Testing subjects before the effects of salmeterol were maximal may explain this (i.e., salmeterol has a slower onset of action); subjects were administered the drugs 30 min before exercise testing. Robertson and colleagues postulated that because salmeterol has a higher beta-2/beta-1 ratio than albuterol, the effects of these two drugs on fat and carbohydrate utilization differ. Two other studies of albuterol did not reveal any effect on lactate concentrations (Ienna and McKenzie 1997; Sandsund et al. 1998). None of these four studies demonstrated an ergogenic effect.

Clenbuterol, however, may be unique among the beta-agonists. It is a very potent, long-acting, beta-2 receptor agonist that is used in Europe. Some athletes in the United States abuse clenbuterol, which is not approved for human use in this country. These athletes believe clenbuterol is a "repartitioning agent," and they use it to enhance fat burning while simultaneously promoting lean body mass. (Physiologically, epinephrine, the body's natural beta-agonist, is an important stimulator of lipolysis.) Indeed, although clenbuterol has been used for this purpose in livestock, Prather and colleagues reviewed the literature on clenbuterol in 1995 and concluded that there are no human studies, particularly at the enormous doses being administered to animals.

The mobilization of free fatty acids (FFAs) from adipocytes appears to be a beta-1 process, and the breakdown of muscle triglycerides appears to be mainly a beta-2 process (Cleroux et al. 1989). Epinephrine is an agonist at both receptor types. Choo and colleagues (1992), in a series of tests, showed that high-dose oral clenbuterol in rats does increase skeletal muscle mass while simultaneously decreasing fat mass. These effects were blocked by propranolol only when this beta-blocker was given in extremely high doses. MacLennan and Edwards (1989) showed, in rats, that propranolol could block the anabolic effects of clenbuterol on muscle mass. In addition, oral albuterol did not produce effects similar to clenbuterol unless it was given in high oral doses or as a continuous IV infusion. The investigators concluded that clenbuterol possesses an anabolic action, which is mediated via the beta-2 receptor. Albuterol has the potential for producing anabolism, but since it is less potent at the beta-2 receptor and shorter acting than clenbuterol, it must be given continuously and in very high doses (Choo et al. 1992). According to a study by Martineau and colleagues (1992), an extended-release form of oral albuterol did not increase lean body mass in 12 males taking this drug for 21 consecutive days. Because salmeterol is more potent and longer-acting than albuterol, salmeterol should be studied for anabolic properties similar to clenbuterol.

As for the effects of bronchodilators on metabolic function, theophylline again needs to be considered. Because of the structural similarity of caffeine and theophylline, the two agents might be expected to produce similar metabolic effects. Marsh and colleagues (1993) found that theophylline delayed the onset of intracellular metabolic acidosis, suggesting that it enhances the oxidative capacity of skeletal muscle. The ability of theophylline to antagonize adenosine receptors brings up some interesting scenarios, even if the significance is as yet unclear. By antagonizing adenosine receptors, theophylline, at least in theory, might attenuate the beneficial aspects of adenosine. Simpson and Phillis (1992) contend that adenosine is a critical regulator of the skeletal-muscle circulatory response to exercise. They propose that drugs such as NSAIDs, which potentiate adenosine, could augment athletic performance. Since theophylline is an antagonist of adenosine, logically it should do the opposite. No data exist to confirm or refute this action.

Clinical data reveal that theophylline can suppress erythropoietin output (Bakris et al. 1990). The relevance of this effect of theophylline to sports medicine, however, remains to be determined.

In brief, antihistamines with potent anticholinergic properties may affect temperature regulation during exercise, but typically these effects are not significant.

Musculoskeletal Actions

The respiratory agents have effects on musculoskeletal function that should be discussed, at least briefly. For example, animal data reveal that 14 consecutive days of ingesting clenbuterol increases contractile

Table 5.4   Contractile Properties for Control and Clenbuterol-Treated Animals

Treatment	Absolute tension (g)	P_o $(g \cdot g^{-1})$	$\dot{V}$max $(mm \cdot s^{-1})$	Fatigue times (s)
Control	2,137 ± 107	930 ± 42	127.9 ± 5.1	57.7 ± 1.7
Clenbuterol	2,442 ± 99*	931 ± 37	151.2 ± 3.7*	47.0 ± 2.0*

* Significantly different from control ($p = 0.05$).
Values are means ± SE. P_o = peak tetanic tension; $\dot{V}$max = maximal shortening
velocity (expressed as $mm \cdot s^{-1}$ since there were no differences in muscle lengths).
Adapted from Dodd et al. 1996.

strength of skeletal muscle. However, expressed per gram of muscle,
power output was similar between animals receiving the beta-agonist
clenbuterol and those receiving placebo. The authors, Dodd and colleagues (1996), concluded that clenbuterol increased muscle strength
and muscle size due to hypertrophy of both slow-twitch and fast-twitch
fibers (see table 5.4).

Theophylline has been shown to stimulate diaphragmatic contractility in asthmatics, but just how this action impacts the exercise response
is unclear. Intravenous aminophylline had no effect on respiratory
muscle strength, ventilatory endurance, or exercise performance in
nonasthmatics during treadmill exercise (Violante et al. 1989).

How Respiratory Agents Affect
Exercise Performance

In general, the lungs do not limit exercise performance (Sutton 1992). To
accurately determine the true effects of the pulmonary drugs on athletic
performance, however, requires differentiating normal subjects from
those with asthma or EIB. In the average untrained subject, exercise is
limited by cardiac output and peripheral $\dot{V}O_2$, not by ventilation or
pulmonary gas diffusion (Hsia 1998). Nevertheless, some elite athletes
experience decreases in arterial oxygenation and desaturate at $\dot{V}O_2$max
or when cardiac output exceeds 25 L/min (Dempsey, Hanson, and
Henderson 1984). Elderly athletes and asthmatic athletes may be other
populations among whom exercise intensity is limited by lung function
(Dempsey, Johnson, and Saupe 1990).

Since ventilation usually delivers more than enough oxygen to meet
a person's needs during exercise, it is doubtful that any of the drugs

discussed in this chapter (except, perhaps, the beta-agonists) would augment performance in patients without pulmonary disease. Babb and colleagues (1991) demonstrated a close relationship between $\dot{V}O_2$max and FEV-1 when patients with mild-to-moderate airflow limitations were compared with controls. Dempsey (1986), too, has reviewed this concept. To facilitate discussion, various drug categories should be considered before guidelines for their use are developed.

Beta-Agonists and Athletic Performance

Because beta-agonists are sympathomimetics, ergogenic effects might occur with their use; these effects are more likely to appear after systemic administration (e.g., oral, intravenous) and are unlikely after inhalation. Of the more than a dozen clinical studies of the effect of beta-agonist bronchodilators on athletic performance, the vast majority showed that, when administered via inhalation, beta-agonists are not ergogenic. This was the case in both trained subjects (Fleck et al. 1993; Lemmer et al. 1995; McKenzie et al. 1983; Meeuwisse et al. 1992; Sandsund et al. 1998) and untrained subjects (Ingemann-Hansen et al. 1980; Freeman, Packe, and Cayton 1989). It was true as well in subjects with a history of asthma (Freeman, Packe, and Cayton 1989; Ingemann-Hansen et al. 1980; Robertson et al. 1994; Schmidt et al. 1988) and those without such a history of asthma (Fleck et al. 1993; Lemmer et al. 1995; McKenzie et al. 1983; Meeuwisse et al. 1992; Sandsund et al. 1998). It even held true when higher-than-recommended doses were tested (Fleck et al. 1993; Lemmer et al. 1995; Sandsund et al. 1998). In all of these studies, cycle ergometry or treadmill running was used as the exercise test.

Only two groups of investigators concluded that beta-agonists are ergogenic when administered by inhalation. Bedi, Gong, and Horvath (1988) found that elite nonasthmatic cyclists could exercise for 37 s longer during an all-out maximum cycle test after inhaling albuterol. It is unclear why these investigators were able to document an ergogenic effect, whereas three other, nearly identical studies (Fleck et al. 1993; Lemmer et al. 1995; Meeuwisse et al. 1992), also using elite nonasthmatic cyclists, found no benefit. Signorile and colleagues (1992) showed that inhaled albuterol provided an ergogenic effect on power output during a 15 s, all-out effort on a cycle ergometer by untrained nonasthmatics, but other investigators (Lemmer et al. 1995; Meeuwisse et al. 1992) have criticized the research design of this study.

Robertson and colleagues (1994) compared albuterol to the long-acting salmeterol and found no improvement by either drug, compared with placebo, on maximum workload, $\dot{V}O_2$max, or perceived exertion (using the Borg scale) in asthmatic men.

In summary, most of the clinical data indicate that beta-2 receptor agonists, when administered via inhalation, do not provide an ergogenic effect. Now, someone needs to inform competitive triathletes of this (see "Triathletes and Bronchodilators").

■ *Triathletes and Bronchodilators*

Clinical research has estimated that roughly 10-15% of Olympic athletes have EIB (Storms 1999). If that's true, then why do 98% of triathletes claim they are asthmatic? Les McDonald, head of the International Triathlon Union (ITU), insists the figure is accurate, since his office in Vancouver, British Columbia, is where these athletes must send their medical paperwork. McDonald suspects that many of the world's top triathletes are not actually asthmatic, but have registered as such to justify use of inhaled bronchodilator drugs in hopes of enhancing their race performance. At the World Cup stop in Sydney, athletes were seen on camera walking down to the start of the race taking one last "hit" from their inhalers before jumping in the water. As each finished with the inhaler, he or she would pass it on to a competitor. This is not only embarrassing to the sport, but pointless as well. William W. Storms, MD, a Colorado Springs allergist and member of the USOC, has studied inhaled bronchodilators and found no physiologic effect—just a psychological effect (T. Farrey, 14 June 1999, Triathletes suck, ESPN.com).

Twenty-one days of oral extended-release albuterol increased strength in quadriceps and hamstring muscle, but not grip strength, in 12 healthy males. Eight weeks of oral albuterol improved both concentric and eccentric strength variables after isokinetic resistance exercise in quadriceps muscle of nonasthmatic normal volunteers (Caruso et al. 1995). Intravenous administration of salbutamol (i.e., albuterol) did not enhance exercise performance or ratings of perceived exertion (RPE) in nonasthmatics (Violante et al. 1989).

The effects of clenbuterol appear to be more pronounced on untrained muscles than trained (Murphy et al. 1996). In healthy males undergoing knee surgery, 4 weeks of clenbuterol provided a very modest benefit in enhancing rate of strength gain in knee extensors, but the absolute amount of strength gained was not greater than in the group receiving placebo (see figure 5.2; Maltin et al. 1993). These limited data suggest that beta-agonists, when administered systemically, may enhance strength performance, but not endurance performance.

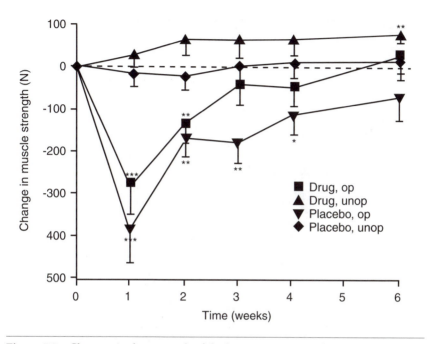

Figure 5.2 Changes in the strength of the knee extensors in drug-treated and placebo-treated patients. The values are means with bars indicating *SEMs*. * = $p < 0.05$; ** = $p < 0.01$; *** = $p < 0.001$ compared with zero. Op = operated leg; unop = unoperated leg.

Reproduced with permission from C.A. Maltin, M.I. Delday, J.S. Watson, S.D. Heys, I.M. Nevison, I.K. Ritchie, and P.H. Gibson, 1993, *Clinical Science*, 84, 651-654. © the Biochemical Society and the Medical Research Society.

Theophylline, Caffeine, and Performance

Caffeine and theophylline both produce significantly diverse metabolic effects. Although the actions of theophylline closely mimic those of caffeine, the two drugs are not identical and one should not assume that theophylline will have the same effects on athletic performance as caffeine does. While such properties as the inhibition of bronchoconstriction, enhanced FFA mobilization, increased circulating epinephrine, increased cardiac output, increased diaphragmatic contractility, and CNS stimulation would be expected to be ergogenic, other properties such as the diuretic effect, adenosine antagonism, and decreased erythropoietin secretion would seem to be ergolytic. The impact of theophylline on active (e.g., athletic) performance probably represents the sum total of all of its actions. Oral, sustained-release theophylline has been shown to significantly increase forearm endurance and maximal muscular power (see figure 5.3) in healthy volunteers (Marsh et al. 1993), but exerted no effect on maximal

Sport and Exercise Pharmacology

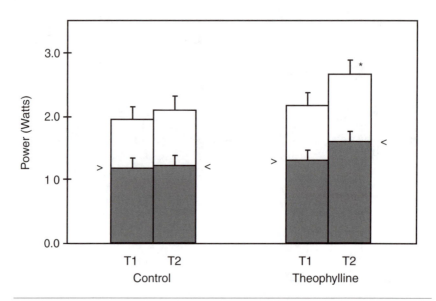

Figure 5.3   Changes (arrows) in maximal power (open bars) and intracellular threshold (IT) power (hatched bars) during repeated exercise testing of the control and theophylline-treated subjects. T1 represents the initial test condition; T2 represents the repeat test given 72 h later. Values are mean ± SD. Theophylline treatment significantly (asterisk indicates $p < 0.05$) increased maximal exercise capacity of the subjects and delayed the onset of the IT. Neither the maximal power achieved nor the power at the onset of the IT was altered in the control group.

From G.D. Marsh, R.G. McFadden, R.L. Nicholson, D.J. Leasa, and R.T. Thompson, 1993, "Theophylline delays skeletal muscle fatigue during progressive exercise," *American Review of Respiratory Disease* 147 (4): 876-879. Official Journal of the American Thoracic Society. © American Lung Association.

oxygen consumption, muscular endurance, muscular power, muscular strength, or reaction time in elite, nonasthmatic athletes (Morton et al. 1989). The elite athletes were tested with a Cybex isokinetic dynamometer while performing leg extension, while the normal volunteers performed wrist flexion. It is possible that the highly developed thigh muscles of the elite athletes masked any benefit provided by theophylline on muscular performance.

Caffeine (see chapter 13), which exerts diverse effects on exercise physiology and performance, has been studied more in relation to athletic competition than has theophylline. Caffeine is clearly ergogenic (Berglund and Hemmingsson 1982); theophylline is not, despite the fact that it can produce substantial increases in circulating epinephrine (Vestal et al. 1983). Although caffeine has been shown to increase the strength and duration of contractions of both skeletal and cardiac muscle, theophylline is less potent in this regard (Morton, Scott, and

Fitch 1989). Caffeine is known to improve reaction time, but theophylline does not appear to do so (Morton et al. 1989).

Other Agents and Exercise Performance

Only limited data are available for the other pulmonary drugs. Nebulized ipratropium appears not to be ergogenic on maximal exercise performance in either asthmatics or nonasthmatics (Freeman, Javaid, and Cayton 1992). Baraldi and colleagues (1994) found that pretreatment of children aged 8 to 14 years with inhaled cromolyn prior to their treadmill running decreased the energy cost of exercise (see figure 5.4).

Of the leukotriene modifiers, zileuton has been shown to effectively attenuate bronchospasm induced by cold air (Israel et al. 1990) and exercise (Meltzer et al. 1996). Its effects on performance, however, were not assessed in these studies.

Montgomery and Deuster (1991, 1992, 1993) studied diphenhydramine (a commonly used type-1 histamine receptor antagonist available in the U.S. without a prescription) and terfenadine (a prescription drug that was removed from the U.S. market in 1998 because of concerns over

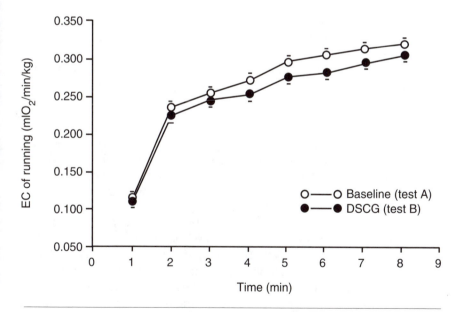

Figure 5.4 Energy cost (EC) of running in asthmatic children at corresponding work rates. The EC of running was higher in test A (without premedication) than in test B (with DSCG [disodium cromoglycate] premedication) at comparable work rates ($p < 0.001$). Values are mean ± *SEM*.

Adapted from Baraldi et al. 1994.

drug-induced arrhythmias). They found that neither agent affected muscle strength (Montgomery and Deuster 1991), muscle endurance (Montgomery and Deuster 1991), or treadmill running performance at various intensities (Montgomery and Deuster 1992) when evaluated 2 h after single doses. Clinicians should note that there is a poor correlation between the timing of peak therapeutic effects (e.g., antihistaminic effect) and peak side effects (e.g., drowsiness) with these drugs. In addition, terfenadine does not cause drowsiness since it does not penetrate the CNS. Thus, it would be inaccurate to extrapolate observations with terfenadine to all antihistamines in general. In their review of the literature, Montgomery and Deuster (1993) did not find data that predicted a detrimental effect of antihistamines on exercise performance.

Avoiding Potential Complications

With the exception of theophylline, all the respiratory drugs discussed in this chapter are extremely safe. Exercising while taking these drugs should pose no problems, with a few notable exceptions:

- Exercise can affect the pharmacokinetics of theophylline.
- Antihistamines with strong anticholinergic properties may affect temperature regulation.
- Antihistamines that induce drowsiness can affect exercise performance.
- Beta-agonists can induce hand tremor, which may be detrimental in shooting events.

The body cools itself by transferring heat to the skin, where it leaves the body by one of four mechanisms: conduction, convection, radiation, or evaporation. It is quite possible for the body temperature of a marathon runner to reach 39 to 41 °C. Drugs with anticholinergic properties, including some antihistamines, can interfere with the sweating response, and thereby inhibit heat loss from evaporation. Thus, exercising in a hot, humid environment while taking certain antihistamines can be detrimental. The type-1 histamine antagonists with the strongest and the least anticholinergic activity are listed in table 5.5.

Antihistamines with minimal anticholinergic activity may be preferred if drying effects are intolerable during exercise. Still, it is important to remind individuals that astemizole has been associated with abnormalities of cardiac conduction (e.g., Q-T prolongation) and cardiac arrhythmias (e.g., torsade de pointes); it is an extremely long-acting agent.

In general, administration of corticosteroids via inhalation is thought

Table 5.5   H-1 Receptor Antagonists and Their Anticholinergic Effects

H-1 blockers with strong anticholinergic activity	H-1 blockers with little or no anticholinergic activity
Carbinoxamine (various combination products)	Astemizole (Hismanal)
	Cetirizine (Zyrtec)
Clemastine (Tavist)	Fexofenadine (Allegra)
Dimenhydrinate (Dramamine)	Loratadine (Claritin)
Diphenhydramine (Benadryl)	
Hydroxyzine (Atarax, Vistaril)	
Methdilazine (Tacaryl)	
Phenyltoloxamine (various combination products)	
Promethazine (Phenergan)	

This listing does not include all H-1 antagonists. Only the agents with the strongest and the least amount of anticholinergic activity are listed.

to greatly reduce the many serious toxic effects of these drugs when they must be used chronically. Detectable reductions in bone mineral density (BMD), however, have been documented in adult women with asthma (Wisniewski et al. 1997) and in children with asthma (Boot et al. 1997) who used inhaled corticosteroids over a period of 3 to 8 years. Another study in children concluded inhaled corticosteroids did not adversely affect BMD (Agertoft and Pedersen 1998), but this study evaluated budesonide; the unique pharmacokinetics of this agent may be partially responsible for an absence of systemic toxicity. Investigators who have extensively reviewed this topic conclude that when excessive doses are avoided, inhaled corticosteroids are extremely safe, even when used for many years (Efthimiou and Barnes 1998; Woodcock 1998). If these drugs allow the asthmatic to exercise, conceivably the beneficial effects of exercise on BMD may offset the detrimental effects of corticosteroid therapy.

NCAA and USOC Status

Note first that the NCAA and the USOC ban all the beta-receptor agonists listed in table 5.1 for use during competition when administered systemically (e.g., oral tablets, oral solution, parenteral injection). Since beta-agonists are sympathomimetics, they are regarded as stimulants. However, some beta-agonists are not banned if administered by inhalation. The NCAA permits use of any beta-agonist when administered by inhalation; however, the USOC permits inhaled albuterol, salmeterol, and terbutaline only with prior written permission. Fortunately, all of the beta-agonists (except for salmeterol) have short half-lives; discontinuation 2 to 3 days prior to competition should allow sufficient time to completely clear these drugs from the body. Clenbuterol, banned by both the NCAA and USOC, is *not licensed for human use* in the United States. Ipratropium and theophylline are not banned by either governing body.

The NCAA places no restriction on the use of corticosteroid anti-inflammatory agents; however, the USOC bans the use of corticosteroids by most routes of administration. With prior written permission, the USOC allows the use of inhaled corticosteroids. The USOC bans the use of sedating antihistamines for sports involving riflery. Note that antihistamines are frequently found in drug-combination products for coughs and cold or flu symptoms, and some of these drug combinations may contain other types of banned substances (e.g., sympathomimetics). The status of the newer drugs (e.g., zileuton, zafirlukast) is still unclear, but judging by their actions and side effects, it seems unlikely that these drugs would be banned.

Guidelines for Exercisers

Exercisers should keep in mind the following points:

- Avoid herbal products or dietary supplements that contain ephedra or ephedrine.
- Avoid antihistamines with significant anticholinergic activity during endurance activities.
- While inhaled beta-2 receptor agonists are the preferred type of drug for preventing EIB, the USOC does not permit the use of this type of medication without written permission.

Guidelines for Trainers and Coaches

These are tips for helping active individuals in managing EIB:

- If the individual has been prescribed an inhaler containing cromolyn or a rapid-onset beta-agonist (e.g., albuterol), it can be used just prior to beginning exercise.
- Not all inhalers for EIB are alike: beta-agonist drugs (e.g., albuterol) are effective with the first dose, but if the inhaler is salmeterol, it should be used at least 30 min prior to beginning exercise because salmeterol has a slower onset than albuterol.
- If the individual has been prescribed a steroid inhaler, encourage daily use; single doses (i.e., episodic use) of corticosteroid inhalers

just prior to exercise are ineffective in preventing EIB. Inhaled corticosteroids require daily use to be effective (Hansen-Flaschen and Schotland 1998).

• Remember that both the NCAA and the USOC prohibit systemic use of beta-agonists.

• Since EIB does not lead to long-term deterioration of lung function, generally there is no need for continuous (i.e., daily) drug therapy (McFadden and Gilbert 1994); theophylline, however, must be administered daily to be effective.

If exercise readily provokes bronchospasm in asthmatics, what advice should you give a person with asthma who wants to exercise or compete in sports? First, keep in mind that though exercise (certain types at least) can induce bronchospasm in susceptible individuals, the response to long-term training is a decrease in symptoms. Postexercise bronchodilation has actually been documented in elite athletes (Todaro 1996). Note that some Olympic athletes have asthma; so a diagnosis of asthma should not deter any athlete from setting lofty goals or cause him or her to shy away from intense exercise. Second, symptoms do not occur during exercise but rather immediately *after completion;* they then reach a peak within 5 to 10 min. Recovery is usually complete in some 30 to 60 min postexercise (McFadden and Gilbert 1994).

Third, not all sports or types of exercise induce EIB. Intense, short bouts of activity are less of a problem than are prolonged events or exercise sessions. Furthermore, running is worse than jogging, and jogging is worse than walking. Exercise during winter months is worse than during the fall, and the fall months are worse than the summer months (McFadden and Gilbert 1994). Finally, despite uncertainty about the pathophysiology of EIB, exposure to cold, dry air is a known stimulus to the condition.

References

Agertoft, L., and Pedersen, S. 1998. Bone mineral density in children with asthma receiving long-term treatment with inhaled budesonide. *Am J Respir Crit Care Med* 157:178-183.

Babb, T.G., Viggiano, R., Hurley, B., Staats, B., and Rodarte, J.R. 1991. Effect of mild-to-moderate airflow limitation on exercise capacity. *J Appl Physiol* 70:223-230.

Bakris, G.L., Sauter, E.R., Hussey, J.L., Fisher, J.W., Gaber, A.O., and Winsett, R. 1990. Effects of theophylline on erythropoietin production in normal subjects and in patients with erythrocytosis after renal transplantation. *N Engl J Med* 323:86-90.

Baraldi, E., Pierantonio, S., Magagnin, G., Filippone, M., and Zacchello, F. 1994. Effect of disodium cromoglycate on ventilation and gas exchange during exercise in asthmatic children with a postexertion FEV-1 fall less than 15 percent. *Chest* 106:1083-1088.

Bedi, J.F., Gong Jr., H., and Horvath, S.M. 1988. Enhancement of exercise performance with inhaled albuterol. *Can J Sport Sci* 13:144-148.

Berglund, B., and Hemmingsson, P. 1982. Effects of caffeine ingestion on exercise performance at low and high altitudes in cross country skiers. *Int J Sports Med* 3:234-236.

Boot, A.M., de Jongste, J.C., Verberne, A.A., Pols, H.A., and de Muinck Keizer-Schrama, S.M. 1997. Bone mineral density and bone metabolism of prepubertal children with asthma after long-term treatment with inhaled corticosteroids. *Pediatr Pulmonol* 24:379-384.

Briner Jr., W.W. 1993. Physical allergies and exercise. Clinical implications for those engaged in sports activities. *Sports Med* 15:365-373.

Bronsky, E.A., Kemp, J.P., Zhang, J., Guerreiro, D., and Reiss, T.F. 1997. Dose-related protection of exercise bronchoconstriction by montelukast, a cysteinyl leukotriene-receptor antagonist, at the end of a once-daily dosing interval. *Clin Pharmacol Ther* 62:556-561.

Bundgaard, A. 1985. Exercise and the asthmatic. *Sports Med* 2:254-266.

Caruso, J.F., Signorile, J.F., Perry, A.C., Leblanc, B., Williams, R., Clark, M., and Bamman, M.M. 1995. The effects of albuterol and isokinetic exercise on the quadriceps muscle group. *Med Sci Sports Exerc* 27:1471-1476.

Choo, J.J., Horan, M.A., Little, R.A., and Rothwell, N.J. 1992. Anabolic effects of clenbuterol on skeletal muscle are mediated by beta 2-adrenoceptor activation. *Am J Physiol* 263(1 Pt. 1):E50-56.

Cleroux, J., Van Nguyen, P., Taylor, A.W., and Leenen, F.H.H. 1989. Effects of beta-1 vs. beta-1+beta-2-blockade on exercise endurance and muscle metabolism in humans. *J Appl Physiol* 66:548-554.

Dempsey, J.A. 1986. J.B. Wolffe memorial lecture. Is the lung built for exercise? *Med Sci Sports Exerc* 18:143-155.

Dempsey, J.A., Hanson, P.G., and Henderson, K.S. 1984. Exercise-induced arterial hypoxaemia in healthy human subjects at sea level. *J Physiol* 355:161-175.

Dempsey, J.A., Johnson, B.D., and Saupe, K.W. 1990. Adaptations and limitations in the pulmonary system during exercise. *Chest* 97(3 suppl):81S-87S.

Dodd, S.L., Powers, S.K., Vrabas, I.S., Criswell, D., Stetson, S., and Hussain, R. 1996. Effects of clenbuterol on contractile and biochemical properties of skeletal muscle. *Med Sci Sports Exerc* 28:669-676.

Duffull, S.B., and Begg, E.J. 1992. Terfenadine ineffective in the prophylaxis of exercise-induced pruritus. *J Allergy Clin Immunol* 89:916-917.

Efthimiou, J., and Barnes, P.J. 1998. Effect of inhaled corticosteroids on bones and growth. *Eur Respir J* 11:1167-1177.

Fleck, S.J., Lucia, A., Storms, W.W., Wallach, J.M., Vint, P.F., and Zimmerman, S.D. 1993. Effects of acute inhalation of albuterol on submaximal and maximal VO_2 and blood lactate. *Int J Sports Med* 14:239-243.

Freeman, W., Javaid, A., and Cayton, R.M. 1992. The effect of ipratropium bromide on maximal exercise capacity in asthmatic and non-asthmatic men. *Respir Med* 86:151-155.

Freeman, W., Packe, G.E., and Cayton, R.M. 1989. Effect of nebulized salbutamol on maximal exercise performance in men with asthma. *Thorax* 44:942-947.

Godfrey, S., and Konig, P. 1975. Suppression of exercise-induced asthma by salbutamol, theophylline, atropine, cromolyn, and placebo in a group of asthmatic children. *Pediatrics* 56(5 pt 2 suppl):930-934.

Haas, F., Pasierski, S., Levine, N., Bishop, M., Axen, K., Pineda, H., and Haas, A. 1987. Effect of aerobic training on forced expiratory airflow in exercising asthmatic humans. *J Appl Physiol* 63:1230-1235.

Hansen-Flaschen, J., and Schotland, H. 1998. New treatments for exercise-induced asthma. *N Engl J Med* 339:192-193.

Helenius, I.J., Tikkanen, H.O., and Haahtela, T. 1998. Occurrence of exercise induced bronchospasm in elite runners: Dependence on atopy and exposure to cold air and pollen. *Br J Sports Med* 32:125-129.

Helenius, I.J., Tikkanen, H.O., Sarna, S., and Haahtela, T. 1998. Asthma and increased bronchial responsiveness in elite athletes: Atopy and sport event as risk factors. *J Allergy Clin Immunol* 101:646-652.

Hendeles, L., and Marshik, P.L. 1996. Zileuton: A new therapy for asthma or just the first of a new class of drugs? *Ann Pharmacother* 30:873-875.

Hsia, C.C.W. 1998. Respiratory function of hemoglobin. *N Engl J Med* 338:239-247.

Ienna, T.M., and McKenzie, D.C. 1997. The asthmatic athlete: Metabolic and ventilatory responses to exercise with and without pre-exercise medication. *Int J Sports Med* 18:142-148.

Ingemann-Hansen, T., Bundgaard, A., Halkjaer-Kristensen, J., Siggaard-Andersen, J., and Weeke, B. 1980. Maximal oxygen consumption rate in patients with bronchial asthma: The effect of beta 2-adrenoreceptor stimulation. *Scand J Clin Lab Invest* 40(2):99-104.

Inman, M.D., and O'Byrne, P.M. 1996. The effect of regular inhaled albuterol on exercise-induced bronchoconstriction. *Am J Respir Crit Care Med* 153:65-69.

Israel, E., Dermarkarian, R., Rosenberg, M., Sperling, R., Taylor, G., Rubin, P., and Drazen, J.M. 1990. The effects of a 5-lipoxygenase inhibitor on asthma induced by cold, dry air. *N Engl J Med* 323:1740-1744.

Kivity, S., Ben Aharon, Y., Man, A., and Topilsky, M. 1990. The effect of caffeine on exercise-induced bronchoconstriction. *Chest* 97:1083-1085.

Kobayashi, R.H., and Mellion, M.B. 1991. Exercise-induced asthma, anaphylaxis, and urticaria. *Primary Care* 18:809-831.

Kukafka, D.S., Lang, D.M., Porter, S., Rogers, J., Ciccolella, D., Polansky, M., and D'Alonzo Jr., G.E. 1998. Exercise-induced bronchospasm in high school athletes via a free running test: Incidence and epidemiology. *Chest* 114:1613-1622.

Larsson, K., Ohlsen, P., Larsson, L., Malmberg, P., Rydstrom, P., and Ulriksen, H. 1993. High prevalence of asthma in cross country skiers. *Br Med J* 307:1326-1329.

Leff, J.A., Busse, W.W., Pearlman, D., Bronsky, E.A., Kemp, J., Hendeles, L., Dockhorn, R., Kundu, S., Zhang, J., Seidenberg, B.C., and Reiss, T.F. 1998. Montelukast, a leukotriene-receptor antagonist, for the treatment of mild asthma and exercise-induced bronchoconstriction. *N Engl J Med* 339:147-152.

Lemmer, J.T., Fleck, S.J., Wallach, M., Fox, S., Burke, E.R., Kearney, J.T., and Storms, W.W. 1995. The effects of albuterol on power output in non-asthmatic athletes. *Int J Sports Med* 16:243-249.

MacLennan, P.A., and Edwards, R.H. 1989. Effects of clenbuterol and propranolol on muscle mass. Evidence that clenbuterol stimulates muscle beta-adrenoceptors to induce hypertrophy. *Biochem J* 264:573-579.

Magnussen, H., Reuss, G., and Jorres, R. 1988. Methylxanthines inhibit exercise-induced bronchoconstriction at low serum theophylline concentration and in a dose-dependent fashion. *J Allergy Clin Immunol* 81(3):531-537.

Maltin, C.A., Delday, M.I., Watson, J.S., Heys, S.D., Nevison, I.M., Ritchie, I.K., and Gibson, P.H. 1993. Clenbuterol, a beta-adrenergic agonist, increases relative muscle strength in orthopedic patients. *Clin Sci (Colch)* 84:651-654.

Mannix, E.T., Farber, M.O., Palange, P., Galassetti, P., and Manfredi, F. 1996. Exercise-induced asthma in figure skaters. *Chest* 109:312-315.

Marsh, G.D., McFadden, R.G., Nicholson, R.L., Leasa, D.J., and Thompson, R.T. 1993. Theophylline delays skeletal muscle fatigue during progressive exercise. *Am Rev Respir Dis* 147:876-879.

Martineau, L., Horan, M.A., Rothwell, N.J., and Little, R.A. 1992. Salbutamol, a beta 2-adrenoceptor agonist, increases skeletal muscle strength in young men. *Clin Sci (Colch)* 83:615-621.

McFadden, E.R., and Gilbert, I.A. 1994. Exercise-induced asthma. *N Engl J Med* 330:1362-1367.

McKenzie, D.C., Rhodes, E.C., Stirling, D.R., Wiley, J.P., Dunwoody, D.W., Filsinger, I.B., Jang, F., and Stevens, A. 1983. Salbutamol and treadmill performance in non-atopic athletes. *Med Sci Sports Exerc* 15(6):520-522.

Meeuwisse, W.M., McKenzie, D.C., Hopkins, S.R., and Road, J.D. 1992. The effect of salbutamol on performance in elite nonasthmatic athletes. *Med Sci Sports Exerc* 24:1161-1166.

Meltzer, S.S., Hasday, J.D., Cohn, J., and Bleecker, E.R. 1996. Inhibition of exercise-induced bronchospasm by zileuton: A 5-lipoxygenase inhibitor. *Am J Respir Crit Care Med* 153(3):931-935.

Montgomery, L.C., and Deuster, P.A. 1991. Acute antihistamine ingestion does not affect muscle strength and endurance. *Med Sci Sports Exerc* 23:1016-1019.

Montgomery, L.C., and Deuster, P.A. 1992. Ingestion of an antihistamine does not affect exercise performance. *Med Sci Sports Exerc* 24:383-388.

Montgomery, L.C., and Deuster, P.A. 1993. Effects of antihistamine medications on exercise performance. *Sports Med* 15:179-195.

Morton, A.R., and Fitch, K.D. 1992. Asthmatic drugs and competitive sport. An update. *Sports Med* 14:228-242.

Morton, A.R., Scott, C.A., and Fitch, K.D. 1989. The effects of theophylline on the physical performance and work capacity of well-trained athletes. *J Allergy Clin Immunol* 83:55-61.

Murphy, R.J., Beliveau, L., Seburn, K.L., and Gardiner, P.F. 1996. Clenbuterol has a greater influence on untrained than on previously trained skeletal muscle in rats. *Eur J Appl Physiol* 73:304-310.

Nelson, J.A., Strauss, L., Skowronski, M., Ciufo, R., Novak, R., and McFadden Jr., E.R. 1998. Effect of long-term salmeterol treatment on exercise-induced asthma. *N Engl J Med* 339:141-146.

O'Byrne, P.M., Israle, E., and Drazen, J.M. 1997. Antileukotrienes in the treatment of asthma. *Ann Intern Med* 127:472-480.

Pierson, W.E., Covert, D.S., Koenig, J.Q., Namekata, T., and Kim, Y.S. 1986. Implications of air pollution effects on athletic performance. *Med Sci Sports Exerc* 18:322-327.

Prather, I.D., Brown, D.E., North, P., and Wilson, J.R. 1995. Clenbuterol: A substitute for anabolic steroids? *Med Sci Sports Exerc* 27:1118-1121.

Prefaut, C., Anselme-Poujol, F., and Caillaud, C. 1997. Inhibition of histamine release by nedocromil sodium reduces exercise-induced hypoxemia in master athletes. *Med Sci Sports Exerc* 29:10-16.

Robertson, W., Simkins, J., O'Hickey, S.P., Freeman, S., and Cayton, R.M. 1994. Does single dose salmeterol affect exercise capacity in asthmatic men? *Eur Respir J* 7:1978-1984.

Sandsund, M., Sue-Chu, M., Helgerud, J., Reinertsen, R.E., and Bjermer, L. 1998. Effect of cold exposure (–15° C) and salbutamol treatment on physical performance in elite nonasthmatic cross-country skiers. *Eur J Appl Physiol* 77:297-304.

Schlaeffer, F., Engelberg, I., Kaplanski, J., and Danon, A. 1984. Effect of exercise and environmental heat on theophylline kinetics. *Respiration* 45:438-442.

Schmidt, A., Diamant, B., Bundgaard, A., and Madsen, P.L. 1988. Ergogenic effect of inhaled beta 2-agonists in asthmatics. *Int J Sports Med* 9(5):338-340.

Signorile, J.F., Kaplan, T.A., Applegate, B., and Perry, A.C. 1992. Effects of acute inhalation of the bronchodilator, albuterol, on power output. *Med Sci Sports Exerc* 24(6):638-642.

Silvers, W.S. 1992. Exercise-induced allergies: The role of histamine release. *Ann Allergy* 68:58-63.

Simpson, R.E., and Phillis, J.W. 1992. Adenosine in exercise adaptation. *Br J Sports Med* 26:54-58.

Smith, L.J., Greenberger, P.A., Patterson, R., Krell, R.D., and Bernstein, P.R. 1985. The effect of inhaled leukotriene D4 in humans. *Am Rev Resp Dis* 131:368-372.

Somani, S.M., Gupta, S.K., Frank, S., and Corder, C.N. 1990. Effect of exercise on disposition and pharmacokinetics of drugs. *Drug Dev Res* 20:251-275.

Sorensen, E.V., Jensen, H.K., and Faergeman, O. 1991. Comparison of the effects of xamoterol, atenolol and propranolol on breathlessness, fatigue and plasma electrolytes during exercise in healthy volunteers. *Eur J Clin Pharmacol* 41(1):51-55.

Storms, W.W. 1999. Exercise-induced asthma: Diagnosis and treatment for the recreational or elite athlete. *Med Sci Sports Exerc* 31(suppl):S33-S38.

Sutton, J.R. 1992. $\dot{V}O_2$max: New concepts on an old theme. *Med Sci Sports Exerc* 24:26-29.

Tan, R.A., and Spector, S.L. 1998. Exercise-induced asthma. *Sports Med* 25:1-6.

Todaro, A. 1996. Exercise-induced bronchodilation in asthmatic athletes. *J Sports Med Phys Fitness* 36:60-66.

Vestal, R.E., Eriksson, C.E., Musser, B., Ozaki, L.K., and Halter, J.B. 1983. Effect of intravenous aminophylline on plasma levels of catecholamines and related cardiovascular and metabolic responses in man. *Circulation* 67:162-171.

Violante, B., Pellegrino, R., Vinay, C., Selleri, R., and Ghinamo, G. 1989. Failure of aminophylline and salbutamol to improve respiratory muscle function and exercise tolerance in healthy humans. *Respiration* 55:227-236.

Wisniewski, A.F., Lewis, S.A., Green, D.J., Maslanka, W., Burrell, H., and Tattersfield, A.E. 1997. Cross sectional investigation of the effects of inhaled corticosteroids on bone density and bone metabolism in patients with asthma. *Thorax* 52:853-860.

Woodcock, A. 1998. Effects of inhaled corticosteroids on bone density and metabolism. *J Allergy Clin Immunol* 101(4 pt 2):S456-S459.

Yerg, J.E., Seals, D.R., Hagberg, J.M., and Holloszy, J.O. 1985. Effect of endurance exercise training on ventilatory function in older individuals. *J Appl Physiol* 58:791-794.

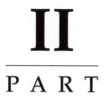

PART II

Hormonal Agents

6
CHAPTER

Human Growth Hormone

■ *CASE*   Tony is a good defensive lineman on a college football team and wants to do everything he can to increase his chances of being drafted into the National Football League (NFL). His older brother Ron has been encouraging him to use growth hormone. Ron claims it has helped him in his bodybuilding work; he tells Tony that since the substance cannot be detected, Tony need not worry. Tony would never use anabolic steroids, because he knows that not only are they easily detected, but that serious long-term consequences are associated with their use. Since he has not heard anything bad about growth hormone, he decides to try it. You discover several months later that he has been using growth hormone. What do you tell him?

■ *COMMENT*   Even if there were no long-term health consequences (and there are!), Tony first needs to realize how serious an error in judgment he has made. Growth hormone is a peptide hormone and, as such, is banned by the NCAA. And even without this restriction, it is illegal to use a prescription drug outside of an appropriate medical need. Tony has broken the law. Unfortunately, these legal issues do not seem to deter overzealous athletes from using drugs they believe will enhance performance. If that reasoning doesn't work with Tony, explain that although growth hormone may have helped his older brother in bodybuilding or body composition, it does not enhance *athletic performance*. Tony is risking it all for, really, no good reason whatsoever.

It has been more than 30 years since the IOC published its first list of banned substances in 1968 and began testing for them that same year at the Mexico City Olympics. How far have we come considering that the 1996 Atlanta Olympics were nicknamed the "Growth Hormone Games"? Ironically, better detection of performance-enhancing substances seems to have contributed to the rise in use (abuse) of growth hormone (GH). Although peptide hormones constituted a relatively small percentage of positive drug tests obtained from sanctioned IOC laboratories between 1993 and 1996 (Mottram 1999), use of human growth hormone (hGH) is increasing owing to its known anabolic actions. With better detection of anabolic steroids, many athletes quit using the steroids and began substituting GH, thinking that similar improvements in performance would occur. Abuse of agents like GH and erythropoietin (see chapter 9), because they are endogenous hormones, is very difficult for athletic officials to detect. The low number of positive tests for peptide hormones is likely a function of the inability to reliably detect abuse of these substances, and should not be misinterpreted as an accurate reflection of the prevalence of their use (Mottram 1999).

Somatrem and Somatropin

Growth hormone—specifically, human growth hormone (hGH), since the amino acid structure of GH differs among different species—is an anabolic hormone that affects all body systems and is important in muscle growth. The endogenous hormone is composed of 191 amino acids. It is secreted from the anterior pituitary at a rate of 0.4-1.0 mg/day in adult males, with higher rates in adolescents and females (Macintyre 1987). Originally, pharmaceutical companies produced GH injection from the pituitary glands of cadavers. The use of human cadavers for GH was discontinued in 1984 when this source was linked to the development of a viral disease known as Creutzfeldt-Jakob disease.

In 1985, the first *bioengineered version* of hGH, somatrem (Protropin), was approved for use, although the endogenous hormone itself had been originally isolated in 1956 and its structure identified in 1972. In 1987, another recombinant product, somatropin, was released. Somatrem contains 191 amino acids, while somatropin contains 192. Several manufacturers produce somatropin, and, as a result, it has been assigned multiple trade names in the United States: Genotropin, Humatrope, Norditropin, Nutropin, Serostim.

Although hGH has a very limited use in clinical medicine, it is reportedly the most highly sought drug among athletes (Macintyre 1987). Because athletes believe hGH has anabolic properties, and because urine testing is an unreliable screen for hGH abuse, the use of hGH

Table 6.1 Pharmacologic and Physiologic Agents That Affect hGH Production

Stimulate output	Suppress output
Bromocriptine	Beta-2 receptor agonists (i.e., isoproterenol)
Clonidine	Corticosteroids (glucocorticoids)
Corticotropin (ACTH)	Cyproheptadine
Estrogen	Imipramine
Glucagon	Octreotide
Levodopa	Phenothiazines
Propranolol	Phentolamine
Vasopressin	Progesterone

by athletes is on the rise (Mottram 1999). It's important to question any individual who is using one of these drugs without having a clear medical indication to do so. There are reports that athletes spend up to $30,000 per year to obtain hGH and use it in amounts 20-fold higher than recommended doses, but, unfortunately, the substance they receive in return may not even be hGH (Smith and Perry 1992). Since the legal distribution of hGH is tightly controlled, what is available on the black market may actually be human chorionic gonadotropin (HCG) or, in some cases, anabolic steroids (Smith and Perry 1992).

Other drugs and hormones can affect the production of endogenous hGH (see table 6.1).

In addition to the interest in GH because of its use (abuse) by athletes, there is increasing interest in the role of GH in the elderly, specifically with regard to muscle strength, bone density, and body composition (Pyka, Taaffe, and Marcus 1994; Taaffe et al. 1994; Yarasheski et al. 1995; Yarasheski, Campbell, and Kohrt 1997). The clinical medicine uses of GH have been recently reviewed by Tritos and Mantzoros (1998). Other authors have reviewed the topic of GH in sports (Jenkins 1999; Macintyre 1987; Roemmich and Rogol 1997; Zachwieja and Yarasheski 1999).

How Exercise Affects the Action of Growth Hormone

Researchers have not studied how exercise affects either the pharmacology or the pharmacokinetics of exogenous hGH. It is known, however, that exercise stimulates endogenous hGH output acutely (see

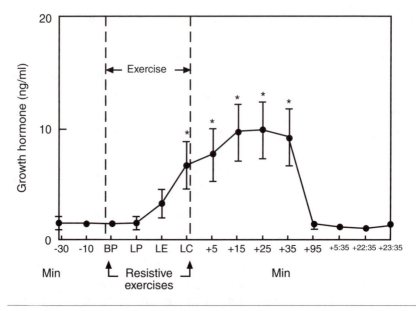

Figure 6.1   Alteration of growth hormone concentrations before, during, and after resistive exercise. Results are corrected for plasma volume change. Values are mean ± *SEM*; $n = 8$. * = $p < 0.05$ compared with –10 value. BP = bench press; LP = leg press; LE = leg extension; LC = leg curl.

Adapted from Kraemer et al. 1992.

figure 6.1). This has been reported in both males and females (Bunt et al. 1986), and after both resistance exercise (Kraemer et al. 1992; Kraemer et al. 1991) and aerobic exercise, such as treadmill running (Bunt et al. 1986). There is some evidence (see figure 6.2) that hGH output is related to intensity of resistance exercise (Kraemer et al. 1991; Pritzlaff et al. 1999; Weltman et al. 1997). Obesity (Kanaley et al. 1999) and advanced age (Zaccaria et al. 1999) attenuate exercise-induced increases in GH output, although GH levels have been documented to increase substantially in elderly men immediately after resistance exercise (Nicklas et al. 1995). Women who take oral contraceptives have an increased response (Bernardes and Radomski 1998).

How Growth Hormone Affects Exercisers

Growth hormone really works quite differently than anabolic steroids do: GH causes hyperplasia (i.e., increased cell number), whereas anabolic steroids tend to cause hypertrophy (i.e., increased size) of some tissues. Growth hormone facilitates the transport of amino acids across

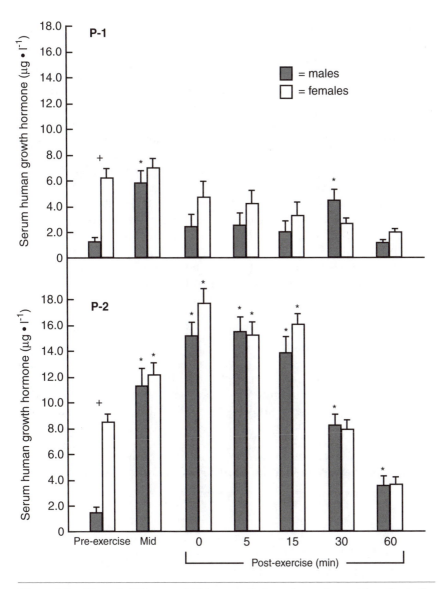

Figure 6.2 Mean (+ SE) serum hGH concentrations for males and females to P-1 and P-2 HREPs (heavy resistance exercise protocol). P-1 = exercise protocol utilizing longer rest and heavier weight. P-2 = exercise protocol utilizing shorter rest and more repetitions. * = $p < 0.05$ from corresponding preexercise values and + = $p < 0.05$ from corresponding female values.

Adapted from Kraemer et al. 1991.

the cell membrane, which results in increased amounts of RNA, ultimately leading to increased protein synthesis. The effects of GH on skeletal muscle are thought to be mediated through the effects of insulinlike growth factor (IGF-1) activity (Kraemer et al. 1992). While many of the effects of anabolic steroids wear off after use is discontinued, with GH the effects persist. When endogenous GH levels are excessive, a condition known as acromegaly results. Acromegaly is associated with left ventricular hypertrophy and a diminished exercise capacity (Giustina et al. 1995).

In contrast to the data that indicate widespread use of GH by athletes, data regarding the effects of hGH on the physiology of exercisers and athletes are somewhat limited. Administration of GH has been shown to decrease body fat and produce significant increases in fat-free mass in weightlifters (see table 6.2; Crist et al. 1988), healthy normal subjects (Yarasheski et al. 1992), elderly subjects (Papadakis et al. 1996; Taaffe et al. 1994), and GH-deficient subjects (Jorgensen et al. 1996). Other investigators have found that body composition changes during weight training with hGH are not different from changes during weight training without hGH (Deyssig et al. 1993).

Although the physiologic effect of GH is anabolic, Yarasheski and colleagues reported that a 14-day regimen of GH did not augment muscle protein synthesis in 7 power athletes currently enrolled in a weight-training program (Yarasheski et al. 1993), and 16 weeks of GH did not augment improvements in bone mineral density related to weight-training in elderly subjects (Yarasheski, Campbell, and Kohrt

Table 6.2   FFW, % Fat, and FFW/FW in Subjects Before and After Six Weeks Treatment With Placebo and Met-hGH During Weight Training

Body composition	Placebo		Met-hGH	
	Pre	Post	Pre	Post
FFW, kg	60.8 ± 4.5	61.8 ± 4.0	61.8 ± 4.0	$64.5 \pm 3.9^*$
% fat	13.4 ± 1.6	13.0 ± 0.9	12.8 ± 1.0	$11.3 \pm 1.2^*$
FFW/FW	7.8 ± 1.9	6.9 ± 0.6	7.3 ± 0.7	$9.1 \pm 1.7^*$

* Significant difference between pre- and posttest means ($p < 0.05$)

Values are means $\pm$ SE; n = 8 subjects. FFW = fat-free weight; % fat = percent body fat; FFW/FW = ratio of fat-free weight to fat weight; met-hGH = methionyl-human growth hormone.

Adapted from Crist et al. 1988.

1997). Deyssig and colleagues found that 6 weeks of injecting hGH daily in male power athletes undergoing weight training significantly decreased thyroxine levels (Deyssig et al. 1993).

Cuneo and colleagues showed that exogenous hGH improved $\dot{V}O_2$max (oxygen uptake) measured via cycle ergometry, but they studied GH-deficient subjects, not athletes (Cuneo et al. 1991b).

How Growth Hormone Affects Exercise Performance

Administration of GH to individuals who produce inadequate endogenous quantities has been associated with an improvement in exercise performance; however, GH does not appear to be ergogenic in subjects who are not GH-deficient. A human's lack of endogenous hGH produces a condition known in clinical medicine as dwarfism, and supplementary hGH corrects the diminished growth rate in people having this condition. In GH-deficient adults, muscle mass (Cuneo et al. 1991a), muscle strength (Cuneo et al. 1991a), and exercise performance (Cuneo et al. 1991b; Jorgensen et al. 1996) have all been shown to improve after hGH supplementation. Cuneo and colleagues showed that hGH improved muscle strength in hip flexors in GH-deficient adults but not in any of the other eight muscle groups tested, and they concluded that these patients may have a proximal myopathy. Thus, data obtained in GH-deficient subjects should not be extrapolated to subjects who are not GH-deficient.

When non-GH-deficient subjects are studied, regardless of their level of fitness, the combination of GH plus weight training does not produce further improvements in muscle strength over weight training alone. This has been documented in male power athletes (Deyssig et al. 1993) and healthy untrained males (Yarasheski et al. 1992) (see table 6.3). When elderly subjects were studied, GH was not shown to improve muscle strength regardless of whether GH and weight training began simultaneously (Yarasheski et al. 1995) or if, instead, GH was added after several months of weight training had already occurred (Taaffe et al. 1994). Even when GH was given to elderly subjects in the absence of weight training, no improvements in muscle strength were seen (Papadakis et al. 1996).

To summarize, while GH produces a generalized anabolic action on many tissues of the body, its actual anabolic and lipolytic actions in adults depend on the preexisting state of GH output and amount of body fat. Regardless of its physiologic actions and effects on body composition, GH does not augment improvements in muscle strength more than the response from weight training alone.

Table 6.3   Effect of Growth Hormone on Muscle Strength Response to Resistance Exercise

Exercise	Exercise + placebo		Exercise + GH	
	Delta	% change	Delta	% change
Shoulder press	5.3 ± 0.5	53 ± 6	6.5 ± 0.9	60 ± 10
Bench press	6.1 ± 0.7	43 ± 6	6.2 ± 1.3	43 ± 11
Deltoids	4.4 ± 0.5	47 ± 7	4.5 ± 0.4	50 ± 6
Bicep curl	4.4 ± 0.3	36 ± 3	4.2 ± 0.6	33 ± 4
Latissimus	6.5 ± 0.4	59 ± 5	6.3 ± 0.5	60 ± 8
Flys	6.5 ± 0.4	73 ± 8	6.4 ± 0.5	66 ± 10
Knee extension	9.7 ± 0.9	63 ± 10	8.8 ± 1.2	65 ± 16
Leg press	4.9 ± 0.7	26 ± 4	4.8 ± 0.5	34 ± 5
Knee flexion	4.1 ± 0.4	47 ± 8	5.0 ± 0.8	71 ± 17
Average	5.8 ± 0.6	50 ± 4.8	5.9 ± 0.5	54 ± 4.7

Values are means ± SE. Final strength score greater ($p < 0.01$) than initial for all exercises in both groups. Delta scores represent absolute increase in number of 4.5 kg weights lifted. Average and individual delta and % change scores were not different between groups.

Adapted from Yarasheski et al. 1992.

Avoiding Potential Complications

Whereas androgenic-anabolic steroids (AASs) stimulate the growth of only muscle, hGH stimulates the growth of *all* tissues, including internal organs. Even more worrisome, while some of the effects of AASs are reversible, the effects of long-term administration of hGH are not. Acromegaly is a syndrome affecting many organ systems as a result of overproduction of endogenous hGH. The disease affects the skeleton, soft tissues, heart, glucose metabolism, and sexual function, and it can cause hypertension. Acromegaly is irreversible, and individuals with the condition typically die by the sixth decade of life. Further, acromegalics have been shown to develop left ventricular hypertrophy and have a diminished exercise capacity (Giustina et al. 1995). Although the effects of long-term, exogenous hGH are not clear, it seems likely that many of these same consequences would occur. In several studies of non-GH-deficient subjects, carpal tunnel syndrome and pain and edema of the fingers were reported in several subjects in the active drug group

(Deyssig et al. 1993; Yarasheski et al. 1992). Individuals with acromegaly are noted to have thick hands and fingers. Is carpal tunnel syndrome a warning that anatomical changes similar to acromegaly are occurring?

Even without the health consequences associated with the use of hGH, athletes risk disqualification and, worse, arrest for illicitly using a prescription-only drug. Further, since hGH is administered only by injection, sharing needles is still another risk—and another reason to avoid abusing this drug.

NCAA and USOC Status

Since it is a peptide hormone, hGH (or GH from any animal source) is banned by both the NCAA and the USOC. In his book *Drugs, Sport, and Politics* (1991) Robert Voy, MD and former chief medical officer for the USOC, has summarized many of the issues of hGH abuse by athletes and what should be done to stop the overuse.

Guidelines for Use

The entire sports medicine community, including coaches, athletic trainers, and sports medicine physicians, should universally discourage individuals from using GH. Tell athletes especially that the claims regarding performance-enhancement are not supported by scientific studies. Warn them that the drug has serious, irreversible effects. Remind them that the drug is banned and its use is illegal!

References

Bernardes, R.P., and Radomski, M.W. 1998. Growth hormone responses to continuous and intermittent exercise in females under oral contraceptive therapy. *Eur J Appl Physiol* 79:24-29.

Bunt, J.C., Boileau, R.A., Bahr, J.M., and Nelson, R.A. 1986. Sex and training differences in human growth hormone levels during prolonged exercise. *J Appl Physiol* 61:1796-1801.

Crist, D.M., Peake, G.T., Egan, P.A., and Waters, D.L. 1988. Body composition response to exogenous GH during training in highly conditioned adults. *J Appl Physiol* 65:579-584.

Cuneo, R.C., Salomon, F., Wiles, C.M., Hesp, R., and Sonksen, P.H. 1991a. Growth hormone treatment in growth hormone-deficient adults. I. Effects on muscle mass and strength. *J Appl Physiol* 70:688-694.

Cuneo, R.C., Salomon, F., Wiles, C.M., Hesp, R., and Sonksen, P.H. 1991b. Growth hormone treatment in growth hormone-deficient adults. II. Effects on exercise performance. *J Appl Physiol* 70:695-700.

Deyssig, R., Frisch, H., Blum, W.F., and Waldhor, T. 1993. Effect of growth hormone treatment on hormonal parameters, body composition and strength in athletes. *Acta Endrocrinol* 128:313-318.

Giustina, A., Boni, E., Romanelli, G., Grassi, V., and Giustina, G. 1995. Cardiopulmonary performance during exercise in acromegaly, and the effects of acute suppression of growth hormone hypersecretion with octreotide. *Am J Cardiol* 75:1042-1047.

Jenkins, P.J. 1999. Growth hormone and exercise. *Clin Endocrinol (Oxf)* 50:683-689.

Jorgensen, J.O., Vahl, N., Hansen, T.B., Thuesen, L., Hagen, C., and Christiansen, J.S. 1996. Growth hormone versus placebo treatment for one year in growth hormone deficient adults: Increase in exercise capacity and normalization of body composition. *Clin Endocrinol (Oxf)* 45:681-688.

Kanaley, J.A., Weatherup-Dentes, M.M., Jaynes, E.B., and Harman, M.L. 1999. Obesity attenuates the growth hormone response to exercise. *J Clin Endocrinol Metab* 84:3156-3161.

Kraemer, R.R., Kilgore, J.L., Kraemer, G.R., and Castrancane, V.D. 1992. Growth hormone, IGF-I, and testosterone responses to resistive exercise. *Med Sci Sports Exerc* 24:1346-1352.

Kraemer, W.J., Gordon, S.E., Fleck, S.J., Marchitelli, L.J., Mello, R., Dziados, J.E., Friedl, K., Harman, E., Maresh, C., and Fry, A.C. 1991. Endogenous anabolic hormonal and growth factor responses to heavy resistance exercise in males and females. *Int J Sports Med* 12:228-235.

Macintyre, J.G. 1987. Growth hormone and athletes. *Sports Med* 4:129-142.

Mottram, D.R. 1999. Banned drugs in sport: Does the International Olympic Committee (IOC) list need updating? *Sports Med* 27:1-10.

Nicklas, B.J., Ryan, A.J., Treuth, M.M., Harman, S.M., Blackman, M.R., Hurley, B.F., and Rogers, M.A. 1995. Testosterone, growth hormone and IGF-I responses to acute and chronic resistive exercise in men aged 55-70 years. *Int J Sports Med* 16:445-450.

Papadakis, M.A., Grady, D., Black, D., Tierney, M.J., Gooding, G.A., Schambelan, M., and Grunfeld, C. 1996. Growth hormone replacement in healthy older men improves body composition but not functional ability. *Ann Intern Med* 124:708-716.

Pritzlaff, C.J., Wideman, L., Weltman, J.Y., Abbott, R.D., Gutgesell, M.E., Hartman, M.L., Veldhuis, J.D., and Weltman, A. 1999. Impact of acute exercise intensity on pulsatile growth hormone release in men. *J Appl Physiol* 87:498-504.

Pyka, G., Taaffe, D.R., and Marcus, R. 1994. Effect of a sustained program of resistance training on the acute growth hormone response to resistance exercise in older adults. *Horm Metab Res* 26:330-333.

Roemmich, J.N., and Rogol, A.D. 1997. Exercise and growth hormone: Does one affect the other? *J Pediatr* 131(1 pt 2):S75-S80.

Smith, D.A., and Perry, P.J. 1992. The efficacy of ergogenic agents in athletic competition. Part II: Other performance-enhancing agents. *Ann Pharmacother* 26:653-659.

Taaffe, D.R., Pruitt, L., Reim, J., Nintz, R.L., Butterfield, G., Hoffman, A.R., and Marcus, R. 1994. Effect of recombinant human growth hormone on the muscle strength response to resistance exercise in elderly men. *J Clin Endocrinol Metab* 79:1361-1366.

Tritos, N.A, and Mantzoros, C.S. 1998. Recombinant human growth hormone: Old and novel uses. *Am J Med* 105:44-57.

Voy, R. 1991. *Drugs, sport, and politics.* Champaign, IL: Leisure Press, Human Kinetics.

Weltman, A., Weltman, J.Y., Womack, C.J., Davis, S.E., Blumer, J.L., Gaesser, G.A., and Hartman, M.L. 1997. Exercise training decreases the growth hormone (GH) response to acute constant-load exercise. *Med Sci Sports Exerc* 29:669-676.

Yarasheski, K.E., Campbell, J.A., and Kohrt, W.M. 1997. Effect of resistance exercise and growth hormone on bone density in older men. *Clin Endocrinol (Oxf)* 47:223-229.

Yarasheski, K.E., Campbell, J.A., Smith, K., Rennie, M.J., Holloszy, J.O., and Bier, D.M. 1992. Effect of growth hormone and resistance exercise on muscle growth in young men. *Am J Physiol* 262:E261-E267.

Yarasheski, K.E., Zachwieja, J.J., Angelopoulos, T.J., and Bier, D.M. 1993. Short-term growth hormone treatment does not increase muscle protein synthesis in experienced weight lifters. *J Appl Physiol* 74:3073-3076.

Yarasheski, K.E., Zachwieja, J.J., Campbell, J.A., and Bier, D.M. 1995. Effect of growth hormone and resistance exercise on muscle growth and strength in older men. *Am J Physiol* 268(2 pt 1):E268-E276.

Zaccaria, M., Varnier, M., Piazza, P., Noventa, D., and Ermolao, A. 1999. Blunted growth hormone response to maximal exercise in middle-aged versus young subjects and no effect of endurance training. *J Clin Endocrinol Metab* 84:2303-2307.

Zachwieja, J.J., and Yarasheski, K.E. 1999. Does growth hormone therapy in conjunction with resistance exercise increase muscle force production and muscle mass in men and women aged 60 years or older? *Phys Ther* 79(1):76-82.

7

CHAPTER

Androgenic-Anabolic Steroids

■ *CASE*   Ben Johnson exploded out of the blocks in the 100-meter dash in 1988, easily beating the field in Seoul to win the gold medal and set a new world record. The medal was later taken away when a urine test confirmed the presence of the anabolic steroid stanozolol, a substance banned under IOC rules. Do anabolic steroids really improve athletic performance?

■ *COMMENT*   Anabolic steroids appear to enhance improvements in muscular strength that occur in response to weight training, but no direct beneficial effect on aerobic exercise has been demonstrated. Regarding the 100-meter dash, specifically, improvements in performance are likely due to enhanced muscular strength. An indirect benefit might be realized from an enhanced ability to train longer and harder. Although the effects of anabolic steroids in sport settings have been studied for decades, the results are varied and interpretations of them are controversial. A major obstacle in determining how these drugs affect athletes in various competitive venues is the fact that many athletes consume multiple drugs simultaneously, often in enormous excess of the recommended medical dose. Designing a controlled study to mimic these conditions would be unethical. Nevertheless, the NCAA, USOC, IOC, NFL, and the U.S. Powerlifting Federation all ban anabolic steroids in competitions.

Anabolic steroids, simply put, are derivatives of testosterone. Technically, these drugs are best called *androgenic-anabolic steroids* (AASs). They produce both masculinizing (i.e., androgenic) and tissue-building (i.e., anabolic) effects. Since no steroid has been produced that is purely anabolic (i.e., totally devoid of androgenic properties), however, it is more accurate to refer to these drugs as androgenic-anabolic steroids. The term *steroids* is loosely applied to several different groups of hormonal agents. To athletes, the term *steroids* usually refers to AASs, but in clinical medicine, the term more often refers to adrenal corticosteroids (i.e., glucocorticoids). The female hormones estrogen and progestin and related molecules are yet other examples of steroid hormones.

This chapter discusses only androgenic-anabolic steroids. Many authors have thoroughly reviewed anabolic steroids (see Bahrke, Yesalis, and Brower 1998; Clarkson and Thompson 1997; Smith and Perry 1992; Sturmi and Diorio 1998, Mottram 1988; Voy 1991; Wadler and Hainline 1989; Yesalis 1993; Yesalis and Cowart 1998). Readers are especially encouraged to consult *Anabolic Steroids in Sport and Exercise (2nd ed.)* (Yesalis 2000) for a very thorough review of all aspects of anabolic steroid use in sports.

Testosterone was first isolated in 1935 and was synthesized shortly after. Synthetic anabolic steroids were later developed in an attempt to produce purely anabolic compounds without androgenic properties. These compounds have additional advantages over testosterone, which is not bioavailable after oral administration and has a short biologic half-life.

Anabolic steroids have had a colorful history of varied usage. First employed in the 1930s to promote positive nitrogen balance in starvation victims, anabolic steroids were used in the 1940s by German troops to improve muscle strength and increase aggressiveness. The earliest reports of use for a sport edge appeared by 1954, when Russian athletes used anabolic steroids to increase their weight and power loads. Rumors of the effectiveness of these drugs began to circulate, which led some competitors in weightlifting and throwing events to use them during the 1956 Olympic Games in Melbourne, Australia. This attracted the attention of clinical investigators, who in the 1960s and 1970s attempted to determine the impact of anabolic steroids in sports. Androgenic-anabolic steroids were included on the original list of banned substances compiled in the late 1960s. Urine tests became available in 1976, and the International Olympic Committee (IOC) immediately began testing for anabolic steroids in the 1976 Olympics in Montreal, Canada. In 1983, seven athletes were disqualified from the Pan American Games when anabolic steroids were detected in their urine. Not long after, the public's attention was riveted when Ben Johnson ran a spectacular 100 m dash to win the gold medal in the 1988 Seoul Olympics, only to have it taken away when stanozolol was detected in his urine. Johnson subsequently tested positive a second time in 1993, garnering him a lifetime ban from competition. A more comprehensive review of the history of anabolic steroid use in sports can be found in *Anabolic Steroids in Sport and Exercise (2nd ed.)* (Yesalis 2000).

With the Johnson incident in 1988, people worldwide learned of the use of AASs in sports. On 27 February 1991, AASs were reclassified in the United States into Schedule III of the Controlled Substances Act in an attempt to better control the distribution of these drugs in the clinical setting. Gradually, the use of AASs by elite athletes appeared to be on the decline—owing to better and more rigorous testing (Smith and Perry 1992); indeed, this may be one reason for the growing abuse in sport and bodybuilding of growth hormone (chapter 6) and epoetin alfa (erythropoietin; chapter 9). These latter hormones are discussed in other chapters.

Several facts should concern the sports medicine community. It is believed that between 3% and 12% of male high school students and 1% of female high school students (see table 7.1) have used anabolic steroids during their lives (Lukas 1993). The user incidence increases to roughly 14% among Division I college athletes and 30% to 75% among competitive bodybuilders (Lukas 1993). In 1984, a Michigan State University study of NCAA athletes reported that 9% of football players acknowledged using anabolic steroids in the prior year, as did 4% of athletes from basketball, tennis, and track. In the United Kingdom, even among "regular" gymnasium users (i.e., nonelite athletes), 38.8% admitted to using anabolic steroids (Perry, Wright, and Littlepage 1992)! Based on data from the first nationwide evaluation of steroid use among adults in the United States, Yesalis and colleagues (1993) reported that as of 1991 more than one million people were current or former AAS users (and more than 300,000 had then used AASs in the past year). Additional data regarding the incidence and prevalence of anabolic steroid use has been summarized by Yesalis (1993).

Even more ominous, among adolescents and young adults, taking AASs is associated with a higher use of other illicit substances, such as cocaine, alcohol, tobacco, and marijuana (DuRant et al. 1993; Yesalis et al. 1993). Yet, despite the increased scrutiny and the increased public awareness of the risks of these drugs, elite athletes are continuing to use—and get caught. In July 1998, shot-putter Randy Barnes and Olympic sprinter Dennis Mitchell were suspended, pending a hearing, for testing positive for use of testosterone-related substances (*USA Today*, 28 July 1998); in August 1998, British athletes Gary Edwards (track cyclist) and Paul Supple (weightlifter) had testosterone-to-epitestosterone (T:E) ratios above the acceptable limit; a third British athlete, Andrew Goswell (weightlifter), is alleged to have taken stanozolol (*Times* [London], 27

Table 7.1 Prevalence of Androgenic-Anabolic Steroid Abuse

Population	n	Prevalence (%)*
Bodybuilders	380	
Male		59/108 (54.6)
Female		7/68 (10.3)
College students	NA	
Athletes: 1970		(15)
1976		(20)
1980		(20)
1984		(20)
Nonathletes: 1984		(1)
Male bodybuilders	138	53 (38.4)
High school students	NA	
Male		(5)
Female		(1)
12th grade male students	3403	226 (6.6)
11th grade male students	853	95 (11.1)
High school students	1010	
Male		23/462 (5.0)
Female		6/439 (1.4)
High school students	3047	
Male		67/1028 (6.5)
Female		27/1085 (2.5)

*Includes only those subjects who completed the surveys.
NA = not available.

Adapted from Smith and Perry 1992.

August 1998), the same drug that got Ben Johnson into trouble. Nor is the economic cost of this use slight. Athletes spend an estimated $100 million annually for anabolic steroids: 20% for legal prescriptions and the rest for drugs obtained through illicit channels. They risk the potentially severe adverse reactions of these drugs, especially unfortunate considering that the performance advantage conveyed by anabolic steroids may be quite modest.

Anabolic steroids really have no place in sports. They are used in clinical medicine for hypogonadism, as palliative therapy in the treat-

Table 7.2   Androgenic-Anabolic Steroids Available in the United States

Oral agents	Parenteral agents
Danazol (Danocrine)	Nandrolone decanoate (Deca-Durabolin)
Fluoxymesterone (Halotestin)	
Methyltestosterone (Android, Virilon)	Nandrolone phenpropionate (Durabolin)
Oxandrolone (Oxandrin)	Testosterone aqueous suspension (Andro-100)
Oxymetholone (Anadrol)	
Stanozolol (Winstrol)	Testosterone cypionate in oil (Depo-Testosterone, Virilon IM)
	Testosterone enanthate in oil (Delatestryl)
	Testosterone propionate in oil (no trade names)

ment of breast cancer, and for the treatment of angioneurotic edema. At one time anabolic steroids, specifically testosterone decanoate (Deca-Durabolin), were used to stimulate erythropoiesis in patients with renal failure; however, with the marketing of recombinant erythropoietin, their use for this purpose has faded. In the late 1990s, there is renewed interest in testosterone for the management of AIDS-related cachexia.

All anabolic steroids are derivatives of testosterone. Their modification for use of the testosterone molecule essentially follows two approaches: (a) esterification of the 17-beta-hydroxyl group with different carboxylic acids to increase lipid solubility and create slow-release injectables; and (b) alkylation of 17-alpha position to decrease hepatic metabolism, thereby increasing the effectiveness of oral administration. Other testosterone derivatives (e.g., danazol, a drug used to treat endometriosis) can possess anabolic or ergogenic actions (or both) and, thus, are also considered banned substances for use in competitive sports. Table 7.2 lists anabolic steroids that are commercially available in the United States.

How Exercise Affects the Action of Androgenic-Anabolic Steroids

Testosterone and its derivatives are short-lived compounds. Testosterone has a plasma half-life of only minutes, but this value is somewhat misleading, since, like the corticosteroids, testosterone exerts biologic effects longer than its plasma half-life would suggest. At the cellular level, steroid hormones readily pass through the cell wall of the target tissue where they exert their effects. Testosterone is reduced to dihydrotestosterone, which is the principle intracellular mediator of hormonal action.

In comparison, fluoxymesterone, a synthetic AAS, has a plasma half-life of 9.2 hours. Oral dosage forms are generally administered daily. Parenteral agents, however, vary in their administration, depending on how they are formulated: aqueous testosterone injection is administered 3 times weekly, but testosterone injections formulated in an oil vehicle release drug more slowly and are administered (at least, in clinical medicine!) every 2 to 4 weeks. A relevant footnote to the pharmacokinetics of AAS is that estradiol is an active metabolite of testosterone. When supraphysiologic doses of testosterone are ingested, enough estradiol is generated in the male to lead to gynecomastia and a heightened voice. See figure 12.1 (page 257) for a summary of the metabolic pathways for testosterone.

How exercise affects the pharmacokinetics of AASs has not been studied much. Some AASs undergo significant first-pass metabolism by the liver after oral administration. Since exercise diverts blood flow away from the liver acutely, one would expect exercise, therefore, to affect the pharmacokinetics of AASs. Unfortunately, a recent text (Somani 1996) on the effects of exercise on drug pharmacokinetics simply ignores this issue.

The effects of exercise on endogenous testosterone levels have been attributed to exercise mode and intensity, but they may be more a function of exercise-induced changes in plasma volume. Some data show that a single session of heavy resistance exercise increases the levels of postexercise endogenous testosterone (Kraemer et al. 1991), but in a similar study where testosterone levels were corrected for changes in postexercise plasma volume, no significant change in testosterone levels was detected (Kraemer et al. 1992). Another study involved 8 weeks of resistance exercise and found no changes in testosterone levels (Hickson et al. 1994). Intense (3.3 min/km), long-term (45 min) running (but not maximal short runs) produced a substantial decrease in serum testosterone levels in young healthy males (Kuoppasalmi et al. 1980); however, these values were not corrected for changes in plasma volume.

How Androgenic-Anabolic Steroids Affect Exercisers

The main problem associated with research on the effects of AASs on athletes and exercisers is that doses used in the studies do not match the doses that many athletes and bodybuilders actually ingest. The relevant issues are effects on skeletal muscle mass, metabolic effects, and cardio-vascular effects. Kochakian (1993) has reviewed the effects of testosterone on human physiology.

The physiologic effects of testosterone and synthetic anabolic steroids are mediated through a steroid-receptor complex. Separate receptor complexes exist for adrenal corticosteroids (e.g., glucocorticoids), estrogen, and testosterone in skeletal muscle. The reduced form of testosterone, dihydrotestosterone, is the principal intracellular mediator of the hormone's actions.

General pharmacologic principles dictate that drugs must first bind to a receptor to exert a physiologic effect. Any remaining drug that is unbound is more readily metabolized, excreted, or both. It is thought that in skeletal muscle the steroid receptor complex can be saturated. Data from human subjects show that anabolic steroids affect lean body mass in a typical dose-response curve. This observation is consistent with the concept of saturation of available (testosterone) receptors at high doses and further calls into question the validity of using supraphysiologic doses of these drugs. For example, the recommended dosage of methandrostenolone—an extremely potent anabolic steroid formerly marketed in the United States as Dianabol— was in the range of 2.5 to 5.0 mg a day. Yet some athletes have, within a 2-week period, taken as much as 6000 mg of this drug (Wadler and Hainline 1989).

When assessing whether there is a dose-response relationship with anabolic steroids, one needs to differentiate effects on lean body mass (LBM) from those on muscular strength. Both physiologic (Kuipers et al. 1991) and supraphysiologic (Forbes 1985) doses of anabolic steroids have been shown to increase LBM, leading one group of investigators (Forbes 1985) to conclude that there is a dose-response relationship (see figure 7.1). There does not appear to be as good a relationship between dose of anabolic steroids and increases in muscle strength. In 1996, Bhasin and colleagues published a report in the *New England Journal of Medicine* showing supraphysiologic doses of testosterone were associated with greater improvements in muscle size and strength compared to placebo; however, only a single dose was assessed. Elashoff and colleagues (1991), in a meta-analysis, found no clear relationship between the dose, potency, and duration of anabolic steroid ingestion and percent change in muscle strength (Elashoff et al. 1991; figure 7.2). Finally, it is worth noting that resistance exercise has been associated with increases in output of growth hormone (Kraemer et al. 1992), and an increase in testosterone receptors has been proposed to occur in relationship to anabolic steroid use (Hickson and Kurowski 1986). Either of these two physiologic adaptations may influence the dose-response curve to anabolic steroids.

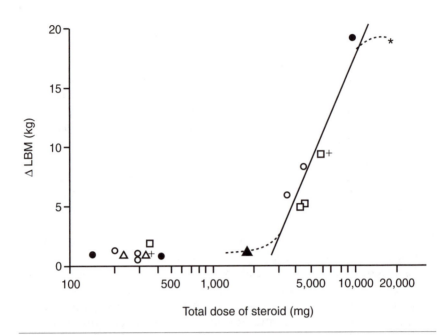

Figure 7.1 Semilogarithmic plot of increment in LBM against total dose of anabolic steroid. ○ = testosterone; ● = oxandrolone; □ = Dianabol; ▲ = andro-stalone; △ = nandrolone; + = also testosterone. Equation for the regression line for total dose of 3500 mg and greater is $y = 29.1 \log x - 99$ (r 0.91). Point (★) represents estimate of the effect of endogenous testosterone production by males during the teen years; this point was not used in calculating the regression line.

Adapted from Forbes 1985.

Hickson and Kurowski (1986) believed that skeletal muscle repre-sented a relatively minor target for anabolic steroids, based on the density of androgen receptors in this tissue and assuming that receptor binding does represent a rate-limiting step in steroid action. Males with hypogonadism and females in general are more sensitive to anabolic steroids, owing to the increased availability of unsaturated receptors (Hickson and Kurowski 1986). Further, heavy resistance training in humans increases muscle size without any significant increase in endog-enous testosterone levels (Hickson et al. 1994). The fact that the number of steroid receptors in tissues increases in response to forced muscle hypertrophy may explain why additional pharmacologic effect is seen with supraphysiologic doses of AASs (Hickson and Kurowski 1986).

Ultimately, testosterone increases the size of muscle cells, but it does not increase cell number. In this it differs from growth hormone, which produces hyperplasia not only of skeletal muscle but of other tissues as well. Further, the effects of testosterone wear off after its administration

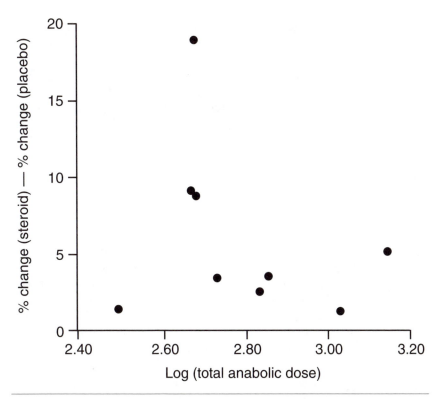

Figure 7.2 Relation of steroid effect to total anabolic dosage in trained athletes. Over nine studies on trained athletes, percent mean improvement of the steroid-treated subjects minus mean percent improvement of placebo-treated subjects is plotted against the log of the total anabolic dosage calculated.

Adapted from Elashoff et al. 1991, p. 391.

ceases, but this is not the case with growth hormone. Testosterone receptors exist not only in skeletal muscle, but also in the prostate, testes, seminiferous tubules, heart, and probably the brain. This explains the diversity of physiologic effects of anabolic steroids. Clinically, the normal testosterone surge in puberty leads to enlarged testes and penis, laryngeal enlargement (which, in turn, leads to a deeper voice in males), secondary hair growth, increased height (unless premature closure of the epiphyses occurs), skeletal muscle growth, increased sebaceous gland proliferation (which aggravates acne), and some psychological changes.

Effects on Muscle Size and Fat-Free Mass

Since anabolic steroids act at the cellular level to increase the size of muscle cells, it is easy to predict their effects on muscle size in general (refer to figure 7.4, page 173). In a creative and revealing study, investigators administered 6000 mg of testosterone enanthate over a 10-week period. For comparison, based on the recommended dose range for this agent for the treatment of male hypogonadism, a total dose of 125 to 2000 mg would be administered in a 10-week period. This study showed that the combination of resistance exercise and supraphysiologic doses of testosterone produced greater increases in muscle size than were achieved by either intervention alone.

Metabolic Effects

Unlike endocrine, hepatic, or cardiovascular effects, the metabolic effects of anabolic steroids do not appear to be as significant. Since many of the effects of anabolic steroids are unwanted, they are discussed later under "Avoiding Potential Complications." Male bodybuilders who start taking anabolic steroids do not demonstrate acute metabolic changes during exercise that differ from those experienced by bodybuilders who do not take steroids. Both groups show a metabolic acidosis, with little change in serum glucose. Bodybuilders demonstrate a marked elevation of creatine kinase, but the contribution of anabolic steroids to this phenomenon is uncertain (McKillop et al. 1989).

Cardiovascular Effects

Anabolic steroids can exert many effects on the cardiovascular system, some of which we will examine in the next section. Anabolic steroids increase diastolic blood pressure (Kuipers et al. 1991), but do not significantly affect resting or exercise heart rate. Even though anabolic steroids increase red cell mass, this effect is modest (Yesalis 1993). The resulting impact of this action on maximal oxygen uptake during exercise ($\dot{V}O_2$max) has been variable in clinical studies. Both improvement in $\dot{V}O_2$max and no improvement (Johnson et al. 1975) have been noted in human subjects. Yesalis (1993) has reviewed these data and concluded that tests of $\dot{V}O_2$max are not good predictors of endurance capacity, and the literature on the effects of anabolic steroids on aerobic performance is inconclusive.

How Androgenic-Anabolic Steroids Affect Exercise Performance

Despite decades of research, questions as to the effects of anabolic steroids on athletic performance are still unresolved. Because controlled studies generally evaluate doses much lower than those used by steroid-abusing athletes, it is difficult to determine the true benefit of anabolic steroids. Yesalis (1993) has summarized other issues that contribute to a lack of consensus regarding the effects of anabolic steroids on athletic performance. These issues include

- type of subjects;
- study design (i.e., controlling for diet, training methods, testing methods);
- dose and type of anabolic steroid studied; and
- length of study.

To look at what is known, the effects on performance can be broken down into effects on either strength or aerobic performance.

Effects on Muscle Strength

Much of the controversy regarding the effects of anabolic steroids relates to their effects on muscular strength. Disagreement exists because (a) doses used in the clinical studies do not match the enormous doses some athletes ingest, and (b) steroid abusers often use combinations of drugs, whereas most research assesses the effects of only a single drug. Some 15 years ago Haupt and Rovere (1984) reviewed the literature and concluded that anabolic steroids do increase strength if

- intensive weight training occurs before and during supplementation;
- a high-protein diet is maintained; and
- strength gains are measured with a single repetition maximum using an exercise with which the athlete trains.

Elashoff and colleagues (1991) later analyzed this issue from a different perspective. They concluded that previous reviews had focused on categorizing the studies into those claiming statistical significance and those that did not. Elashoff and colleagues decided to address the question of size and consistency of observed steroid effects. They performed a MEDLINE analysis of the period 1966 to 1990, obtaining 16 studies that met their strict criteria for inclusion (placebo-control, randomization, and objective measurement of strength). Their analysis led them to the following conclusions regarding the effects of anabolic steroids on muscular strength:

- For trained subjects, the improvement in strength gain obtained by comparing active drug group to placebo group ranged from 1.2% to 18.7% (median 5.0%) (see figure 7.4).
- For untrained subjects, the range of improvement was from –14.4% to +12.9% (median 3.4%; see figure 7.3).

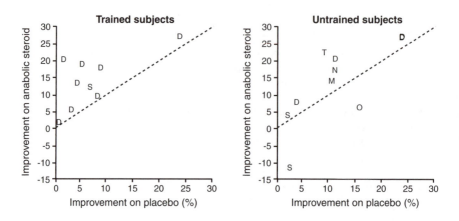

Figure 7.3   Percent mean improvement of the steroid group compared to the placebo group for trained and untrained subjects. Results from each study are plotted using a letter denoting the steroid used. D = methandrostenolone; S = stanozolol; O = oxandrolone; T = methyl testosterone; N = nandrolone decanoate; M = mesterolone.

Adapted from Elashoff et al. 1991.

- There was no evidence of a positive relation between total steroid dose and the effect on strength (although none of the studies they reviewed analyzed the enormous doses some athletes reportedly ingest).
- Well-trained athletes had a greater strength gain with supplemental steroids (compared to well-trained athletes who do not use AASs), but it was not possible to relate this finding to the ability of anabolic steroids to improve overall athletic performance.

These data were based on studies of men younger than 40 years old. The nine studies of trained athletes reviewed by Elashoff and colleagues evaluated only the drug methandrostenolone (Dianabol), an extremely potent anabolic steroid that is no longer marketed in the United States. Also, they included only the bench press as the objective assessment of strength. Finally, these nine studies were heterogenous in design (Elashoff et al. 1991).

In 1996, Bhasin and colleagues assessed the effects of supraphysiologic doses of testosterone enanthate in oil (600 mg intramuscular once weekly) and resistance training for 10 weeks on muscular strength. The study showed that testosterone alone and resistance exercise alone each increased strength independently, but when the two were combined, the strength gains were greater than from either intervention alone (see figure 7.4)

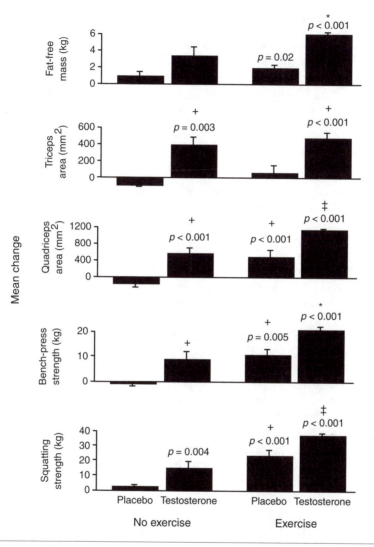

Figure 7.4 Changes from baseline in mean (± *SEM*) fat-free mass, triceps, and quadriceps cross-sectional areas, and muscle strength in bench press and squatting exercises over 10 weeks of treatment. The p values shown are for the comparison between the change indicated and a change of zero. * = $p < 0.05$ for the comparison between the change indicated and that in either no-exercise group; † = $p < 0.05$ for the comparison between the change indicated and that in the group assigned to placebo with no exercise; ‡ = $p < 0.05$ for the comparison between the change indicated and the changes in all three other groups.

Effects on Reflex Time

If skeletal muscles are stronger, does an athlete have faster reflexes? To answer this, Ariel and Saville (1972) used the patellar reflex to show that anabolic steroids decreased reflex latency. These data suggest that anabolic steroids might be beneficial for athletes such as boxers, hockey goalies, and baseball hitters.

Effects on Aerobic Performance

Not only is there a lingering debate about the effects of AASs on muscle strength and related parameters in general, but also the benefit of anabolic steroids on aerobic performance is uncertain. As discussed above, anabolic steroids exert variable effects on $\dot{V}O_2$max (Fahey and Brown 1973; Johnson et al. 1975), and this may partially explain why the data regarding effects of AASs on aerobic performance are also contradictory. Unfortunately, there isn't much new data on this topic. Wadler and Hainline (1989) reviewed this issue and concluded that, in general, anabolic steroids do not enhance aerobic performance. Lombardo also reviewed this issue in 1993 and concluded that the effects of anabolic steroids on aerobic performance are unclear.

On the other hand, those taking anabolic steroids report having a sense of well-being and increased energy, and they demonstrate increased aggressiveness. These psychological elements could perhaps contribute to improved performance during aerobic competition, but documenting the association is not easy. Further, some recent data indicate that nandrolone injections improved running endurance in rats (Van Zyl, Noakes, and Lambert 1995); so it appears this issue will require further investigation before a definitive conclusion is reached.

Avoiding Potential Complications

Adverse reactions of anabolic steroids have been reviewed by Kibble and Ross (1987) and Yesalis (2000). Concerns about the substances go beyond their being banned by a variety of sport organizations, and involve not only legal but physiologic and psychologic aspects.

NCAA and USOC Status

All AASs are banned by the NCAA, USOC, IOC, NFL, and the U.S. Powerlifting Federation. In addition, the FDA classifies AASs as Schedule III controlled substances.

■ *Androstenedione in Sport*

On the verge of breaking the home-run record Roger Maris had set, Mark McGwire of the St. Louis Cardinals in August 1998 admitted to regularly using the dietary supplements androstenedione and creatine. Indeed, these products are sold without prescription, and creatine seems relatively safe for short-term use. Nevertheless, androstenedione should not be considered a benign nutrient. "Andro" is an androgen produced by both the adrenal gland and ovaries, and it is converted into either testosterone or estrogen, depending on the sex of the individual, by peripheral tissues. Thus, taking androstenedione is the equivalent of taking a testosterone precursor. Neither Major League Baseball nor the NBA have banned this "hormone," but both the NFL and IOC do indeed ban it.

Other Legal Issues

On 27 February 1991, all anabolic steroids became Schedule III controlled substances in the United States. Although these drugs do not induce physical dependence in the same manner as benzodiazepines, barbiturates, or opiate agonists, anabolic steroids were reclassified in an attempt to better control their distribution within legitimate medical channels. This law makes distribution of these drugs a felony punishable by up to 5 years imprisonment and a fine of up to $250,000. Possession of these drugs without a prescription is a misdemeanor.

Physiologic Complications

In supraphysiologic doses, many serious reactions to AASs can occur (see table 7.3). In summary, these involve hepatic, endocrine, cardiovascular, skeletal, and subjective responses and have been thoroughly reviewed by Friedl (1993).

Hepatic Effects

Orally administered AASs, which are modified at the C17-alpha position, are associated with a higher incidence of hepatotoxicity than are the injectable preparations (Farrell et al. 1975). Hepatotoxic effects related to anabolic steroid abuse have included cholestatic jaundice, a serious condition of blood-filled cysts known as "peliosis hepatis," and primary hepatic tumors, including malignant hepatocellular carcinoma and hepatic angiosarcoma. Hepatic tumors can be reversible, or can be metastatic and fatal.

Table 7.3   Possible Health Risks Associated With Use of Anabolic/Androgenic Steroids

Cosmetic-related effects	Cardiovascular risk factors and diseases
Facial and body acne	Atherosclerotic serum lipid profile
Female-like breast enlargement in males	Decreased HDL-cholesterol
Premature baldness	Increased LDL-cholesterol
Masculinization in females	High blood pressure
Facial and body hair growth in females	Impaired glucose tolerance
	Stroke
Premature closure of growth centers in adolescents, leading to stunted growth	Heart disease
	Liver function
Deepening of the voice in females	Jaundice
Psychologic effects	Peliosis hepatis (blood-filled cysts)
Increased aggressiveness and possible violent behavior	Liver tumors
	Athletic injuries
Reproductive effects	Tendon rupture
Reduction of testicular size	**AIDS**
Reduction of sperm production	Use of contaminated needles
Decreased libido	
Impotence in males	
Enlargement of the prostate gland	
Enlargement of the clitoris	

Adapted from Williams, M.H. 1998.

Cardiovascular Effects

Athletes who abuse AASs should realize that these drugs affect human physiology in ways that *directly oppose the beneficial cardiovascular aspects* of exercise. Hypertension, ventricular remodeling, myocardial ischemia, unfavorable changes in serum lipid profiles, and sudden cardiac death have all been associated with AAS use in humans—and these effects persist long after AAS use is discontinued (Sullivan et al. 1998). Anabolic steroids can decrease HDL cholesterol and increase LDL cholesterol (Haffner et al. 1983; Kuipers et al. 1991; Webb, Laskarzewski, and Glueck 1984). The degree of change in serum lipids is substantial at "normal" (i.e., therapeutic) AAS doses (Haffner et al. 1983) and is profound at dosage levels bodybuilders are known to use (Webb, Laskarzewski, and Glueck 1984). Friedl has reviewed these data (1993). Anabolic steroids, used chronically, may accelerate atherosclerosis, possibly leading to premature coronary heart disease. This concern is even more real when one considers that resistance strength training, the typical mode of exercise chosen by users of anabolic steroids (Perry, Wright, and Littlepage 1992), does not appear to induce the favorable effects on blood lipids that endurance exercise does (Manning et al. 1991).

Left ventricular hypertrophy (LVH) has been demonstrated in elite athletes. Consider these two facts: normotensive men (not using AASs) with LVH have been shown to demonstrate an exaggerated pressor response to treadmill exercise (Gottdiener et al. 1990), and enormous increases in blood pressure occur during resistance exercise (MacDougall et al. 1985). These facts add to the likelihood that LVH is yet another potential adverse cardiovascular effect of AAS use.

Indeed, because hypertrophic cardiomyopathy is the most common cause of sudden death in young athletes, medical professionals recommend that these individuals avoid intense training and competition (Spirito et al. 1997). Sudden cardiac death has been reported in a 20-year-old bodybuilder who used anabolic steroids. At autopsy he was documented to have a hypertrophic (515 g) heart (Dickerman et al. 1995). When bodybuilders not taking AASs were compared with bodybuilders of similar body mass index who were using AASs, increases in left ventricular posterior-wall thickness and ventricular septal thickness were apparent in the AAS group (Dickerman et al. 1997). Cardiovascular complications of AAS use have been reviewed by Dickerman and colleagues (1996) and Sullivan and colleagues (1998).

Endocrine Effects

By stimulating negative feedback to the brain, testosterone excess causes a *reduction* in the output of endogenous testosterone. This leads to a reduction in sperm production and testicular size. In addition, since testosterone is metabolized (in part) to estradiol, gynecomastia can occur in males. Breast tissue in males can return to normal if AAS use is discontinued, but some athletes instead choose to take additional drugs (see table 7.4) such as estrogen-receptor blockers like tamoxifen to try and treat or prevent this (Friedl 1993).

Women who take AASs develop masculine features, including a deepening of the voice, male-pattern baldness, and enlarged clitoris, to name a few. Adolescents who take AASs can experience premature closing of the epiphyses of the long bones, resulting in short stature.

Psychologic Complications

Bahrke and colleagues (Bahrke, Yesalis, and Wright 1990, 1996; Bahrke, Yesalis, and Brower 1998) have thoroughly reviewed the issue of psy-

Table 7.4 Other Drugs Used by Steroid Abusers

Drug	Reason for use
Cyproheptadine	Ability to stimulate appetite is mistaken for an anabolic action; erroneous belief that the drug increases testosterone production
DHEA	Erroneous belief that it normalizes the T:E ratio
Diuretics	Increases muscular definition; offsets steroid-induced fluid retention
HCG	Used to offset steroid-induced oligospermia and decreased libido
Tamoxifen	Offsets steroid-induced gynecomastia

chological and behavioral effects from AASs. Anecdotal reports of personality changes seen in AAS users have included

- depression and euphoria;
- hypomania;
- aggression, hostility, and anger;
- increased alertness;
- anxiety;
- paranoia and psychotic episodes; and
- violent rages.

They conclude that the behavioral effects, overall, of anabolic steroids are variable and appear to be related to type and dose of anabolic steroid (Bahrke, Yesalis, and Wright 1996). While most reports reveal a pattern of association between these personality changes and AAS use, some do not (Bahrke, Yesalis, and Brower 1998).

Clearly, the negative aspects of anabolic steroids outweigh any potential benefit, but that does not seem to prevent some athletes from abusing these drugs.

Guidelines for Sports Medicine Specialists

If the acute- and long-term toxicities of these drugs are not enough to deter users, specialists should work to communicate to these individuals that AASs are Schedule III controlled substances in the United States. Distribution of these drugs without a legal prescription is a felony punishable by up to 5 years imprisonment and a fine of up to $250,000. Possession of these drugs (i.e., not involving distribution) without a legal prescription is a misdemeanor. Coaches and athletic trainers especially must educate their athletes on this serious issue.

All AASs are banned substances. Athletes need to realize that testing for these substances occurs and that many of the strategies for masking detection of these substances don't work.

While many of the adverse effects of AAS use disappear after the drug is discontinued, some do not. The health consequences are extremely serious—in some cases, they are fatal. Individuals should avoid these drugs at all costs.

Finally, the true medical uses of AASs are very limited. Health care professionals who distribute these drugs to athletes without a bona fide medical need are behaving unethically, as are the bodybuilders and athletes who use them.

References

Ariel, G., and Saville, W. 1972. The effect of anabolic steroids on reflex components. *Med Sci Sports* 4:120.

Bahrke, M.S., Yesalis, C.E., and Brower, K.J. 1998. Anabolic-androgenic steroid abuse and performance-enhancing drugs among adolescents. *Child Adolesc Psych Clin N Amer* 7:821-838.

Bahrke, M.S., Yesalis, C.E., and Wright, J.E. 1990. Psychological and behavioural effects of endogenous testosterone levels and anabolic-androgenic steroids among males. *Sports Med* 10:303-337.

Bahrke, M.S., Yesalis, C.E., and Wright, J.E. 1996. Psychological and behavioural effects of endogenous testosterone and anabolic-androgenic steroids. *Sports Med* 22:367-390.

Bhasin, S., Storer, T.W., Berman, N., Callegari, C., Clevenger, B., Phillips, J., Bunnell, T.J., Tricker, R., Shirazi, A., and Casaburi, R. 1996. The effects of supraphysiologic doses of testosterone on muscle size and strength in normal men. *N Engl J Med* 335:1-7.

Clarkson, P.M., and Thompson, H.S. 1997. Drugs and sport. Research findings and limitations. *Sports Med* 24:366-384.

Dickerman, R.D., McConathy, W.J., Schaller, F., and Zachariah, N.Y. 1996. Cardiovascular complications and anabolic steroids. *Eur Heart J* 17:1912.

Dickerman, R.D., Schaller, F., Prather, I., and McConathy, W.J. 1995. Sudden cardiac death in a 20-year-old bodybuilder using anabolic steroids. *Cardiology* 86:172-173.

Dickerman, R.D., Schaller, F., Zachariah, N.Y., and McConathy, W.J. 1997. Left ventricular size and function in elite bodybuilders using anabolic steroids. *Clin J Sport Med* 7:90-93.

DuRant, R.H., Rickert, V.I., Ashworth, C.S., Newman, C., and Slavens, G. 1993. Use of multiple drugs among adolescents who use anabolic steroids. *N Engl J Med* 328:922-926.

Elashoff, J.D., Jacknow, A.D., Shain, S.G., and Braunstein, G.D. 1991. Effects of anabolic-androgenic steroids on muscular strength. *Ann Intern Med* 115:387-393.

Fahey, T.D., and Brown, C.H. 1973. The effects of an anabolic steroid on the strength, body composition, and endurance of college males when accompanied by a weight training program. *Med Sci Sports* 5:272-276.

Farrell, G.C., Joshua, D.E., Uren, R.F., Baird, P.J., Perkins, K.W., and Kronenberg, H. 1975. Androgen-induced hepatoma. *Lancet* 1:430-432.

Forbes, G.B. 1985. The effect of anabolic steroids on lean body mass: The dose response curve. *Metabolism* 34:571-573.

Friedl, K.E. 1993. Effects of anabolic steroids on physical health. In *Anabolic steroids in sport and exercise*, edited by C.E. Yesalis. Champaign, IL: Human Kinetics.

Gottdiener, J.S., Brown, J., Zoltick, J., and Fletcher, R.D. 1990. Left ventricular hypertrophy in men with normal blood pressure: Relation to exaggerated blood pressure response to exercise. *Ann Intern Med* 112:161-166.

Haffner, S.M., Kushwaha, R.S., Foster, D.M., Applebaum-Bowden, D., and Hazzard, W.R. 1983. Studies on the metabolic mechanism of reduced high density lipoproteins during anabolic steroid therapy. *Metabolism* 32:413-420.

Haupt, H.A., and Rovere, G.D. 1984. Anabolic steroids: A review of the literature. *Am J Sports Med* 12:469-484.

Hickson, R.C., Hidaka, K., Foster, C., Falduto, M.T., Chatterton Jr., R.T. 1994. Successive time courses of strength development and steroid hormone responses to heavy-resistance training. *J Appl Physiol* 76:663-670.

Hickson, R.C., and Kurowski, T.G. 1986. Anabolic steroids and training. *Clin Sports Med* 5:461-469.

Johnson, L.C., Roundy, E.S., Allsen, P.E., Fisher, A.G., and Silvester, L.F. 1975. Effect of anabolic steroid treatment on endurance. *Med Sci Sports* 7:287-289.

Kibble, M.W., and Ross, M.B. 1987. Adverse effects of anabolic steroids in athletes. *Clin Pharm* 6:686-692.

Kochakian, C.D. 1993. Androgenic-anabolic steroids: A historical perspective and definition. In *Anabolic steroids in sport and exercise*, edited by C.E. Yesalis. Champaign, IL: Human Kinetics.

Kraemer, R.R., Kilgore, J.L., Kraemer, G.R., and Castracane, V.D. 1992. Growth hormone, IGF-I, and testosterone responses to resistive exercise. *Med Sci Sports Exerc* 24:1346-1352.

Kraemer, W.J., Gordon, S.E., Fleck, S.J., Marchitelli, L.J., Mello, R., Dziados, J.E., Friedl, K., Harman, E., Maresh, C., and Fry, A.C. 1991. Endogenous anabolic hormonal and growth factor responses to heavy resistance exercise in males and females. *Int J Sports Med* 12:228-235.

Kuipers, H., Wijnen, J.A.G., Hartgens, F., and Willems, S.M.M. 1991. Influence of anabolic steroids on body composition, blood pressure, lipid profile and liver functions in body builders. *Int J Sports Med* 12:413-418.

Kuoppasalmi, K., Naveri, H., Harkonen, M., and Adlercreutz, H. 1980. Plasma cortisol, androstenedione, testosterone and luteinizing hormone in running exercise of different intensities. *Scand J Clin Lab Invest* 40:403-409.

Lombardo, J. 1993. The efficacy and mechanisms of action of anabolic steroids. In *Anabolic steroids in sport and exercise*, edited by C.E. Yesalis. Champaign, IL: Human Kinetics.

Lukas, S. 1993. Current perspectives on anabolic-androgenic steroid abuse. *Trends Pharmacol Sci* 14:61-65.

MacDougall, J.D., Tuxen, D., Sale, D.G., Moroz, J.R., and Sutton, J.R. 1985. Arterial blood pressure response to heavy resistance exercise. *J Appl Physiol* 58:785-790.

Manning, J.M., Dooly-Manning, C.R., White, K., Kampa, I., Silas, S., Kesselhaut, M., and Ruoff, M. 1991. Effects of a resistive training program on lipoprotein: Lipid levels in obese women. *Med Sci Sports Exer* 23:1222-1226.

McKillop, G., Ballantyne, F.C., Borland, W., and Ballantyne, D. 1989. Acute metabolic effects of exercise in bodybuilders using anabolic steroids. *Br J Sports Med* 23:186-187.

Mottram, D.R., ed. 1988. *Drugs in sports.* Champaign, IL: Human Kinetics.

Perry, H.M., Wright, D., and Littlepage, B.N.C. 1992. Dying to be big: A review of anabolic steroid use. *Br J Sports Med* 26:259-261.

Sahelian, R., and Tuttle, D. 1997. *Creatine: Nature's muscle builder.* Garden City Park, NY: Avery.

Smith, D.A., and Perry, P.J. 1992. The efficacy of ergogenic agents in athletic competition. Part I: Androgenic-anabolic steroids. *Ann Pharmacother* 26:520-528.

Somani, S.M. 1996. *Pharmacology in exercise and sports.* Boca Raton, FL: CRC Press.

Spirito, P., Seidman, C.E., McKenna, W.J., and Maron, B.J. 1997. The management of hypertrophic cardiomyopathy. *N Engl J Med* 336:775-785.

Sturmi, J.E., and Diorio, D.J. 1998. Anabolic agents. *Clin Sports Med* 17:261-282.

Sullivan, M.L., Martinez, C.M., Gennis, P., and Gallagher, E.J. 1998. The cardiac toxicity of anabolic steroids. *Prog Cardiovasc Dis* 41:1-15.

Van Zyl, C.G., Noakes, T.D., and Lambert, M.I. 1995. Anabolic-androgenic steroid increases running endurance in rats. *Med Sci Sports Exerc* 27:1385-1389.

Voy, R. 1991. *Drugs, sports, and politics.* Champaign, IL: Human Kinetics.

Wadler, G.I., and Hainline, B. 1989. Anabolic steroids. In *Drugs and the athlete.* Philadelphia: F.A. Davis.

Webb, O.L., Laskarzewski, P.M., and Glueck, C.J. 1984. Severe depression of high-density lipoprotein cholesterol levels in weight lifters and body builders by self-administered exogenous testosterone and anabolic-androgenic steroids. *Metabolism* 33:971-975.

Yesalis, C.E., ed. 2000. *Anabolic steroids in sport and exercise (2nd ed.).* Champaign, IL: Human Kinetics.

Yesalis, C.E., and Cowart, V.S, eds. 1998. *The steroids game: An expert's look at anabolic steroid use in sports.* Champaign, IL: Human Kinetics.

Yesalis, C.E., Kennedy, N.J., Kopstein, A.N., and Bahrke, M.S. 1993. Anabolic-androgenic steroid use in the United States. *JAMA* 270:1217-1221.

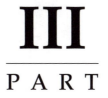

PART

Metabolic Agents

8

CHAPTER

Creatine

CASE STUDY

■ *CASE*   Steve participates in triathlons. He remembers seeing Olympic decathlete Dan O'Brien on television, proclaiming the benefits of creatine supplementation. Subsequently, he read that St. Louis Cardinals slugger Mark McGwire had also used creatine regularly. Steve wants your opinion of using creatine supplements. How do you respond?

■ *COMMENT*   Does creatine improve athletic performance? Yes and no. It depends on what kind of exercise is involved. Many well-designed scientific studies have been conducted to answer this question. It appears that exogenous creatine monohydrate does improve exercise performance, but this has mostly been demonstrated in laboratory tests of extremely short periods of maximal effort (e.g., anaerobic power, anaerobic endurance), separated by limited recovery time. An ergogenic effect has also been demonstrated in field tests involving similar short-duration events; however, in events that do not place such extreme, short-term demands on muscle energy metabolism, creatine's benefits are less evident. In some cases, such as sprint swimming, an ergolytic effect has been documented. Creatine might possibly be beneficial during intense weight training, which, in turn, might enhance performance in another athletic event. Even if it is not officially regarded as a banned substance, since creatine does possess ergogenic properties, its use in competitive athletics should be discouraged. Potential side effects should also be considered. Weight gain, mostly due to fluid retention, can occur, and the long-term effects of daily creatine supplementation are still unclear.

Interest in "nontraditional" forms of health care in the United States exploded in the mid-1990s; the general public's use of herbal medications has skyrocketed. Demand for these products has proved lucrative: the market for *nutraceuticals* (i.e., nutritional supplements used like pharmaceuticals) likely will exceed $12 billion by the year 2001. And this is in addition to the already pervasive use of other nutritional supplements by athletes seeking anything that will provide an extra 2% or 3% improvement in performance. Creatine and androstenedione are just two examples of supplements that are being widely used in sports. It has been estimated that up to 80% of athletes at the 1996 Olympic Games in Atlanta used creatine (Williams, Kreider, and Branch 1999).

While the role of phosphocreatine in muscle energy metabolism has been investigated for many decades, interest in creatine supplements as a potential ergogenic aid has occurred only recently. Creatine supplements were first used in Europe in the mid-1980s, and they became popular in the United States in the early 1990s. Endorsements by high-profile athletes, such as Dan O'Brien and Mark McGwire, plus the public's intense interest in dietary supplements, make it likely that use of creatine supplements in sports will increase in the near future.

Creatine (or, intracellularly, phosphocreatine [PCr] or creatine phosphate) is a nitrogenous compound (see figure 8.1) that participates in the production and maintenance of ATP, the major energy source for anaerobic and aerobic metabolism. Because of its ability to assist in the regeneration of ATP, creatine has been called a "metabolic buffer." Creatine can be synthesized by the body from the amino acids arginine, glycine, and methionine. Individuals can also ingest it directly by consuming fish and meats. A single 5 g dose of creatine, for example, corresponds to the creatine content of 1.1 kg of fresh, uncooked steak (Harris, Soderlund, and Hultman 1992). Vegetarians may have lower serum concentrations of creatine, but not necessarily lower tissue concentrations when compared to meat eaters (Harris, Soderlund, and Hultman 1992). Even though the creatine your body needs can be obtained from foods, some individuals (mostly athletes) experiment with the supplement creatine monohydrate.

How Exercise Affects the Action of Creatine Supplements

Endogenous PCr gives up its phosphate molecule in order to facilitate the regeneration of ATP. During extreme energy demands, reserves of PCr within the mitochondria of skeletal muscle can be depleted within seconds, despite the fact that concentrations of PCr are some three times

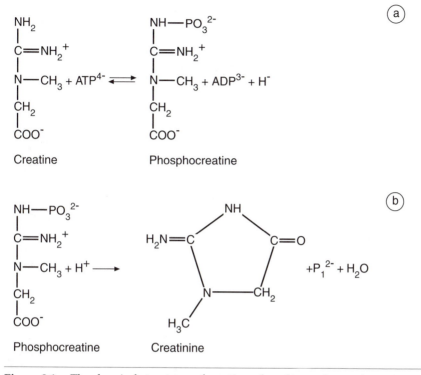

Figure 8.1   The chemical structures of creatine, phosphocreatine, and creatinine. (*a*) Creatine to phosphocreatine; (*b*) phosphocreatine to creatinine.

greater than concentrations of ATP (Green 1995). Even with the assistance of PCr, ATP stores can meet the anaerobic energy demands of intense exercise for only the initial 15 s (see figure 8.2). After this, other pathways, specifically anaerobic glycolysis and oxidation of other substrates, must provide the necessary ATP. These additional pathways for generating ATP prevent depletion of ATP by more than 20% to 25% during voluntary exercise (Green 1995). Ingestion of creatine supplements, even in doses that raise serum creatine concentrations substantially, does not increase tissue ATP concentrations (Harris, Soderlund, and Hultman 1992).

Data describing the effects of exercise on the actions or pharmacokinetics of creatine supplements are limited. Harris and colleagues (1992) examined this issue by having subjects taking creatine exercise one leg on a stationary cycle for 60 min; vastus lateralis muscle concentrations were measured both before and after the exercise session. The researchers found that creatine concentrations increased after exercise in both the exercised and the stationary leg, but tissue creatine increased more in the exercised leg compared to the sedentary leg.

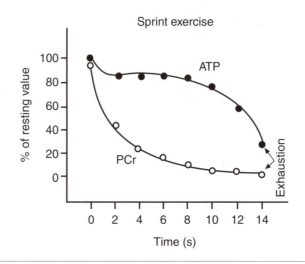

Figure 8.2   Changes in muscle ATP and PCr during the first seconds of maximal muscular effort.

Adapted from Wilmore and Costill 1994.

The PCr content averaged 103.1 mmol/kg dry muscle in the exercised leg, 93.8 in the control leg, and 81.9 in the presupplementation, preexercise phase (Harris, Soderlund, and Hultman 1992) (see figure 8.3).

Dosing Strategies and Effects on Tissue Concentrations of Creatine

It has been estimated that the dietary needs of creatine for an average 70 kg male are in the range of 2 g/day (Harris, Soderlund, and Hultman 1992). The total amount of creatine ingested per day is important to achieving increases in tissue concentrations of creatine and improving performance. Some data support a direct relationship between tissue concentrations of creatine and performance (Casey et al. 1996) (see figure 8.4).

Single doses of just 1 g produced only a modest rise in the plasma creatine concentration; but single 5 g doses produced a marked, though short-lived, increase in plasma creatine concentrations (Harris, Soderlund, and Hultman 1992) (see figure 8.5). In another study, doses of 2 g/day for 6 weeks in elite female swimmers did not change the creatine-to-choline ratios in the calf muscle during plantar flexion (Thompson et al. 1996). In this latter study, not surprisingly, no improve-

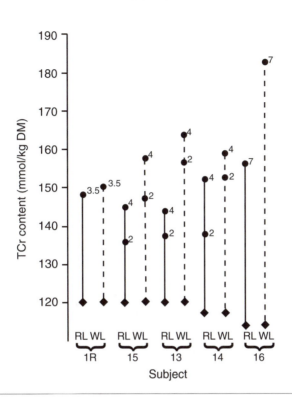

Figure 8.3   Effect of exercise and creatine supplementation on the total creatine (TCr) content of the quadriceps femoris. During supplementation, subjects performed 1 h of strenuous exercise on a bicycle ergometer using one leg only; the control leg rested. For the rest of the time, the subjects went about their normal daily activities. Doses used were 4 × 5 g for 3.5 days (subject 1R); 6 × 5 g for 4 days (subjects 13-15) with biopsies on days 2 and 4; and 6 × 5 g for 7 days (subject 16). One biopsy from the rest leg was taken before supplementation and was assumed to describe also the presupplementation TCr content of the other leg. Subjects are arranged in order of increasing initial TCr content. RL = rest leg; WL = work leg; ◆ = before supplementation; ● = after supplementation. Numbers denote the days of supplementation at the time of the biopsy.

Reproduced with permission of R.C. Harris, K. Soderlund, and E. Hultman, 1992, *Clinical Science* 83, 367-374. © the Biochemical Society and the Medical Research Society.

ment in performance was seen. In another study where plasma creatine did not increase and tissue concentrations increased only slightly, total work during a 30 s maximum cycling test was not enhanced during creatine supplementation (Odland et al. 1997).

Clinical studies of creatine monohydrate supplementation generally evaluate multiple daily-dosing regimens—for example, doses taken 4 times a day (Dawson et al. 1995) or 5 times a day for 5 to 7 days (Schneider et al. 1997). Although frequent doses administered at short dosing

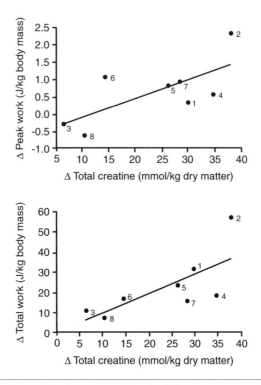

Figure 8.4   Relationship between individual changes in mixed-muscle total creatine (Σ phosphocreatine and creatine) concentration and cumulative changes in peak ($r = 0.71$, $p < 0.05$; A, $y = -0.65 + 0.05x$) and total ($r = 0.71$, $p < 0.05$; B, $y = -0.29 + 0.96x$) work production over two bouts of exercise. Values are given precreatine and postcreatine supplementation for 5 days (4×5 g/day).
Adapted from Casey et al. 1996.

intervals seems logical, given the extremely short-lived nature of endogenous PCr, there is no evidence that giving 20 to 25 g/day of creatine monohydrate in divided doses benefits users more than ingesting the total amount in one single, daily dose.

Increases in muscle PCr occurred within 5 days after beginning supplementation (Casey et al. 1996; Rossiter, Cannell, and Jakeman 1996; Vandenberghe et al. 1996), with uptake greatest during the first 2 days (Harris, Soderlund, and Hultman 1992). Doses of 5 g ingested 4 to 6 times per day for 2 or more days produced a significant increase in the total creatine content of the quadriceps femoris muscle in normal subjects (Harris, Soderlund, and Hultman 1992). Other investigators found that doses of 0.25 g/kg/day for 5 days (Rossiter, Cannell, and Jakeman 1996) and 0.5 g/kg/day for 6 days (Vandenberghe et al. 1996) produced significant elevations in muscle PCr content. One group of

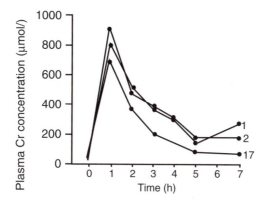

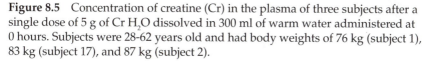

Figure 8.5 Concentration of creatine (Cr) in the plasma of three subjects after a single dose of 5 g of Cr H$_2$O dissolved in 300 ml of warm water administered at 0 hours. Subjects were 28-62 years old and had body weights of 76 kg (subject 1), 83 kg (subject 17), and 87 kg (subject 2).

Reproduced with permission of R.C. Harris, K. Soderlund, and E. Hultman, 1992, *Clinical Science* 83, 367-374. © the Biochemical Society and the Medical Research Society.

investigators administered creatine 18.75 g/day for 5 days, followed by 2.25 g/day during the testing phase, and demonstrated a significant ergogenic effect (Prevost, Nelson, and Morris 1997).

Thus, a "loading dose" for several days appears to be logical, although it is possible that the benefit of a loading dose is minimized after a week or more of continual, daily, low-dose administration. Hultman and colleagues (1996) showed that muscle creatine was similar after either a "rapid" protocol (20 g/day for the first 6 days, followed by 2 g/day until day 28) or a slower protocol (3 g/day for 28 days). And just as tissue concentrations of creatine accumulate gradually during administration, they also decline gradually after administration ceases. Vandenberghe and colleagues (1997) demonstrated that after the individual ceased creatine intake, muscle PCr returned to baseline in 4 weeks. Other studies suggest that the ergogenic effect of creatine supplementation can persist for 1 week after discontinuation (Jacobs, Bleue, and Goodman 1997).

Thus, some predictable relationships have been seen between dosing regimens and the resulting tissue concentrations of creatine. Harris, Soderlund, and Hultman (1992) concluded that increases in tissue concentrations of creatine appear to be less dependent on the amount of creatine ingested than on the initial tissue creatine content. They found that the greatest increases in tissue creatine content occurred in subjects with the lowest initial content. How tissue concentrations of creatine relate to athletic performance will be examined in greater detail below.

How Creatine Supplements Affect Exercisers

Some studies have focused on the effects that creatine supplements have on the physiology of the individuals ingesting them. They have looked in particular at whether changes resulted in postexercise lactate concentrations and body composition. The effects on oxygen uptake ($\dot{V}O_2$) and heart rate are also briefly discussed.

Heart Rate and Oxygen Uptake

Generally, creatine supplements do not affect either resting or exercise heart rate (Engelhardt et al. 1998). In addition, creatine supplements did not directly affect $\dot{V}O_2$ in elite triathletes during sustained cycle ergometry (Engelhardt et al. 1998). It is theoretically possible, however, that by increasing an athlete's ability to train longer and harder, creatine supplementation indirectly leads to an increase in $\dot{V}O_2$.

Postexercise Lactate Concentrations

If creatine supplementation allows the athlete to exercise harder, it seems likely that postexercise lactate concentrations would also be higher. However, there is no apparent relationship between the effects of creatine on performance and the resulting postexercise plasma lactate concentrations. Studies of trained athletes where a beneficial effect of creatine on performance was seen showed that lactate concentrations were higher after intense bench press exercise (Volek et al. 1997), but no difference in lactate concentrations was seen in trained athletes after a maximum cycling effort (Engelhardt et al. 1998), although a lower dose of creatine was used in this latter study. In untrained subjects, no increases in lactate concentrations were found in several studies of short-duration sprint cycling (Dawson et al. 1995; Odland et al. 1997; Schneider et al. 1997). In these three studies, the dose of creatine was 20 to 25 g/day for 3 to 7 days (table 8.1).

Body Composition

A number of bodybuilders apparently believe that creatine, because of its participation in muscle physiology, has anabolic (i.e., muscle-building) properties. Unfortunately, research has not yet yielded a clear answer on this issue. Total body mass does appear to increase; most studies show that short-term use of creatine leads to an increase in body mass in diverse groups of individuals. Creatine taken at 20 g/day for 5 days had no effect on body weight of elite male runners (Terrillion et al. 1997). However, one study looked at "active men"

Table 8.1   Power Output, Percent Fatigue, and Blood Lactate Concentration Following a Single 30-Second Bout of Maximal Cycle Exercise in Each of Three Conditions

	Creatine	Placebo	Control
Peak power (W · kg^{-1})	9.96 ± 0.32	10.46 ± 0.35	9.95 ± 0.44
Mean 10 s power (W · kg^{-1})	9.82 ± 0.32	9.97 ± 0.37	9.79 ± 0.40
Mean 30 s power (W · kg^{-1})	7.62 ± 0.23	7.79 ± 0.26	7.58 ± 0.27
Percent fatigue	41.47 ± 1.99	44.33 ± 2.24	40.89 ± 3.65
Blood lactate (mmol · l^{-1})	10.19 ± 0.72	10.74 ± 0.64	10.21 ± 0.95

Adapted from Odland et al. 1997.

doing jump squats and bench press during a regimen of creatine 25 g/ day for 7 days; it found that this combination produced a significant 1.4 kg mean increase in body weight (Volek et al. 1997). Resistance-trained men who received creatine and continued to weight train for 12 weeks demonstrated significantly greater increases in Type I, Type IIA, and Type IIAB muscle fiber cross-sectional area, compared to controls who weight trained but did not receive creatine (Volek et al. 1999) (see figures 8.6 and 8.7). In 19 young female "volunteers" who were given creatine supplementation during 10 weeks of resistance training, fat-free mass remained at a higher level in the group that

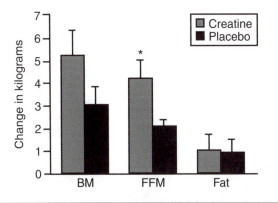

Figure 8.6   Delta changes in body mass (BM), fat-free mass (FFM), and fat mass after 12 weeks of heavy resistance training in creatine and placebo subjects. * = p 0.05 fr om corresponding change in the placebo group. Values are mean ± SE.

Adapted from Volek et al. 1999.

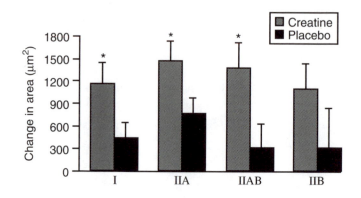

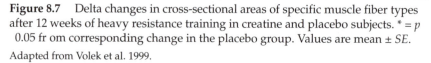

Figure 8.7   Delta changes in cross-sectional areas of specific muscle fiber types after 12 weeks of heavy resistance training in creatine and placebo subjects. $* = p$ 0.05 fr om corresponding change in the placebo group. Values are mean ± *SE*.

Adapted from Volek et al. 1999.

continued creatine after resistance training concluded (Vandenberghe et al. 1997).

In the longer term, a slight increase in fat-free mass can occur (Williams and Branch 1998). In 25 football players from Division I of the NCAA, total body weight and fat/bone-free mass increased after 28 days of creatine 15.75 g/day, but total body water did not change (Kreider et al. 1998). Williams, Kreider, and Branch (1999) have thoroughly reviewed these data and state that, generally, the effect is due to retention of intracellular water, although increased protein synthesis has been documented.

How Creatine Supplements Affect Exercise Performance

Many authors have reviewed the use of creatine supplementation as an ergogenic aid in sports (Demant and Rhodes 1999; Greenhaff 1995; Maughan 1995; Mujika and Padilla 1997; Williams 1995; Williams and Branch 1998; Williams, Kreider, and Branch 1999). Factors that must be considered when determining the effect of creatine on performance are (a) dose, which was discussed above; (b) trained versus untrained subjects; and (c) laboratory study versus field study.

Mujika and Padilla (1997) performed a meta-analysis and concluded that creatine supplementation was beneficial in untrained athletes but had little effect on the athletic performance of trained athletes. Since conditioning optimizes the endogenous production of creatine to meet the individual's needs, the untrained person likely realizes greater benefit from creatine supplements than an elite athlete. As was discussed earlier in this chapter, exercise can augment creatine uptake by exercising muscle tissue. Also, a saturation point may occur with creatine supplementation (Harris, Soderlund, and Hultman 1992) similar to other substrates used by the body. Further, it has been shown that, while creatine supplementation can raise resting muscle PCr concentrations, it does not enhance the rate of PCr resynthesis during and after intermittent isometric muscle contraction (Vandenberghe et al. 1999). Thus, trained athletes may have augmented this metabolic pathway relative to untrained athletes. Next, we will compare laboratory data with data obtained in the field.

Laboratory data on the effects of creatine on performance are not consistent (Williams and Branch 1998; Williams, Kreider, and Branch 1999). Discrepancies have been seen in studies of untrained athletes during maximum-effort cycling. Schneider and colleagues (1997) found that creatine improved performance of untrained males in a 15 s maximal cycling effort, while a similar study of untrained males in a 10 s cycling effort showed no benefit (Barnett, Hinds, and Jenkins 1996). The dosing regimen of creatine in these two studies was nearly identical. In another study utilizing a 30 s effort, no benefit was observed (Odland et al. 1997). In another study, the degree of improvement with creatine supplementation was inversely proportional to the duration of the exercise test. Marines were subjected to high-intensity cycling for various periods of time. Performance improved 61.0% when the test duration was 60 s; it improved 61.9% in the 20 s test; and improved by >100% in the 10 s test (Prevost, Nelson, and Morris 1997). Bosco and colleagues (1997) tested trained jumpers in a 45 s maximum continuous-jumping exercise. Performance improved significantly with creatine supplementation in both the first and the second 15 s phases, but not in the third.

Thus, some laboratory data support the premise that the benefit of creatine supplementation is most apparent in exercises requiring short, intense bursts of activity; this conclusion is consistent with the known physiology of endogenous PCr. However, inconsistencies in the data are perplexing.

Field studies of creatine also provide contradictory results. Elite swimmers given creatine improved their swim times in freestyle sprints in one study (Grindstaff et al. 1997), but two other groups of investigators did not see any benefit in sprint swimmers given the same dose of creatine (Burke, Pyne, and Telford 1996; Mujika et al. 1996). Similar discrepancies have been noted in running, skating, and resistance exercise (Williams and Branch 1998; Williams, Kreider, and Branch 1999). To properly assess the impact of creatine on performance, one needs to consider the duration of the activity, as Williams and colleagues have done. A summary of their findings is presented below.

Williams and Branch (1998) first classified studies of the effects of creatine on performance into three groups, based on the duration of the exercise test that they equated to the respective energy pathway most involved: (A) 4 to 30 s (ATP-plasma creatine system); (B) 30 to 150 s (anaerobic glycolysis); and (C) >150 s (aerobic glycolysis). According to these researchers, studies of group A revealed the following effects of creatine supplements:

- They may improve isotonic strength and endurance.
- They may improve isokinetic torque.
- A significant improvement is seen in isometric force with their use.
- Arm and cycle ergometer studies of 30 s duration or less show mixed results, although the majority of individuals in group A show benefit from creatine.

When the testing lasted 30 to 150 s (group B) or > 150 s (group C), the majority of both laboratory studies and field studies did not support any benefit of creatine.

The 1999 book *Creatine: The Power Supplement* provides the most extensive review yet of the scientific literature on creatine. Williams, Kreider, and Branch reviewed 80 studies of the effect of creatine on performance. A greatly condensed summary of their findings follows. With regard to the effect of creatine on anaerobic power (defined as activity lasting 30 s or less)

- in cycle ergometry studies, 18 of 24 studies documented an ergogenic effect;
- in isokinetic torque studies, 7 of 14 studies documented an ergogenic effect;
- in isotonic force studies, 17 of 23 studies documented an ergogenic effect;
- in isometric strength/endurance studies, 5 of 9 studies documented an ergogenic effect; and
- in "field" studies, 9 of 19 studies documented an ergogenic effect.

With regard to effects on anaerobic endurance (defined as activity lasting 30-150 s)

- in cycle ergometry studies, 4 of 7 reported an ergogenic effect;
- in laboratory or field-based running studies, 4 of 5 reported an ergogenic effect; and
- in swimming studies, 1 of 6 reported an ergogenic effect.

In general, roughly half of the laboratory-based studies and roughly half of the field-based studies of activities thought to rely most heavily on the anaerobic system have documented an ergogenic effect of creatine supplementation. In the remaining studies, generally no effect, either positive or negative, was observed—with the notable exception of studies of swimmers, where some studies revealed an ergolytic effect. In the setting of 25 to 50 m sprint swimming, some data showed that creatine was associated with an ergolytic effect. Williams and colleagues postulate that this may be due to increased body mass and an associated increase in body drag. The reader is encouraged to review this comprehensive text, as only a portion of it can be summarized here.

Flaws in research design may explain some of the divergence in studies of creatine. The fact that in one investigation no ergogenic effect was observed can be explained by the use of very low doses (e.g., 2 g/day) (Thompson et al. 1996). On the other hand, dietary factors in the study subjects (e.g., carbohydrate intake, caffeine intake, vegetarian status) may have affected the response to creatine. Uncontrolled dietary influences may explain why some studies show improved performance with creatine supplementation, whereas others do not. Some of the dietary factors associated with creatine supplementation and effects on performance will now be considered.

Dietary Factors and Their Effects on the Response to Creatine

Some dietary factors are known to influence the clinical response to creatine supplementation. Uncontrolled dietary factors—such as caffeine or carbohydrate or animal protein intake (or lack of it)—might explain why different results were obtained from nearly identical studies of creatine supplements. Vegetarians may have a more dramatic response to creatine supplements than meat eaters, since, in theory, vegetarians have a lower baseline intake of dietary creatine (Maughan 1995), and there is some evidence that muscle uptake of creatine is greatest in individuals with the lowest baseline levels (Harris, Soderlund, and Hultman 1992). Carbohydrate loading may augment the beneficial effects of creatine. Muscle creatine levels were higher in young, healthy males when each creatine dose was given with a sugar solution; this study, however, did not evaluate the effects on exercise performance (Green et al. 1996). Conversely, 5 mg/kg/day of caffeine ingested for 6 days completely *eliminated the beneficial effects* of creatine supplementation in a maximal, intermittent-exercise fatigue test of the knee extensors—despite the fact that muscle PCr content increased whether or not subjects ingested caffeine along with creatine supplements (Vandenberghe et al. 1996). Assuming a 70 kg adult, this dose of caffeine would be equivalent to the amount in about three cups of coffee.

In conclusion, several factors may influence whether or not creatine supplementation is associated with performance enhancement: training level of the subjects; dose administered; dietary factors; and type of exercise studied.

Avoiding Potential Complications

From 7 November to 9 December 1997, three healthy collegiate wrestlers in different states died unexpectedly (Centers for Disease Control and Prevention 1998). Although one of the wrestlers was found to have elevated levels of creatine, these deaths were attributed to an overly rapid loss of fluid and weight and not to creatine ingestion. Creatine supplementation is not known to be toxic, despite the relatively large amounts that athletes ingest (Harris, Soderlund, and Hultman 1992; Maughan 1995). In *Creatine: Nature's Muscle Builder* (1997), Ray Sahelian, MD, and Dave Tuttle claim that no significant side effects occur with moderate (e.g., 2-5 g/day) doses of creatine, but they go on to note that muscle cramping, loose stools, and nausea can occur. Weight gain has been noted in many studies of creatine supplementation, and this may be an undesirable factor in weight-based sports such as boxing or wrestling, or in events such as swimming or running where increased weight could hinder performance (Williams, Kreider, and Branch 1999).

It is worth pointing out that, since creatine is a nitrogenous compound, detrimental effects on renal function might be a concern when creatine is ingested chronically in high doses. Since muscle cells are limited in the amount of creatine they can store, excess must be eliminated via the kidneys (Crim, Calloway, and Margen 1975). Derek Bell, outfielder for the Houston Astros, contends that misuse of creatine supplements may have contributed to kidney problems that hospitalized him (Williams, Kreider, and Branch 1999). Unfortunately, data regarding the effect of creatine on renal function are limited. Several groups of investigators (Harris, Soderlund, and Hultman 1992; Poortmans et al. 1997) found that 3-7 days of creatine in doses of 20-30 g/day did not have any detrimental effect on the renal responses in healthy males; however, one should be careful not to extrapolate any conclusions about long-term safety from these short-term studies. Acute renal dysfunction has been reported in a 25-year-old male several months after he began creatine supplements. This individual, however, had preexisting renal disease and was taking a known nephrotoxic drug (cyclosporine) concomitantly (Pritchard and Kaira 1998). While it would be somewhat unusual for athletes to be taking cyclosporine, many do take NSAIDs and these drugs, too, are potentially nephrotoxic. The effects of creatine and NSAIDs combined, however, are still unknown.

Individuals who take large quantities of creatine may also be taking protein supplements. Both substances are sources of nitrogenous products that are eliminated renally (for creatine, the metabolic end product is creatinine; for protein, it is urea). The relationship of "nitrogen load" (in terms of urea nitrogen) to renal function has been studied in clinical medicine (Holm and Solling 1996). Some investigators believe that to properly answer this question, at least a 2-year study must be conducted (Parving 1997). Glomerular function was not affected in young, healthy males by a single amino acid load (Solling et al. 1986). However, a 4-month study of 88 healthy volunteers with normal renal function, including 28 bodybuilders taking protein supplements, revealed that chronic intake of protein was a crucial control variable for glomerular filtration rate. The investigators in the 4-month study concluded that these observations were due, in part, to structural changes in the glomerulus and tubules, and these changes were related to chronic protein intake (Brandle, Sieberth, and Houtmann 1996). These data are difficult to interpret, however, since exercise itself has been shown to disrupt the handling of protein by the kidney in healthy males (Poortmans, Rampaer, and Wolfs 1989) and females (Poortmans and Vancalck 1978). In addition, urea is more active osmotically than is creatinine.

Recently, some data regarding long-term use of creatine in athletes and the effect on renal function were published. Eight men and 1 woman who were track-and-field and volleyball athletes were examined after 1-5 years of creatine use and compared with a control group. No significant differences in renal function were noted in the group of creatine users compared to the control group (Poortmans and Francaux 1999).

NCAA and USOC Status

No athletic body currently bans creatine supplements. Since creatine is a naturally occurring compound, qualitative urine testing for its presence is impractical. But because creatine does possess ergogenic effects when ingested in amounts that greatly exceed the amounts one would obtain from food sources alone, in this author's opinion some quantitative limit should be established, much like the approach taken for caffeine. The fact that creatine is a "natural substance" should not imply that it is immune from restriction. Indeed, erythropoietin, adrenalin, growth hormone, and testosterone are all naturally occurring substances. The IOC has stated that a physiologic substance, when taken in abnormal quantities with the intention of artificially and unfairly increasing performance, should be construed as *doping* (Williams 1994). Thus, it would seem that routine ingestion of creatine as supplements and in supranormal amounts violates the *ethics* of sport and fair competition.

Guidelines for Use

The short-term use of creatine monohydrate supplements in conjunction with exercising appears to be safe. Whether the use in sanctioned events is *ethical* is another question. Enough data exist to demonstrate that creatine supplements are ergogenic in some athletes and events. Because of this, sports medicine specialists and athletic trainers are well advised to discourage athletes from using creatine supplementation during sanctioned events.

Since creatine is found naturally in many foods, testing outright for its supplemental use is impractical. Perhaps limits of tolerance may be adopted in the future for creatine, as they currently are for caffeine. For the weekend exerciser who wants an extra boost while lifting weights or playing softball, there are no contraindications to short-term use of creatine supplements. Indeed, one might even consider recommending creatine supplements for the deconditioned vegetarian who anticipates an abrupt increase in exercise routine.

Individuals who do not want to antagonize the performance-enhancing effects of creatine should avoid caffeine. Daily ingestion of high doses of creatine chronically, particularly in athletes taking protein supplements, appears unwise until the effects of creatine on renal function have been thoroughly investigated. For a thorough review of creatine's use in sports, see reviews by Williams and Branch (1998) and Kreider (1998) and the book *Creatine: The Power Supplement* (Williams, Kreider, and Branch 1999).

References

Barnett, C., Hinds, M., and Jenkins, D.G. 1996. Effects of oral creatine supplementation on multiple sprint cycle performance. *Aust J Sci Med Sport* 28:35-39.

Bosco, C., Tihanyi, J., Pucspk, J., Kovacs, I., Gabossy, A., Colli, R., Pulvirenti, G., Tranquilli, C., Foti, C., Viru, M., and Viru, A. 1997. Effect of oral creatine supplementation on jumping and running performance. *Int J Sports Med* 18(5):369-372.

Brandle, E., Sieberth, H.G., and Houtmann, R.E. 1996. Effect of chronic dietary protein intake on the renal function in healthy subjects. *Eur J Clin Nutr* 50:734-740.

Burke, L.M., Pyne, D.B., and Telford, R.D. 1996. Effect of oral creatine supplementation on single-effort sprint performance in elite swimmers. *Int J Sport Nutr* 6:222-233.

Casey, A., Constantin-Teodosiu, D., Howell, S., Hultman, E., and Greenhaff, P.L. 1996. Creatine ingestion favorably affects performance and muscle metabolism during maximal exercise in humans. *Am J Physiol* 271(1 pt 1):E31-E37.

Centers for Disease Control and Prevention. 1998. Hyperthermia and dehydration-related deaths associated with intentional rapid weight loss in three collegiate wrestlers—North Carolina, Wisconsin, and Michigan, November-December 1997. *Morbid Mortal Wkly Rep* 47:105-108.

Crim, M.C., Calloway, D.H., and Margen, S. 1975. Creatine metabolism in men: Urinary creatine and creatinine excretions with creatine feeding. *J Nutr* 105:428-438.

Dawson, B., Cutler, M., Moody, A., Lawrence, S., Goodman, C., and Randall, N. 1995. Effects of oral creatine loading on single and repeated maximal short sprints. *Aust J Sci Med Sport* 27:56-61.

Demant, T.W., and Rhodes, E.C. 1999. Effects of creatine supplementation on exercise performance. *Sports Med* 28:49-60.

Engelhardt, M., Neumann, G., Berbalk, A., and Reuter, I. 1998. Creatine supplementation in endurance sports. *Med Sci Sports Exerc* 30:1123-1129.

Green, A.L., Hultman, E., Macdonald, I.A., Sewell, D.A., and Greenhaff, P.L. 1996. Carbohydrate ingestion augments skeletal muscle creatine accumulation during creatine supplementation in humans. *Am J Physiol* 271(5 pt 1):E821-E826.

Green, H.J. 1995. Metabolic determinants of activity induced muscular fatigue. In *Exercise metabolism*, edited by M. Hargreaves. Champaign, IL: Human Kinetics.

Greenhaff, P.L. 1995. Creatine and its application as an ergogenic aid. *Int J Sport Nutr* 5(suppl):S100-S110.

Grindstaff, P.D., Kreider, R., Bishop, R., Wilson, M., Wood, L., Alexander, C., and Almada, A. 1997. Effects of creatine supplementation on repetitive sprint performance and body composition in competitive swimmers. *Int J Sport Nutr* 7:330-346.

Harris, R.C., Soderlund, K., and Hultman, E. 1992. Elevation of creatine in resting and exercised muscle of normal subjects by creatine supplementation. *Clin Sci* 83:367-374.

Holm, E.A., and Solling, K. 1996. Dietary protein restriction and the progression of chronic renal insufficiency: A review of the literature. *J Intern Med* 239:99-104.

Hultman, E., Soderland, K., Timmons, J.A., Cederblad, G., and Greenhaff, P.L. 1996. Muscle creatine loading in men. *J Appl Physiol* 81:232-237.

Jacobs, I., Bleue, S., and Goodman, J. 1997. Creatine ingestion increases anaerobic capacity and maximum accumulated oxygen deficit. *Can J Appl Physiol* 22:231-243.

Kreider, R.B. 1998. Creatine supplementation: Analysis of ergogenic value, medical safety, and concerns. *JEP Online* 1:1-6 (viewed on 2 June 1998).

Kreider, R.B., Ferreira, M., Wilson, M., Grindstaff, P., Plisk, S., Reinardy, J., Cantler, E., and Almada, A.L. 1998. Effects of creatine supplementation on body composition, strength, and sprint performance. *Med Sci Sports Exerc* 30:73-82.

Maughan, R.J. 1995. Creatine supplementation and exercise performance. *Int J Sport Nutr* 5:94-101.

Mujika, I., Chatard, J.C., Lacoste, L., Barale, F., and Geyssant, A. 1996. Creatine supplementation does not improve sprint performance in competitive swimmers. *Med Sci Sports Exerc* 28:1435-1441.

Mujika, I., and Padilla, S. 1997. Creatine supplementation as an ergogenic aid for sports performance in highly trained athletes: A critical review. *Int J Sports Med* 18:491-496.

Odland, L.M., MacDougall, J.D., Tarnopolsky, M.A., Elorriaga, A., and Borgmann, A. 1997. Effect of oral creatine supplementation on muscle [PCr] and short-term maximum power output. *Med Sci Sports Exerc* 29:216-219.

Parving, H-H. 1997. Effects of dietary protein on renal disease [Letter to the editor]. *Ann Intern Med* 126:330-331.

Poortmans, J.R., Auquier, H., Renaut, V., Durussel, A., Saugy, M., and Brisson, G.R. 1997. Effect of short-term creatine supplementation on renal responses in men. *Eur J Appl Physiol* 76:566-567.

Poortmans, J.R., and Francaux, M. 1999. Long-term oral creatine supplementation does not impair renal function in healthy athletes. *Med Sci Sports Exerc* 31:1108-1110.

Poortmans, J.R., Rampaer, L., and Wolfs, J.C. 1989. Renal protein excretion after exercise in man. *Eur J Appl Physiol* 58:476-480.

Poortmans, J.R., and Vancalck, B. 1978. Renal glomerular and tubular impairment during strenuous exercise in young women. *Eur J Clin Invest* 8:175-178.

Prevost, M.C., Nelson, A.G., and Morris, G.S. 1997. Creatine supplementation enhances intermittent work performance. *Res Q Exerc Sport* 68:233-240.

Pritchard, N.R., and Kaira, P.A. 1998. Renal dysfunction accompanying oral creatine supplements. *Lancet* 351:1252-1253.

Rossiter, H.B., Cannell, E.R., and Jakeman, P.M. 1996. The effect of oral creatine supplementation on the 1000-m performance of competitive rowers. *J Sports Sci* 14:175-179.

Sahelian, R., and Tuttle, D. 1997. *Creatine: Nature's muscle builder.* Garden City Park, NY: Avery.

Schneider, D.A., McDonough, P.J., Fadel, P.J., and Berwick, J.P. 1997. Creatine supplementation and the total work performed during 15-s and 1-min bouts of maximal cycling. *Aust J Sci Med Sport* 29:65-68.

Solling, K., Christensen, C.K., Solling, J., Christiansen, J.S., and Mogensen, C.E. 1986. Effect on renal haemodynamics, glomerular filtration rate and albumin excretion of high oral protein load. *Scand J Clin Lab Invest* 46:351-357.

Terrillion, K.A., Kolkhorst, F.W., Dolgener, F.A., and Joslyn, S.J. 1997. The effect of creatine supplementation on two 700-m maximal running bouts. *Int J Sport Nutr* 7:138-143.

Thompson, C.H., Kemp, G.J., Sanderson, A.L., Dixon, R.M., Styles, P., Taylor, D.J., and Radda, G.K. 1996. Effect of creatine on aerobic and anaerobic metabolism in skeletal muscle in swimmers. *Br J Sports Med* 30:222-225.

Vandenberghe, K., Gillis, N., Van Leemputte, M., Van Hecke, P., Vanstapel, F., and Hespel, P. 1996. Caffeine counteracts the ergogenic action of muscle creatine loading. *J Appl Physiol* 80:452-457.

Vandenberghe, K., Goris, M., Van Hecke, P., Van Leemputte, M., Vangerven, L., and Hespel, P. 1997. Long-term creatine intake is beneficial to muscle performance during resistance training. *J Appl Physiol* 83:2055-2063.

Vandenberghe, K., Van Hecke, P., Van Leemputte, M., Vanstapel, F., and Hespel, P. 1999. Phosphocreatine resynthesis is not affected by creatine loading. *Med Sci Sports Exerc* 31:236-242.

Volek, J.S., Duncan, N.D., Mazzetti, S.A., Staron, R.S., Putukian, M., Gomez, A.L., Pearson, D.R., Fink, W.J., and Kraemer, W.J. 1999. Performance and muscle fiber adaptations to creatine supplementation and heavy resistance training. *Med Sci Sports Exerc* 31:1147-1156.

Volek, J.S., Kraemer, W.J., Bush, J.A., Boetes, M., Incledon, T., Clark, K.L., and Lynch, J.M. 1997. Creatine supplementation enhances muscular performance during high-intensity resistance exercise. *J Am Diet Assoc* 97(7):765-770.

Williams, M.H. 1994. The use of nutritional ergogenic aids in sports: Is it an ethical issue? *Int J Sport Nutr* 4:120-131.

Williams, M.H. 1995. Nutritional ergogenics in athletics. *J Sports Sci* 13 (spec no):S63-S74.

Williams, M.H., and Branch, J.D. 1998. Creatine supplementation and exercise performance: An update. *J Am Coll Nutr* 17:216-234.

Williams, M.H., Kreider, R.B., and Branch, J.D. 1999. *Creatine: The power supplement.* Champaign, IL: Human Kinetics.

9
CHAPTER

Iron and Erythropoietin (Epoetin Alfa)

CASE STUDY

■ *CASE* On 11 July 1998, border guards discovered 400 vials of the hormone epoetin alfa (erythropoietin, EPO) in the car of the Festina cycling team en route to the Tour de France. The team manager then admitted that Festina riders used the drug, which prompted expulsion of the entire Festina team several days later. Because no testing was done of any of the cyclists, remaining cyclists protested the expulsion, initiating the biggest scandal in the history of the Tour. Many cyclists have long known that some of their colleagues were using epoetin alfa. Why did it take this incident to provoke an investigation?

■ *COMMENT* Epoetin alfa is a bioengineered version of erythropoietin, which is a naturally occurring hormone. Since erythropoietin can be detected in all individuals, testing for its presence is not helpful unless blood tests are conducted within hours of its being injected, due to its relatively short half-life. In lieu of testing for erythropoietin, testing of hematocrit is used. When hematocrit is >50%, epoetin alfa use is suspected. In fact, just weeks after the Tour de France, this test was the basis for banning several Italian cyclists from the 1998 Tour de Portugal. Until the 1998 Tour de France, punishment amounted only to several months of suspension from competition. Researchers are also developing other types of tests. Ironically, very little is known regarding the effects of EPO on performance in elite cyclists.

Hematinic agents stimulate erythrocyte formation or increase the amount of hemoglobin in red blood cells (RBC). The production of RBC is controlled by erythropoietin (EPO), a hormone produced by the kidney. Iron is a critical atom in the hemoglobin molecule, and iron stores must be adequate if EPO is to work properly. Athletes use (abuse) hematinic drugs in hopes that these agents will increase the oxygen-carrying capacity of their blood and, in turn, improve exercise endurance and athletic performance. This chapter discusses the effects of iron supplementation and epoetin alfa. *Erythropoietin, EPO,* will be used to refer to the endogenous hormone, while *epoetin alfa* will refer to the bioengineered drug for parenteral administration. Since the amino acid sequence of the bioengineered product is essentially the same as that of the endogenous hormone (Erslev 1991), the pharmacologic effects of the two are identical.

Hematinic Agents

In 1972, Ekblom, Goldbarg, and Gullbring demonstrated that blood loss and subsequent reinfusion of RBC increased maximal oxygen uptake ($\dot{V}O_2$max) by 9% and improved running performance by 23%. This physiologic principle eventually became abused in athletic competition, and the practice came to be known as "blood doping." In 1985 the gene for EPO was cloned, setting the stage for the production of a bioengineered form of this endogenous hormone—epoetin alfa (Epogen, Procrit). It was eventually approved for human use in 1989 for treating anemia in patients who have renal disease. Overzealous athletes found that this hormone was an ideal substitute for autologous transfusions or even high-altitude training to increase the oxygen-carrying capacity of the blood. Even the astronomical cost of epoetin alfa apparently has not prevented widespread abuse of this drug in sports (see the case study at the beginning of this chapter).

Nonetheless, some athletes may have justifiable, clinical reasons for using a hematinic agent. For example, increased gastrointestinal (GI) bleeding has been demonstrated in marathon runners (McMahon et al. 1984; Stewart et al. 1984) and triathletes (Rudzki, Hazard, and Collinson 1995). After a competitive race, most runners develop an increase in stool heme, and in some 20% of them fecal hemoglobin reaches clinically detectable levels (Buckman 1984). Paradoxically, Pahor and colleagues (1994) found that the risk of GI bleeding is reduced in elderly subjects who engage in vigorous exercise (compared with sedentary elderly). Both elite athletes (McMahon et al.

1984) and elderly subjects (Chrischilles et al. 1990) are populations that routinely use nonsteroidal anti-inflammatory drugs (NSAIDs); this factor would only increase the risk of gastropathy. Researchers have reviewed sports anemia and GI bleeding in athletes, concluding that intestinal ischemia, physical trauma, and medications most likely are the etiology (Balaban 1992; Mechrefe, Wexler, and Feller 1997; Moses 1993). Nevertheless, while blood loss might justify the need for iron supplementation, the use of epoetin alfa is not justified in subjects without renal failure.

Clement and colleagues (1987) evaluated 92 Winter Olympic athletes and found 7% of men and 8% of women were anemic; however, it was unclear if this represented true anemia. While true anemia (i.e., low RBC mass per kg of body weight) can occur in an athlete, more commonly a low hemoglobin or hematocrit value may simply reflect that the expansion of plasma volume is producing a dilutional "pseudoanemia" (i.e., hemoglobin concentrations decrease as a result of plasma volume expansion). Many cross-sectional and longitudinal studies have shown that endurance athletes display a low hemoglobin concentration. Cross-sectional data reveal that endurance-trained athletes exhibit a 20% to 25% increase in blood volume as compared with untrained subjects; longitudinal studies report a 7% increase. Ferritin levels in soccer players have been reported to decrease during the course of the season (Escanero et al. 1997). Low ferritin levels in distance runners range from 3-5% (Weight et al. 1992) to 16% (Matter et al. 1987). Many sports medicine professionals refer to this as *sports anemia*, and some investigators claim the incidence of this finding is as high as 80% (Dressendorfer et al. 1991). Seen in both males and females, this phenomenon is related to exercise intensity, appears within 24-48 h after a specific exercise period, and occurs independently of age (Bodary et al. 1999) and independently of administration of iron supplements (Dressendorfer et al. 1991). Even when iron stores are found to be reduced in athletes, mean hemoglobin (Weight et al. 1992) and EPO (Remacha et al. 1994) levels can still be within normal limits.

Some people consider "footstrike hemolysis" another cause of true anemia; but since the loss of iron stores among endurance athletes is negligible, this is not a noteworthy explanation of anemia in this population (Eichner 1992). Thus, while anemia (i.e., a true decrease in hemoglobin content) does appear to affect exercise performance (Ekblom 1996), "pseudoanemia" does not (Eichner 1992). Several investigators have reviewed the concept of sports anemia (Balaban 1992; Clarkson and Haymes 1995; Clement and Sawchuk 1984; Convertino 1991; Mechrefe, Wexler, and Feller 1997; Newhouse and Clement 1988; Raunikar and Sabio 1992). Unfortunately, the effects of epoetin alfa on the performance of elite athletes have been studied less well.

How Exercise Affects the Action of Epoetin Alfa and Iron

In healthy athletes, the serum half-life of subcutaneous epoetin alfa is 42.0 ± 34.2 h (Souillard et al. 1996). Erythropoietin serum and urine levels decrease to baseline by 7 and 4 days, respectively, after repeated subcutaneous doses of 200 units per kg (Souillard et al. 1996). The effects of exercise on the pharmacokinetics of epoetin alfa have not been assessed; however, several groups of investigators have assessed the effects of exercise on endogenous EPO serum concentrations. Increases in serum concentrations of endogenous EPO have been seen within hours following a 50 km ski race at 1600 m above sea level (De Paoli Vitali et al. 1988). Distance running has been shown to increase EPO serum concentrations at 3 h and also 31 h postexercise in one study (Schwandt et al. 1991); yet it had no effect on serum EPO concentrations in another study (Remacha et al. 1994). These contradictory findings are unexplained. Vedovato and colleagues (1988) found that postexercise concentrations of serum EPO increased more in distance runners than in cross-country skiers. These investigators attributed this difference to footstrike hemolysis in the runners. But they did not offer enough details in this study to draw firm conclusions. There does not appear to be any diurnal variation in the output of EPO (Roberts and Smith 1996).

Distance running does not appear to affect serum concentrations of endogenous EPO (Bodary et al. 1999; Remacha et al. 1994). The effect of exercise on the pharmacokinetics of exogenous epoetin alfa is less clear. But athletes should note that regular use (abuse) of epoetin alfa may disrupt the normal physiology of endogenous EPO. Repeated preoperative administration of epoetin alfa to patients undergoing elective surgery blunted the normal physiologic EPO response postoperatively, compared with subjects that did not receive epoetin alfa (Tasaki et al. 1992). Perhaps this phenomenon seen in surgical patients also occurs in athletes who routinely abuse epoetin alfa. It would be consistent with the suppressive effects that other exogenous hormones (e.g., corticosteroids and anabolic steroids) have on production of their respective endogenous counterparts.

How exercise affects the pharmacologic actions of epoetin alfa has not yet been adequately studied. It is not clear if exercise augments the effects of epoetin alfa. Low iron stores, however, are known to compromise the clinical response to both EPO and epoetin alfa. If strenuous exercise enhances the GI losses of iron, for example, exercise might be said to indirectly compromise the clinical response to epoetin alfa.

We know more about how exercise affects the use of iron. Roughly 10% of iron is absorbed after oral administration in healthy individuals, and roughly 10% to 30% is absorbed in iron-deficient individuals. Other than enhancing GI iron losses, exercise does not appear to affect either the pharmacology or pharmacokinetics of iron.

How Epoetin Alfa and Iron Supplements Affect Exercisers

Studies have been conducted in three main areas of exercise physiology and how each are affected by iron or epoetin alfa supplements. These areas are hematocrit and oxygen uptake, heart rate, and postexercise lactate levels. We look at each in turn.

Effects on Hematocrit and Oxygen Uptake

Epoetin alfa is indicated in clinical medicine to increase hematocrit in anemic dialysis patients, but among normal volunteers who were administered the supplement for 6 weeks, researchers found increases in hematocrit of 4.6% (Clyne, Berglund, and Egberg 1995) to >11% (Berglund and Ekblom 1991; Casoni et al. 1993). At higher doses, epoetin alfa might produce an even greater response, since (as figure 9.1 shows) hematocrit is proportional to EPO concentrations in both anemic dialysis subjects and normal blood donors (Erslev 1991). A dose-response effect to the hematinic action of epoetin alfa has been documented in both anemic dialysis patients and in normal subjects (Eschbach, Aquiling, et al. 1992).

Do the effects of epoetin alfa on hematocrit translate to effects on oxygen uptake ($\dot{V}O_2$)? The effects on oxygen consumption were not assessed in the studies of nonanemic subjects just described. In anemic dialysis patients, epoetin alfa increased hematocrit from 21% to 35%, and this was associated with a 17% increase in $\dot{V}O_2$max and a decrease in subjective perception of fatigue (Robertson et al. 1990). While an elevated hematocrit may help indicate epoetin alfa abuse, it may not be the most useful parameter to use to predict effects of epoetin alfa on performance. Hematocrit measures the oxygen-carrying cells of the blood, but hemoglobin is the actual oxygen-carrying molecule. Hematocrit, since it is simply a measurement of the percent of RBC in the blood, is susceptible to changes in plasma volume and RBC size. Both animal (Davies et al. 1982) and human (Celsing et al. 1987; Kanstrup and Ekblom 1984) data suggest that hemoglobin is closely related to $\dot{V}O_2$. Casoni and colleagues (1993) showed that hemoglobin content increased by 6.3% after 45 days of epoetin alfa, but these investigators did not assess the impact of this change on performance. Documentation of the effects of epoetin alfa on $\dot{V}O_2$ and performance in cyclists and other endurance athletes is needed.

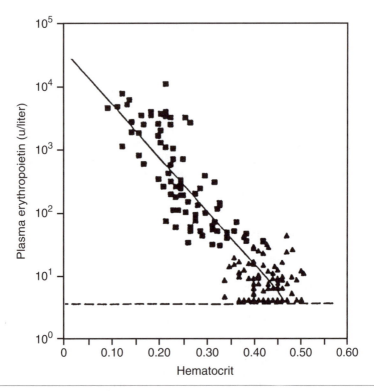

Figure 9.1   Plasma erythropoietin levels in 175 normal blood donors and patients with anemia, according to hematocrit. ▲ = normal blood donors; ■ = patients with various anemias. (Those with anemia due to renal disease, rheumatoid arthritis, or solid tumors are excluded.) The dashed line represents the limit of detection of the assay.

Supplemental iron, according to one study, did not prevent the development of dilutional pseudoanemia in female distance runners (Fogelholm, Jaakkola, and Lampisjarvi 1992). Nor did it affect maximal $\dot{V}O_2$max in female distance runners (Matter et al. 1987) and other female athletes (Fogelholm, Jaakkola, and Lampisjarvi 1992). All of the subjects in these studies demonstrated a normal hemoglobin at baseline, although some of them had low ferritin levels (Matter et al. 1987). These data further reinforce the conclusion that hemoglobin is a more important indicator of oxygen-carrying status than hematocrit.

Effects on Heart Rate

Epoetin alfa decreases exercise heart rate (HR) in both anemic dialysis patients (Robertson et al. 1990) and in normal healthy males (Berglund and Ekblom 1991). In normal healthy males, the exercise HR decreased from 144 ± 15 to 136 ± 8 beats/min. This decrease in exercise HR could be a reflex decrease in response to marked increases in systolic blood pressure (see later discussion) or perhaps improved $\dot{V}O_2$.

In contrast, 10 weeks of iron supplementation had no effect on maximum exercise HR in female marathon runners, regardless of their baseline ferritin or folate status. None of the subjects had low hemoglobin values at the beginning of the study (Matter et al. 1987).

Effects on Postexercise Lactate Levels

Three groups of investigators have assessed the effects of iron supplementation on postexercise lactate levels in female athletes with low serum ferritin levels (Fogelholm, Jaakkola, and Lampisjarvi 1992; Matter et al. 1987; Schoene et al. 1983). Postexercise lactate levels were significantly lower after supplemental iron in women who demonstrated moderately decreased hemoglobin levels at the beginning of the study (Schoene et al. 1983); but no effect was seen on lactate levels if hemoglobin was within normal limits at the beginning of the study (Fogelholm, Jaakkola, and Lampisjarvi 1992; Matter et al. 1987). None of these three studies found effects from iron on the physiology of exercisers and their performance.

How Epoetin Alfa and Iron Supplements Affect Exercise Performance

The belief that the hematinic agents might be ergogenic is based on the possibility that increased RBC mass improves the oxygen-carrying capacity of the blood. This should translate into improved $\dot{V}O_2$ and, ultimately, improved exercise endurance. Ekblom (1996) conducted a unique series of experiments and concluded that hemoglobin content, regardless of the value at baseline—and not hemoglobin concentration (Kanstrup and Ekblom 1984) or iron status (Celsing et al. 1987)—is the critical parameter explaining the effect of anemia on exercise performance. In their experiments, Ekblom and his colleagues studied the relationships between the oxygen-carrying capacity of the blood and exercise performance. Davies and colleagues (1982, 1984) showed in rats that $\dot{V}O_2$ and exercise endurance were not inseparably linked. When rats were fed an iron-deficient diet and then hemoglobin values were corrected, their $\dot{V}O_2$ improved but their exercise duration did not. Davies and colleagues argued that, while hemoglobin content of the blood affects $\dot{V}O_2$, exercise capacity is more closely related to the oxidative capacity of skeletal muscle. Ekblom and colleagues subsequently studied this issue in humans and could not reproduce the findings of Davies and colleagues; they concluded that deficient iron stores did not affect $\dot{V}O_2$, exercise performance, or various enzymes in skeletal muscle (Celsing et al. 1987). As discussed above, iron stores by themselves may not adequately represent the true hematologic picture of endurance athletes. The clinical effects of epoetin alfa and iron supplementation on exercise performance in athletes are summarized a bit later.

What effect does exogenous epoetin alfa have? Does it improve athletic performance? When anemic dialysis patients are studied, the answer is yes. Robertson and colleagues (1990) found clinically significant improvements in aerobic capacity (determined via cycle ergometry) and quadriceps strength, as well as decreased subjective perception of fatigue in these subjects following the administration of epoetin alfa, though none of the 19 subjects (anemic dialysis patients) attained the exercise performance level expected for a sedentary normal subject. The same group of investigators reported in a subsequent paper that epoetin alfa therapy improved both muscular strength and muscular endurance (measured with a Cybex dynamometer) in anemic dialysis patients (Guthrie et al. 1993). These data, however, are not very helpful when the population being evaluated is, for example, world-class cyclists.

It is more difficult to answer the question of the effects of exogenous epoetin alfa for elite athletes. Despite the fact that epoetin alfa has been commercially available since 1989, few scientific data have been generated on how it affects elite athletes. While some investigators suggest epoetin alfa is ergogenic in nonanemic athletes, others feel that normovolemic expansion of red cell mass may not be all that beneficial. Ekblom and Berglund (1991) showed that $\dot{V}O_2$ increased by 8%, and the time to reach exhaustion was delayed by 17% (see figure 9.2) (Ekblom 1996). Erslev (1991) pointed out that elite endurance athletes do not display erythrocytosis, but instead show increased intravascular volume with corresponding pseudoanemia. He therefore questioned claims that the physiologic response to epoetin alfa is ergogenic. In addition, serum levels of endogenous EPO have not been found, in comparisons with control subjects, to be higher in cross-country skiers (Berglund, Birgegard, and Hemmingsson 1988; De Paoli Vitali et al. 1988) or endurance runners (Bodary et al. 1999; Remacha et al. 1994).

Other studies have looked at how iron affects performance. For instance, the effects of iron supplements have been studied in female distance runners with low serum ferritin levels. These investigations were designed over different lengths: for 2 weeks (Schoene et al. 1983), 8 weeks (Fogelholm, Jaakkola, and Lampisjarvi 1992; Newhouse et al. 1989), and 10 weeks (Matter et al. 1987). Despite correcting the low serum ferritin, no positive effect on exercise performance was documented by any of the groups. Schoene and colleagues and Fogelholm and colleagues ex-

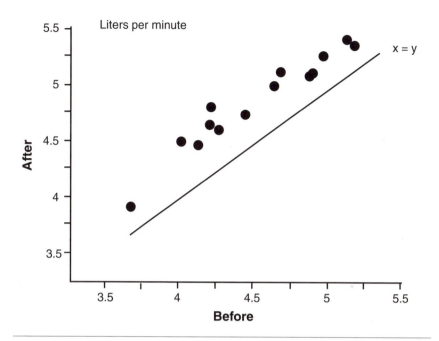

Figure 9.2 Maximal aerobic power (L/min) before and after 6 to 7 weeks of EPO administration in young males.

Adapted from Ekblom 1996.

cluded subjects with low hemoglobin levels at the start of their studies; only a small minority of subjects in the Matter study had an abnormal hemoglobin level. Thus, iron supplementation corrects iron deficiency, but in the setting of a normal hemoglobin content, it does not produce ergogenic responses in female distance runners. The effects of iron on athletic performance have been reviewed (Clement and Sawchuk 1984; Newhouse and Clement 1988; Nielsen and Nachtigall 1998).

Avoiding Potential Complications

Epoetin alfa has a pressor effect in hypertensive patients receiving dialysis (Buckner et al. 1990; Pascual, Teruel, and Ortuno 1991), but this is not seen in subjects with nonrenal anemia (Erslev 1991). The risks of long-term epoetin alfa use in dialysis patients have been reviewed by Eschbach, Haley, and colleagues (1992); it is unclear if these risks apply to athletes. In normal males, 6 weeks of epoetin alfa had no effect on resting blood pressure, but systolic blood pressure during exercise was markedly increased; initial and final values were 177 ± 14.2 mm Hg and 191 ± 19.5 mm Hg, respectively. Increased blood pressure does not appear to be related to increases in hematocrit (Buckner et al. 1990; Pascual, Teruel, and Ortuno 1991).

Another concern with epoetin alfa is the possibility of increased blood viscosity, which might lead to seizures or thrombosis, either of which could be fatal. It is conceivable that a distance cyclist who had used epoetin alfa could start a race with a hematocrit of 50% to 55% and, after several hours, might end the race with a hematocrit of 60% or higher (Eichner 1992). These potential risks are very serious.

Iron overload is well described in medical texts, and it holds risks that also are potentially very serious. No athlete without a clinical need for iron should take the supplement.

NCAA and USOC Status

The NCAA, USOC, and IOC ban use of epoetin alfa; they do not ban iron supplementation. Blood doping with reinfusion of autologous RBC is likewise prohibited (American College of Sports Medicine 1987). Although serum EPO concentrations are easily measured, detection of epoetin alfa abuse is very difficult since it is rapidly cleared from the bloodstream. Unfortunately, the physiologic effects of EPO are long-lived, since induced erythrocytosis persists for many weeks. Measurement of fibrinolytic products has been proposed (Gareau et al. 1992), as has measuring a difference in the electrical charge between endogenous EPO and exogenous epoetin alfa molecules. This latter method allows for a high detection rate in either blood or urine up to 24 h after injection (Wide et al. 1995).

Italian researchers have shown that epoetin alfa induces a hypochromic macrocytosis; they have proposed a value of 0.6% or higher as an indicator of epoetin alfa use (see figure 9.3). They also caution, however, that this strategy needs to be studied further; while none of the nonusers had values >0.6%, this cutoff identified only 50% of the users (Casoni et al. 1993).

Guidelines for Use

Tell athletes to avoid using epoetin alfa, which is banned from use during athletic competition. Although the substance is difficult to detect, some innovative detection methods are being developed. Note that elite athletes generally demonstrate a slightly decreased hematocrit ("pseudoanemia"); in contrast, documentation of an elevated hematocrit in an endurance athlete suggests epoetin alfa use. Since androgens (i.e., nandrolone decanoate) have been shown to potentiate the effects of epoetin alfa in patients with renal disease (Ballal et al. 1991), be aware that an individual who is taking anabolic steroids might also be using

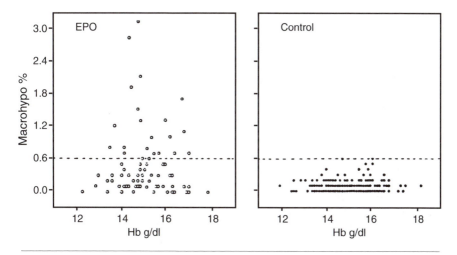

Figure 9.3 Relation between hemoglobin concentration and hypochromic macrocytes (Macrohypo) in EPO-treated and control subjects.

Adapted from Casoni et al. 1993.

epoetin alfa. Remind the exercising individuals that you work with that epoetin alfa is a prescription drug. Use of the drug outside the scope of a legal prescription represents criminal behavior.

Occasionally an athlete, bodybuilder, or other exerciser may develop a true need for iron supplementation. Although the supplement routinely causes GI upset and constipation, iron must be taken regularly for weeks, depending on the severity of iron deficiency. To minimize the risk of stomach cramps or nausea during actual competition, athletes should avoid taking any iron supplement doses for several hours prior to actual competition.

Finally, you should encourage endurance athletes, particularly menstruating females, to eat properly. In addition to losing iron via menstruation, females have only one-third the total body iron stores of males (Clarkson and Haymes 1995). In one study of female marathon runners, 16% had low ferritin levels (indicating iron deficiency), and 33% had low folate levels (Matter et al. 1987). Vitamin C increases the absorption of iron from the GI tract; large quantities of tea or antacids decrease it.

References

American College of Sports Medicine. 1987. Position on blood doping as an ergogenic aid. *Med Sci Sports Exerc* 19:540-543.

Balaban, E.P. 1992. Sports anemia. *Clin Sports Med* 11:313-325.

Ballal, S.H., Domoto, D.T., Polack, D.C., Marciulonis, P., and Martin, K.J. 1991. Androgens potentiate the effects of erythropoietin in the treatment of anemia of end-stage renal disease. *Am J Kidney Dis* 17:29-33.

Berglund, B., Birgegard, G., and Hemmingsson, P. 1988. Serum erythropoietin in cross-country skiers. *Med Sci Sports Exerc* 20:208-209.

Berglund, B., and Ekblom, B. 1991. Effect of recombinant human erythropoietin treatment on blood pressure and some haematological parameters in healthy men. *J Intern Med* 229:125-130.

Bodary, P.F., Pate, R.R., Wu, Q.F., and McMillan, G.S. 1999. Effects of acute exercise on plasma erythropoietin levels in trained runners. *Med Sci Sports Exerc* 31:543-546.

Buckman, M.T. 1984. Gastrointestinal bleeding in long-distance runners. *Ann Intern Med* 101:127-128.

Buckner, F.S., Eschbach, J.W., Haley, N.R., Davidson, R.C., and Adamson, J.W. 1990. Hypertension following erythropoietin therapy in anemic hemodialysis patients. *Am J Hypertens* 3(12 pt 1):947-955.

Casoni, I., Ricci, G., Ballarin, E., Borsetto, C., Grazzi, G., Guglielmini, C., Manfredini, F., Mazzoni, G., Patrecchini, M., De Paoli Vitali, E., et al. 1993. Hematological indices of erythropoietin administration in athletes. *Int J Sports Med* 14:307-311.

Celsing, F., Svedenhag, J., Pihlstedt, P., and Ekblom, B. 1987. Effects of anaemia and stepwise-induced polycythemia on maximal aerobic power in individuals with high and low haemoglobin concentrations. *Acta Physiol Scand* 129:47-54.

Chrischilles, E.A., Lemke, J.H., Wallace, R.B., and Drube, G.A. 1990. Prevalence and characteristics of multiple analgesic drug use in an elderly study group. *J Am Geriatr Soc* 38:979-984.

Clarkson, P.M., and Haymes, E.M. 1995. Exercise and mineral status of athletes: Calcium, magnesium, phosphorus, and iron. *Med Sci Sports Exerc* 27:831-843.

Clement, D.B., Lloyd-Smith, D.R., Macintyre, J.G., Matheson, G.O., Brock, R., and Dupont, M. 1987. Iron status in Winter Olympic sports. *J Sports Sci* 5:261-271.

Clement, D.B., and Sawchuk, L.L. 1984. Iron status and sports performance. *Sports Med* 1:65-74.

Clyne, N., Berglund, B., and Egberg, N. 1995. Treatment with recombinant human erythropoietin induces a moderate rise in hematocrit and thrombin antithrombin in healthy subjects. *Throm Res* 79:125-129.

Convertino, V.A. 1991. Blood volume: Its adaptation to endurance training. *Med Sci Sports Exerc* 23:1338-1348.

Davies, K.J., Donovan, C.M., Refino, C.J., Brooks, G.A., Packer, L., and Dallman, P.R. 1984. Distinguishing effects of anemia and muscle iron deficiency on exercise bioenergetics in the rat. *Am J Physiol* 246(6 pt 1):E535-E543.

Davies, K.J., Maguire, J.J., Brooks, G.A., Dallman, P.R., and Packer, L. 1982. Muscle mitochondrial bioenergetics, oxygen supply, and work capacity during dietary iron deficiency and repletion. *Am J Physiol* 242:E418-E427.

De Paoli Vitali, E., Guglielmini, C., Casoni, I., Vedovato, M., Gilli, P., Farinelli, A., Salvatorelli, G., and Conconi, F. 1988. Serum erythropoietin in cross-country skiers. *Int J Sports Med* 9:99-101.

Dressendorfer, R.H., Keen, C.L., Wade, C.E., Claybaugh, J.R., and Timmis, G.C. 1991. Development of runner's anemia during a 20-day road race: Effect of iron supplements. *Int J Sports Med* 12(3):332-336.

Eichner, E.R. 1992. Sports anemia, iron supplements, and blood doping. *Med Sci Sports Exerc* 24(suppl 9):S315-S318.

Ekblom, B. 1996. Blood doping and erythropoietin. The effects of variation in hemoglobin concentration and other related factors on physical performance. *Am J Sports Med* 24:S40-S42.

Ekblom, B., and Berglund, B. 1991. Effect of recombinant erythropoietin on physical performance and maximal aerobic power in man. *Scand J Med Sci Sports* 1:125-130.

Ekblom, B., Goldbarg, A.N., and Gullbring, B. 1972. Response to exercise after blood loss and reinfusion. *J Appl Physiol* 33:175-180.

Erslev, A.J. 1991. Erythropoietin. *N Engl J Med* 324:1339-1344.

Escanero, J.F., Villanueva, J., Rojo, A., Herrera, A., del Diego, C., and Guerra, M. 1997. Iron stores in professional athletes throughout the sports season. *Physiol Behav* 62:811-814.

Eschbach, J.W., Aquiling, T., Haley, N.R., Fan, M.H., and Blagg, C.R. 1992. The long-term effects of recombinant human erythropoietin on the cardiovascular system. *Clin Nephrol* 38(suppl 1):S98-S103.

Eschbach, J.W., Haley, N.R., Egrie, J.C., and Adamson, J.W. 1992. A comparison of the responses to recombinant human erythropoietin in normal and uremic subjects. *Kidney Internat* 42:407-416.

Fogelholm, M., Jaakkola, L., and Lampisjarvi, T. 1992. Effects of iron supplementation in female athletes with low serum ferritin concentration. *Int J Sports Med* 13:158-162.

Gareau, R., Brisson, G.R., Ayotte, C., Dube, J., and Caron, C. 1992. Erythropoietin doping in athletes: Possible detection through measurement of fibrinolytic products. *Thromb Haemost* 68(4):481-482.

Guthrie, M., Cardenas, D., Eschbach, J.W., Haley, N.R., and Robertson, H.T. 1993. Effects of erythropoietin on strength and functional status of patients on hemodialysis. *Clin Nephrol* 39:97-102.

Kanstrup, I.L., and Ekblom, B. 1984. Blood volume and hemoglobin concentration as determinants of maximal aerobic power. *Med Sci Sports Exerc* 16:256-262.

Matter, M., Stittfall, T., Graves, J., Myburgh, K., Adams, B., Jacobs, P., and Noakes, T.D. 1987. The effect of iron and folate therapy on maximal exercise performance in female marathon runners with iron and folate deficiency. *Clin Sci* 72:415-422.

McMahon, L.F., Ryan, M.J., Larson, D., and Fisher, R.L. 1984. Occult gastrointestinal blood loss in marathon runners. *Ann Intern Med* 100:846-848.

Mechrefe, A., Wexler, B., and Feller, E. 1997. Sports anemia and gastrointestinal bleeding in endurance athletes. *Med Health RI* 80:216-218.

Moses, F.M. 1993. Gastrointestinal bleeding and the athlete. *Am J Gastroenterol* 88:1157-1159.

Newhouse, I.J., and Clement, D.B. 1988. Iron status in athletes: An update. *Sports Med* 5:337-352.

Newhouse, I.J., Clement, D.B., Taunton, J.E., and McKenzie, D.C. 1989. The effects of prelatent/latent iron deficiency on physical work capacity. *Med Sci Sports Exerc* 21:263-268.

Nielsen, P., and Nachtigall, D. 1998. Iron supplementation in athletes. Current recommendations. *Sports Med* 26:207-216.

Pahor, M., Guralnik, J.M., Salive, M.E., Chrischilles, E.A., Brown, S.O., and Wallace, R.B. 1994. Physical activity and risk of severe gastrointestinal hemorrhage in older persons. *JAMA* 272:595-599.

Pascual, J., Teruel, J.L., and Ortuno, J. 1991. Hypertensive effect of erythropoietin. *Ann Intern Med* 114:1063.

Raunikar, R.A., and Sabio, H. 1992. Anemia in the adolescent athlete. *Am J Dis Child* 146(10):1201-1205.

Remacha, A.F., Ordonez, J., Barcelo, M.J., Garcia-Die, F., Arza, B., and Estruch, A. 1994. Evaluation of erythropoietin in endurance runners. *Haematologica* 79:350-352.

Roberts, D., and Smith, D.J. 1996. Erythropoietin does not demonstrate circadian rhythm in healthy men. *J Appl Physiol* 80:847-851.

Robertson, H.T., Haley, N.R., Guthrie, M., Cardenas, D., Eschbach, J.W., and Adamson, J.W. 1990. Recombinant erythropoietin improves exercise capacity in anemic hemodialysis patients. *Am J Kidney Dis* 15:325-332.

Rudzki, S.J., Hazard, H., and Collinson, D. 1995. Gastrointestinal blood loss in triathletes: Its etiology and relationship to sports anaemia. *Aust J Sci Med Sport* 27(1):3-8.

Schoene, R.B., Escourrou, P., Robertson, H.T., Nilson, K.L., Parsons, J.R., and Smith, N.J. 1983. Iron repletion decreases maximal exercise lactate concentrations in female athletes with minimal iron-deficiency anemia. *J Lab Clin Med* 102:306-312.

Schwandt, H.J., Heyduck, B., Gunga, H.C., and Rocker, L. 1991. Influence of prolonged physical exercise on the erythropoietin concentration in blood. *Eur J Appl Physiol* 63:463-466.

Souillard, A., Audran, M., Bressolle, F., Gareau, R., Duvallet, A., and Chanal, J.L. 1996. Pharmacokinetics and pharmacodynamics of recombinant human erythropoietin in athletes. Blood sampling and doping control. *Br J Clin Pharmacol* 42:355-364.

Stewart, J.G., Ahlquist, D.A., McGill, D.B., Ilstrup, D.M., Schartz, S., and Owen, R.A. 1984. Gastrointestinal blood loss and anemia in runners. *Ann Intern Med* 100:843-845.

Tasaki, T., Ohto, H., Hashimoto, C., Abe, R., Saitoh, A., and Kikuchi, S. 1992. Recombinant human erythropoietin for autologous blood donation: Effects on perioperative red-blood-cell and serum erythropoietin production. *Lancet* 339:773-775.

Vedovato, M., De Paoli Vitali, E., Guglielmini, C., Casoni, I., Ricci, G., and Masotti, M. 1988. Erythropoietin in athletes of endurance events. *Nephron* 48:78-79.

Weight, L.M., Klein, M., Noakes, T.D., and Jacobs, P. 1992. 'Sports anemia'—A real or apparent phenomenon in endurance-trained athletes? *Int J Sports Med* 13:344-347.

Wide, L., Bengtsson, C., Berglund, B., and Ekblom, B. 1995. Detection in blood and urine of recombinant erythropoietin administered to healthy men. *Med Sci Sports Exerc* 27:1569-1576.

10
CHAPTER

Antilipemic Agents

■ *CASE*   Harry is a 52-year-old, deconditioned man who is taking lovastatin (Mevacor) to treat hypercholesterolemia. He makes a New Year's resolution to exercise more. During the first week he plays racquetball twice, rides a stationary bicycle, and lifts weights, doing squats and leg extensions. During his second week he tries to jog, but stops after barely getting started, complaining that his legs are sore. The next day his legs are too sore to exercise at all. He calls you (his physician) and states that he read in the *Physician's Desk Reference* that lovastatin can cause muscle soreness; he wants to know if he should stop taking it. You are aware that lovastatin has been reported to cause myopathy, but are puzzled because Harry has been taking this drug for nearly 12 months without any problems. Although you don't believe that the drug is to blame, you wonder if the combined effects of strenuous exercise and lovastatin may have precipitated something more than just normal postexercise muscle soreness.

■ *COMMENT*   At least three possible explanations exist. Strenuous exercise and lovastatin therapy have both been independently associated with myopathy. First, then, it should not be surprising that a deconditioned individual like Harry develops problems after such an abrupt increase in his exercise routine. Even in young, moderately fit males not taking lovastatin, significant elevations of creatine kinase (CK) have been reported. But second, the fact that Harry has been taking lovastatin for a sustained period without any adverse effects should not make you overlook a drug-induced cause. Dozens of cases of lovastatin-induced myopathy—independent of exercise—have been reported in the medical literature. In these cases, the onset of this serious adverse reaction occurred from within a few days of drug therapy to after more than 12 months of drug therapy. Although the patients in most of these reports were receiving other drugs concomitantly, lovastatin-induced myopathy can occur without any concomitant drugs. Third, it is possible that the combination of exercise and lovastatin therapy is to blame (see later discussion for additional details). Whatever the cause, Harry should have a blood test for CK. Until then, he should be instructed to drink plenty of fluids to maintain a dilute urine in case myoglobinuria should develop.

According to the American Heart Association, coronary heart disease killed 466,101 U.S. citizens in 1997 (1997 Heart and Stroke Facts, American Heart Association Web site). Although some individuals debate the overall contribution of exercise in reducing coronary disease risk (see Curfman 1993), substantial data suggest that exercise is beneficial (Lakka et al. 1994; Leon et al. 1987; Morris et al. 1990; Young et al. 1993). However, roughly only one-quarter of the U.S. population exercises regularly (McGinnis and Lee 1995). In addition, when one considers the disappointing exercise level of high schoolers (Heath et al. 1994) and the eating patterns of children and teenagers (Munoz et al. 1997), it appears the problem is far from being resolved.

Hyperlipidemia is a risk factor for cardiovascular disease. After diet and exercise, drug therapy is the primary treatment modality for hyperlipidemias. Nearly 55 million prescriptions were dispensed in 1997 for cholesterol-reducing drugs (Gebhart 1998). This figure is up from 35 million just two years prior (Glaser 1996), making cholesterol-reducing drugs one of the top therapeutic categories driving industry growth (Gebhart 1998). Unfortunately, it appears that these drugs, though effective, are not being used appropriately. A UCLA study revealed that 51% of primary care physicians had not used diet therapy before initiating drug therapy and that 29% did not use diet therapy in conjunction with drug therapy as recommended by the National Cholesterol Education Program (Barnard, DiLauro, and Inkeles 1997). This is unfortunate because diet plus exercise can be just as effective as drug therapy in the management of moderate hypercholesterolemia (Nomura et al. 1996). If we are successful in encouraging more people to exercise, then, considering these statistics, it seems likely that many patients will be exercising while taking antilipemic drugs. Thus, it is clearly worthwhile to consider the implications of the interaction between these therapeutic modalities.

Antilipemic Agents

Drugs available for the treatment of hyperlipidemias fall into the general categories shown in table 10.1.

In clinical medicine, by far the most important group of lipid-lowering drugs are those that inhibit the hepatic enzyme 3-hydroxy-3-methylglutaryl-coenzyme A (HMG-CoA) reductase. These drugs are potent antilipemics that have been associated with reducing cardiovascular mortality and are generally well tolerated. Gemfibrozil, nicotinic acid, and the bile-acid sequesterants are also used regularly, but dextrothyroxine is not. Acipimox and bezafibrate are available in the United Kingdom, but not in the United States. Probucol was removed

Table 10.1   Antilipemic Agents

Bile acid sequesterants	HMG-CoA-reductase inhibitors
Cholestyramine (Questran)	Atorvastatin (Lipitor)
Colestipol (Colestid)	Cerivastatin (Baycol)
Fibric acid derivatives	Fluvastatin (Lescol)
Bezafibrate*	Lovastatin (Mevacor)
Clofibrate (Atromid-S)	Pravastatin (Pravachol)
Fenofibrate (Tricor)	Simvastatin (Zocor)
Gemfibrozil (Lopid)	**Nicotinic acid derivatives**
	Acipimox*
	Nicotinic acid (niacin)
	Other
	Dextrothyroxine (Choloxin)
	Probucol (Lorelco)*

* Not available in the United States

from the U.S. market in 1995 and is mentioned here only for completeness.

How Exercise Affects the Action of Antilipemic Agents

No data are available describing the effects of exercise on the pharmacokinetics of antilipemic agents. The HMG-CoA-reductase inhibitors all undergo a significant "first pass" effect; they can therefore be considered high-extraction-ratio drugs. Plasma concentrations of high-extraction-ratio drugs increase during endurance exercise due to the acute drop in hepatic blood flow. It remains to be determined, however, if exercise actually inhibits the clearance and increases the toxicity of the HMG-CoA-reductase inhibitors.

In general, both exercise and lipid-lowering agents exert beneficial effects on serum lipids. A lot of information is available about the effects of endurance exercise on the pharmacology of antilipemic drugs, but few data exist yet about the effects of strength training. High-density lipoprotein (HDL) cholesterol concentrations in female distance runners, for instance, are proportional to weekly distance run (Williams 1996), but 12 weeks of resistance training did not change lipid levels in obese, sedentary females despite a significant improvement in strength

Table 10.2 Effects of Exercise and Antilipemic Drugs on Plasma Lipids

	Total cholesterol	HDL cholesterol	LDL cholesterol	Triglycerides
Aerobic exercise (athletes)	D	I	D	D
Strength exercise	None	None	None	None
Bile acid sequesterants	D	None	D	None
HMG-CoA-reductase inhibitors	D	I	D	D
Fibric acid derivatives	D	I	D/I	D
Nicotinic acid	D	I	D	D

I = serum concentration is increased
D = serum concentration is decreased
None = no change seen

(Manning et al. 1991). A cross-sectional study of more than 6,000 men and women not currently involved in weight training revealed no association between muscular strength and serum total cholesterol or low-density lipoprotein (LDL) cholesterol, but the researchers did find a direct association between muscle strength and serum triglycerides in males. These authors concluded that muscular strength had no beneficial effect, and perhaps even had a detrimental effect, on lipid and lipoprotein status (Kohl et al. 1992). Table 10.2 summarizes the effects of exercise on plasma lipids. Note that, due to exercise-induced changes in plasma volume (Convertino 1991), some controversy exists about observed changes in serum concentrations of lipid fractions with long-term exercise.

How Antilipemic Agents Affect Exercisers

Complex metabolic pathways mobilize and metabolize lipids for energy. This summary of the actions is intended to help readers understand how antilipemic drugs might affect the utilization of lipids for energy demands during sustained exercise. *Exercise Metabolism* (1995) by Mark Hargreaves is a good source for more information on the topic of lipid metabolism in exercise.

Carbohydrates are the preferential fuel for high-intensity anaerobic work, whereas fats are utilized primarily during very low intensity aerobic exercise (Hagerman 1992). It has been known for some time that the oxidation of free fatty acids (FFAs) provides most of the energy for

Table 10.3   Body Stores of Fuels and Energy

	g	kcal
Carbohydrates		
Liver glycogen	110	451
Muscle glycogen	250	1,025
Glucose in body fluids	15	62
Total	375	1,538
Fat		
Subcutaneous	7,800	70,980
Intramuscular	161	1,465
Total	7,961	72,445

These estimates are based on an average body weight of 65 kg with 12% body fat.
Adapted from Wilmore and Costill 1994.

prolonged submaximal exercise (Hagerman 1992). In contrast to carbohydrate sources, bodily reserves of fat are practically unlimited. Bjorntorp
(1991) calculated that even elite athletes have several kilograms of body
fat, enough to provide energy for many hours of athletic activity (see
table 10.3; Wilmore and Costill 1994) As submaximal exercise progresses,
FFA concentrations increase in response to lipolysis. Eagles and colleagues (Eagles, Kendall, and Maxwell 1996; Eagles and Kendall 1997)
have conducted some revealing studies of the effects of antilipemic
agents on fat oxidation during exercise. These studies clearly show how
reliance on fats as an energy substrate increases as the duration of
submaximal exercise progresses.
    Lipid stores for energy utilization during prolonged exercise are
available as (a) triglycerides in adipose tissue, (b) triglycerides in muscle,
and (c) circulating triglycerides. Some exercise scientists claim that
adipose tissue stores are most important in exercise physiology
(Economos, Bortz, and Nelson 1993). Others point to intramuscular
triglycerides (Turcotte, Richter, and Kiens 1995; Hagerman 1992; Hurley
et al. 1986) or to albumin-bound FFAs (Havel, Pernow, and Jones 1967).
Since plasma FFA oxidation does not match estimates of total lipid
oxidation, however, intramuscular triglycerides must also be an important source of energy during prolonged exercise (Turcotte, Richter, and
Kiens 1995). In addition, since fat stores are more than adequate for any
exercise event, it seems that the mobilization and utilization of energy
from these fat stores are critical factors in meeting energy demands

during prolonged aerobic exercise. When fat stores are broken down for energy, one triglyceride molecule first yields three fatty acids and one molecule of glycerol. Of these two by-products, glycerol is the better parameter to monitor when determining the rate of adipose tissue lipolysis. Glycerol appears in the blood only as a product of lipolysis, while FFAs can be re-esterified. Thus, FFA concentrations represent the dynamic balance between production and re-uptake (Turcotte, Richter, and Kiens 1995).

Lipoprotein lipase (LPL) is an enzyme attached to the luminal endothelial lining of blood vessel cells that facilitates the breakdown and release of triglycerides into FFAs and glycerol. Lipoprotein lipase controls how much fat is captured and stored in adipocytes, but, more importantly, it hydrolyzes the triglyceride core of circulating chylomicrons into smaller units that muscle cells can utilize for energy needs. Much of the glycerol liberated by LPL is transported to the liver and kidney, where it is used to make glucose. Most of the FFAs, on the other hand, are taken up by muscle and adipose cells in the vicinity of the LPL. Muscle cells use the FFAs for energy, while adipose cells re-esterify the FFAs with intracellular glycerol into new triglyceride molecules. This metabolic pathway is highly dynamic, and it reflects both quantity of substrate and activity of enzyme. Higher concentrations of FFAs in the bloodstream lead to greater use of fat as an energy source by muscle. In addition, endurance exercise training stimulates the activity of lipolytic enzymes. A strenuous exercise program (i.e., 6 days a week of alternating cycling and running over 12 weeks) produced a 90% increase in beta-hydroxyacyl-CoA-dehydrogenase activity in the quadriceps muscles of 9 healthy males (Hurley et al. 1986). Kantor and colleagues (1984) found that lipoprotein lipase activity nearly doubled after a 42 km footrace.

Lipoprotein lipase should not be confused with hormone-sensitive lipases (HSLs), which constitute a group of intracellular adipose cell enzymes. Hormone-sensitive lipase liberates fatty acids from storage in adipose cells when fatty acids are needed. Epinephrine, glucagon, growth hormone, and other hormones of minor significance stimulate the activity of HSL. Only catecholamines (in this case, epinephrine) can stimulate lipolysis at physiological concentrations; so it is easy to see why beta-receptor antagonists (e.g., propranolol) would induce detrimental effects on endurance exercise (see chapter 1).

Although the antilipemic drugs exhibit multiple mechanisms of action, and some of their effects are not clearly understood, in general they follow the actions listed in table 10.4.

Several groups of investigators have evaluated how drugs active at each of these sites affect the rate of fat oxidation during sustained exercise. Head and colleagues (1993) compared simvastatin (an inhibi-

Table 10.4　Mechanisms of Action Associated With Specific Drug Groups

Drug group	Mechanism of action	Site
HMG-CoA-reductase inhibitors	Inhibit HMG-CoA reductase	Hepatocyte
Fibric acid derivatives	Stimulate LPL	Vascular endothelial cell surface
Nicotinic acid, acipimox	Inhibit HSL	Adipocyte

LPL = lipoprotein lipase
HSL = hormone sensitive lipase

tor of HMG-CoA reductase), gemfibrozil (a fibric acid derivative that stimulates LPL), and acipimox (a nicotinic acid derivative that inhibits HSL) in young, healthy male volunteers. All three drugs were administered for 5 days continuously. Then subjects were exercised at 50% $\dot{V}O_2$max for 120 min by walking on a treadmill. Investigators found that the HMG-CoA-reductase inhibitor produced no significant changes on fat oxidation. Both gemfibrozil and acipimox impaired fat oxidation; however, only the effects of acipimox were statistically significant (see figures 10.1–10.3). The authors did not relate fat oxidation measurements to any aspect of athletic performance in this study.

Eagles, Kendall, and Maxwell (1996) conducted a similar experiment using a HMG-CoA-reductase inhibitor (fluvastatin) and a fibric acid derivative (bezafibrate) in healthy volunteers. After 21 days of drug administration, fluvastatin had no effect on fat metabolism during 90 min of exercise at 50% $\dot{V}O_2$max, but bezafibrate decreased fat oxidation and decreased FFA concentrations compared to both fluvastatin and to placebo. These metabolic observations did not affect exercise performance; perceived exertion did not differ between treatment groups.

How Antilipemic Agents Affect Exercise Performance

Only two studies have assessed the effects of antilipemic drugs on exercise performance; their findings are consistent with the known metabolic effects of these drugs. Thompson and colleagues (1991) found that exercise performance was not impaired by 4 weeks of lovastatin administration in 20 moderately fit subjects who were exercised to

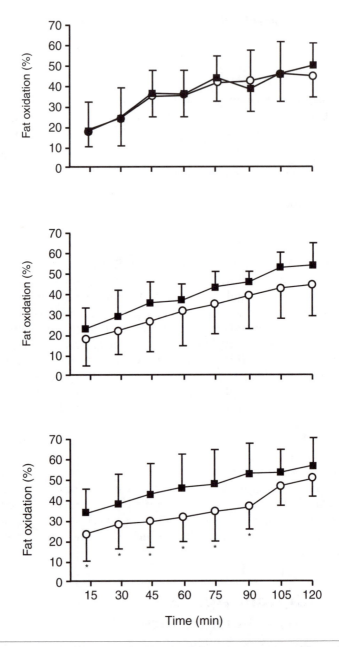

Figure 10.1   Percent fat contribution toward total energy expenditure during 120 min of exercise at 50% $\dot{V}O_2$max with drug (○) and with placebo (■). Values are mean ± *SD*; *n* = 8. *(top)* Simvastatin; *(middle)* gemfibrozil; *(bottom)* acipimox. * = Significantly different between drug and placebo, *p* < 0.05.

Adapted from Head et al. 1993.

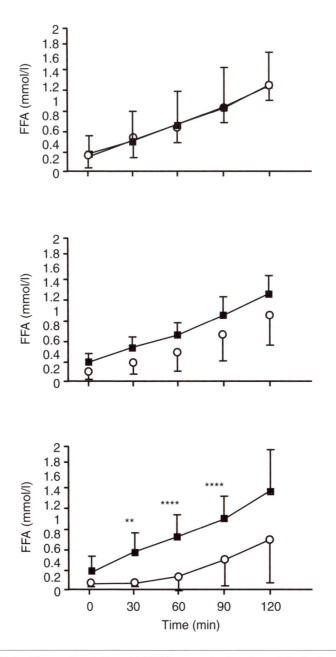

Figure 10.2 Plasma free fatty acid (FFA) concentration (mmol/l) during 120 min of exercise at 50% V̇O₂max with drug (○) and with placebo (■). Values are mean ± *SD*; *n* = 8. *(top)* Simvastatin; *(middle)*, gemfibrozil; *(bottom)* acipimox.
** = $p < 0.01$;
**** = $p < 0.0001$.

Adapted from Head et al. 1993.

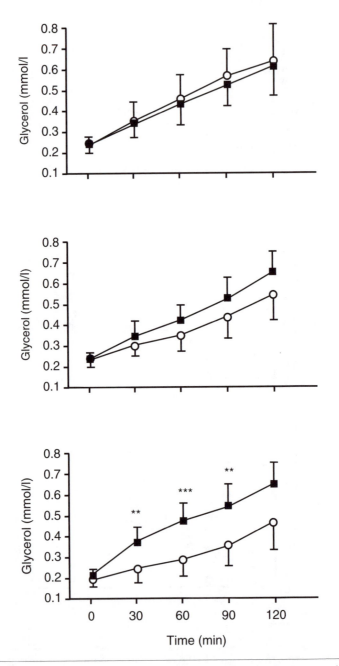

Figure 10.3 Plasma glycerol concentration (mmol/l) during 120 min of exercise at 50% $\dot{V}O_2$max with drug (○) and with placebo (■). Values are mean ± *SD*; *n* = 8. *(top)* Simvastatin; *(middle)* gemfibrozil; *(bottom)* acipimox. ** = *p* < 0.01; *** = *p* < 0.001.

Adapted from Head et al. 1993.

Table 10.5 Exercise Results Before and During Lovastatin Therapy

	Men		Women	
	No drug	Lovastatin	No drug	Lovastatin
Treadmill time (min)	19.7 ± 2.57	19.7 ± 2.70	17.0 ± 4.33	17.0 ± 4.33
MET level	10.8 ± 1.39	10.8 ± 1.39	8.0 ± 1.82	8.0 ± 1.82
Peak HR (bpm)	160 ± 19.7	158 ± 20.1	165 ± 18.0	166 ± 21.8

All values are mean ± SD. There are no significant differences between conditions using a paired *t* test. HR = heart rate; MET = multiple of the resting metabolic rate. Adapted from Thompson et al. 1991.

volitional fatigue after maximal effort on a treadmill (see table 10.5). Although rates of fat oxidation were not measured in this study, the absence of any detrimental effect on exercise performance by lovastatin would be consistent with its (absence of) metabolic effects as described earlier.

Cardiac patients frequently take beta-blocker drugs and antilipemic drugs and are encouraged to walk. Consequently, Eagles and Kendall (1997) later examined the combined effects of beta-blockade and antilipemic agents on fat oxidation in young, healthy volunteers. Subjects were given either atenolol or sustained-release metoprolol in combination with either bezafibrate or fluvastatin. They walked on a treadmill at 50% $\dot{V}O_2$max for 90 min. The investigators found that bezafibrate-containing regimens exerted a greater detrimental effect on fat oxidation than fluvastatin-containing regimens. All four drug combinations exerted negative effects on subjective feelings during exercise, to a significant level compared with placebo (Eagles and Kendall 1997). Thus, this study further implies that drugs that impair fat oxidation may also exert undesirable effects on exercise performance.

Despite these reports, the relationship between the metabolic effects of antilipemic agents and exercise performance has yet to be conclusively demonstrated. Epinephrine is a potent stimulant of adipose tissue lipolysis, and this action is thought to be mediated via beta-1 adrenergic receptors (Turcotte, Richter, and Kiens 1995). Beta-adrenergic blockers interfere with epinephrine binding to beta-receptors. At least this is one clear explanation of how beta-blockers contribute to early fatigue in endurance exercise. Since Eagles and Kendall (1997) assessed the effects of antilipemic agents administered in combination with beta-blockers, however, one cannot be certain that a drug-drug interaction (i.e., a

Table 10.6 Antilipemic Agents and Aerobic Performance

Drug	Performance variable	Effect	Reference
Bezafibrate	Perceived exertion	None	Eagles, Kendall, and Maxwell 1996
Fluvastatin	Perceived exertion	None	Eagles, Kendall, and Maxwell 1996
Lovastatin	Exercise duration	None	Thompson et al. 1991
Lovastatin	Total workload	None	Thompson et al. 1991
Nicotinic acid	Perceived exertion	Worsened	Bergstrom 1969

pharmacokinetic mechanism)—for example, between the beta-blocker and the antilipemic drug—explains the observed physiologic effects in their study. In general, it appears that HMG-CoA-reductase inhibitors do not exert negative effects on endurance exercise, but fibric acid derivatives and nicotinic acid derivatives may. The effects of these drugs on strength have not been studied. Data about the effects of antilipemic agents on aerobic performance are summarized in table 10.6.

The effects of antilipemic agents on exercise performance deserve further study inasmuch as many deconditioned individuals are likely to take these drugs while exercising.

Avoiding Potential Complications

Exercise-induced muscle injury is important to consider in subjects taking antilipemic drugs because some of these agents have been associated with myopathy independently of intense exercise. In addition, Evans and colleagues (1986) showed that postexercise CK levels are higher in untrained than in trained individuals. At least 25 cases of lovastatin-induced myopathy have been reported in the medical literature. The onset of this serious adverse reaction varied, occurring in individuals having continuous drug therapy for just a few days to more than 12 months. Lovastatin-induced myopathy has been reported both with (Wallace and Mueller 1992) and without any concomitant drugs (Thompson et al. 1991). At least three reports attempt to describe the potential for increased risk of myopathy if subjects exercise while taking HMG-CoA-reductase inhibitors. In 1990, Thompson, Nugent, and Herbert observed substantial elevations in CK in 4 subjects who engaged in strenuous exercise while taking either fluvastatin or lovastatin (see table 10.7). All four subjects who were affected were male, but their ages were not

■ *Muscle Injury in Healthy Individuals*

In a bizarre ritual of prison hazing, a 21-year-old deconditioned male had to repeatedly perform deep knee bends to maneuver chess pieces lined up on the floor. After 100 squats, the prisoner could not continue. Within 12 hours, he was bedridden with severe anterior thigh pain. His urine was positive for both protein and occult blood, and his initial creatine phosphokinase (CK) was 160,000 U/L. A diagnosis of exercise-induced rhabdomyolysis and myoglobinuria was made. He was treated and recovered (Frucht 1994).

In another study, investigators observed persistent CK elevations in 10 moderately fit males who had been subjected to jogging for 2 h daily at 78% maximum heart rate for 7 consecutive days (Dressendorfer et al. 1991). These cases demonstrate how abrupt changes in exercise intensity may lead to muscle injury even in young adults or trained athletes.

specified. The other participants were subsequently advised not to engage in strenuous exercise for the duration of the study and no additional problems were noted (Thompson, Nugent, and Herbert 1990).

These chance observations prompted the investigators to conduct a prospective study. Twenty older, moderately fit men and women received lovastatin 20 mg/day for 4 weeks; then they took a maximum treadmill test. In this case, average CK concentrations increased, though

Table 10.7   Increase in Creatine Kinase After Exercise in Four Patients Using HMG-CoA-Reductase Inhibitors

Patient	Average placebo CK, U/L[a]	Post-exercise CK, U/L	Drug[b]	Symptoms
1	60	2050	Fluvastatin, 40 mg	None
2	119	577	Fluvastatin, 40 mg	None
3	49	21,400	Lovastatin, 40 mg	Severe muscle pain
4	53	646	Lovastatin, 20 mg	None

[a] = based on four samples. CK indicates creatine kinase.
[b] = indicates daily dose.
U/L = units per liter
Adapted from Thompson, Nugent, and Herbert 1990.

not significantly, after lovastatin—compared with results from a similar exercise test given prior to lovastatin administration. The increase during lovastatin was due mainly to results from 2 male subjects (ages not specified) who had substantial CK elevations. Neither subject noted symptoms. When data from men were compared with those from women, it appeared CK rose more in the male than in the female patients, although these changes were not statistically significant (see table 10.8; Thompson et al. 1991).

Table 10.8   Total CK and Isoenzyme Levels Relative to Lovastatin Treatment and Exercise

	Change		
	Pre	Post	24 h post
Men			
CK			
No drug	146 ± 69	6 ± 20	4 ± 30
Lovastatin	162 ± 68	10 ± 12	33 ± 115
CK-MM			
No drug	146 ± 66	5 ± 20	4 ± 29
Lovastatin	161 ± 68	10 ± 12	32 ± 114
CK-MB			
No drug	3 ± 3	1 ± 2	0 ± 4
Lovastatin	1 ± 2	0 ± 1	1 ± 4
Women			
CK			
No drug	88 ± 22	6 ± 9	−2 ± 16
Lovastatin	87 ± 22	−1 ± 11	2 ± 31
CK-MM			
No drug	87 ± 21	6 ± 9	−1 ± 15
Lovastatin	86 ± 22	−1 ± 11	2 ± 31
CK-MB			
No drug	1 ± 2	0 ± 0	−1 ± 2
Lovastatin	1 ± 1	0 ± 1	0 ± 1

All values are mean ± SD. There are no significant differences using Wilcoxon's signed rank test for pair-wise comparisons and Bonferroni's correction.

Adapted from Thompson et al. 1991.

Reust, Curry, and Guidry (1991) subjected 10 young males to 1 h of downhill walking after administering lovastatin 40 mg/day for 1 month. With each subject serving as his own control, no changes were seen in postexercise CK values. The age of the men in the Reust study was 27 or 28 years, while the average age of the men in the Thompson study was 52 years. Reust admitted that their subjects were medical residents who were used to walking stairs routinely, and the age and conditioning factors may have played a role in their not observing any difference between the lovastatin and placebo parts of the study.

Fibric acid derivatives have also been associated with myopathy. Nine cases of asymptomatic increases in serum CK were observed in 7 volunteers in a study of bezafibrate, clofibrate, fenofibrate, and probucol (4 with clofibrate, 3 with fenofibrate, 2 with bezafibrate, none with probucol; some subjects took more than one drug). The exercise levels of these subjects were not provided, but all were healthy males, 20 to 30 years old. None were symptomatic (Heller and Harvengt 1983). Clofibrate-induced myopathy has been reported. Only two of five cases were symptomatic in one report. Again, the exercise level was not provided, and the subjects were in their 20s and 30s (Langer and Levy 1968).

In summary, although data are sketchy, it appears that the combination of drug therapy and lipid-lowering agents, particularly HMG-CoA-reductase inhibitors, taken by individuals who engage in strenuous exercise might increase the risk for myopathy, particularly among older males. The antilipemic agents associated with myopathy are bezafibrate, clofibrate, fenofibrate, fluvastatin, lovastatin, and simvastatin. Fibric-acid derivatives have also been associated with myopathy, although it is unclear if exercising while taking these drugs increases this risk.

NCAA and USOC Status

None of the antilipemic agents are banned by the NCAA or USOC (Fuentes and Rosenberg 1999), which might be expected since none of these drugs appear to exhibit any ergogenic properties. Indeed, some of the agents appear to be ergolytic. Due to the potential for muscle injury, however, some individuals (e.g., older males) may want to be cautious about exercising while taking HMG-CoA-reductase inhibitors.

Guidelines for Use

Acipimox, a derivative of nicotinic acid, has been shown to impair fat oxidation more than other types of lipid-lowering agents. Since acipimox's actions and adverse reactions are similar to those of nicotinic acid, it can be assumed that nicotinic acid also exerts detrimental effects on fat oxidation. Both acipimox and nicotinic acid should be avoided if possible in individuals who wish to partake in sustained aerobic exercise, since impairment of fat oxidation may adversely affect exercise performance. These people should also be counseled accordingly. Acipimox is available in the United Kingdom but not in the United States.

While it is always wise to avoid abrupt increases in exercise intensity, deconditioned patients taking HMG-CoA-reductase inhibitors (particularly older males) should be cautioned about weightlifting or any other strenuous exercise in order to minimize the development of myopathy. Sports medicine specialists should consider complaints of muscle soreness from exercising individuals who are taking this type of drug as being potentially serious until proved otherwise. HMG-CoA-reductase inhibitors do not appear to affect exercise performance, however.

Although the combination of exercise and antilipemic drug therapy can cause problems, don't let these overshadow the potential health benefits of exercise. You still should encourage exercise—in appropriate amounts—in all subjects, regardless of whether they are taking antilipemic drugs. Indeed, regular exercise may eliminate the need for antilipemic drugs!

References

Barnard, R.J., DiLauro, S.C., and Inkeles, S.B. 1997. Effects of intensive diet and exercise intervention in patients taking cholesterol-lowering drugs. *Am J Cardiol* 79:1112-1114.

Bergstrom, J., Hultman, E., Jorfeldt, L., Pernow, B., and Wahren, J. 1969. Effect of nicotinic acid on physical working capacity and on metabolism of muscle glycogen in man. *J Appl Physiol* 26(2):170-176.

Bjorntorp, P. 1991. Importance of fat as a support nutrient for energy: Metabolism of athletes. *J Sports Sci* 9:71-76.

Convertino, V.A. 1991. Blood volume: Its adaptation to endurance training. *Med Sci Sports Exerc* 23:1338-1348.

Curfman, G.D. 1993. The health benefits of exercise: A critical reappraisal. *N Engl J Med* 328:574-576.

Dressendorfer, R.H., Wade, C.E., Claybaugh, J., Cucinell, S.A., and Timmis, G.C. 1991. Effects of 7 successive days of unaccustomed prolonged exercise on aerobic performance and tissue damage in fitness joggers. *Int J Sports Med* 12:55-61.

Eagles, C.J., and Kendall, M.J. 1997. The effects of combined treatment with beta 1-selective receptor antagonists and lipid-lowering drugs on fat metabolism and measures of fatigue during moderate intensity exercise: A placebo-controlled study in healthy subjects. *Br J Clin Pharmacol* 43:291-300.

Eagles, C.J., Kendall, M.J., and Maxwell, S. 1996. A comparison of the effects of fluvastatin and bezafibrate on exercise metabolism: A placebo-controlled study in healthy normolipidaemic subjects. *Br J Clin Pharmacol* 41:381-387.

Economos, C.D., Bortz, S.S., and Nelson, M.E. 1993. Nutritional practices of elite athletes. *Sports Med* 16:381-399.

Evans, W.J., Meredith, C.N., Cannon, J.G., Dinarello, C.A., Frontera, W.R., Hughes, V.A., Jones, B.H., and Knuttgen, H.G. 1986. Metabolic changes following eccentric exercise in trained and untrained men. *J Appl Physiol* 61:1864-1868.

Frucht, M. 1994. Challenge, 110 deep knee bends; reward, rhabdomyolysis. *N Engl J Med* 330:1620-1621.

Fuentes, R.J., and Rosenberg, J.M. 1999. *Athletic Drug Reference '99*. Durham, NC: Clean Data.

Gebhart, F. 1998. Annual Rx survey. The new golden age. *Drug Topics*, 16 March, 71-83.

Glaser, M. 1996. Annual Rx survey. *Drug Topics*, 8 April, 97-104.

Hagerman, F.C. 1992. Energy metabolism and fuel utilization. *Med Sci Sports Exerc* 24:S309-S314.

Hargreaves, M., ed. 1995. *Exercise metabolism*. Champaign, IL: Human Kinetics.

Havel, R.J., Pernow, B., and Jones, N.L. 1967. Uptake and release of free fatty acids and other metabolites in the legs of exercising men. *J Appl Physiol* 23:90-99.

Head, A., Jakeman, P.M., Kendall, M.J., Cramb, R., and Maxwell, S. 1993. The impact of a short course of three lipid lowering drugs on fat oxidation during exercise in healthy volunteers. *Postgrad Med J* 69:197-203.

Heath, G.W., Pratt, M., Warren, C.W., and Kann, L. 1994. Physical activity patterns in American high school students: Results from the 1990 Youth Risk Behavior Survey. *Arch Pediatr Adolesc Med* 148:1131-1136.

Heller, F., and Harvengt, C. 1983. Effects of clofibrate, bezafibrate, fenofibrate and probucol on plasma lipolytic enzymes in normolipaemic subjects. *Eur J Clin Pharmacol* 25:57-63.

Hurley, B.F., Nemeth, P.M., Martin, W.H., Hagberg, J.M., Dalsky, G.P., and Holloszy, J.O. 1986. Muscle triglyceride utilization during exercise: Effect of training. *J Appl Physiol* 60:562-567.

Kantor, M.A., Cullinane, E.M., Herbert, P.N., and Thompson, P.D. 1984. Acute increase in lipoprotein lipase following prolonged exercise. *Metabolism* 33:454-457.

Kohl, H.W., Gordon, N.F., Scott, C.S., Vaandrager, H., and Blair, S.N. 1992. Musculoskeletal strength and serum lipid levels in men and women. *Med Sci Sports Exerc* 24:1080-1087.

Lakka, T.A., Venalainen, J.M., Rauramaa, R., Salonen, R., Tuomilehto, J., and Salonen, J.T. 1994. Relation of leisure-time physical activity and cardiorespiratory fitness to the risk of acute myocardial infarction in men. *N Engl J Med* 330:1549-1554.

Langer, T., and Levy, R.I. 1968. Acute muscular syndrome associated with administration of clofibrate. *N Engl J Med* 279:856-858.

Leon, A.S., Connett, J., Jacobs Jr., D.R., and Rauramaa, R. 1987. Leisure-time physical activity levels and risk of coronary heart disease and death: The Multiple Risk Factor Intervention Trial. *JAMA* 258:2388-2395.

Manning, J.M., Dooly-Manning, C.R., White, K., Kampa, I., Silas, S., Kesselhaut, M., and Ruoff, M. 1991. Effect of a resistive training program on lipoprotein-lipid levels in obese women. *Med Sci Sports Exerc* 23:1222-1226.

McGinnis, J.M., and Lee, P.R. 1995. Healthy People 2000 at mid decade. *JAMA* 273:1123-1129.

Morris, J.N., Clayton, D.G., Everitt, M.G., Semmence, A.M., and Burgess, E.H. 1990. Exercise in leisure time: Coronary attack and death rates. *Br Heart J* 63:325-334.

Munoz, K.A., Krebs-Smith, S.M., Ballard-Barbash, R., and Cleveland, L.E. 1997. Food intakes of U.S. children and adolescents compared with recommendations. *Pediatrics* 100:323-329.

Nomura, H., Kimura, Y., Okamoto, O., and Shiraishi, G. 1996. Effects of antihyperlipidemic drugs and diet plus exercise therapy in the treatment of patients with moderate hypercholesterolemia. *Clin Ther* 18:477-482.

Reust, C.S., Curry, S.C., and Guidry, J.R. 1991. Lovastatin use and muscle damage in healthy volunteers undergoing eccentric muscle exercise. *West J Med* 154:198-200.

Thompson, P.D., Gadaleta, P.A., Yurgalevitch, S., Cullinane, E., and Herbert, P.N. 1991. Effects of exercise and lovastatin on serum creatine kinase activity. *Metabolism* 40:1333-1336.

Thompson, P.D., Nugent, A.M., and Herbert, P.N. 1990. Increases in creatine kinase after exercise in patients treated with HMG-CoA reductase inhibitors. *JAMA* 264:2992.

Turcotte, L.P., Richter, E.A., and Kiens, B. 1995. Lipid metabolism during exercise. In *Exercise metabolism*, edited by M. Hargreaves. Champaign, IL: Human Kinetics.

Wallace, C.S., and Mueller, B.A. 1992. Lovastatin-induced rhabdomyolysis in the absence of concomitant drugs. *Ann Pharmacother* 26:190-192.

Williams, P.T. 1996. High-density lipoprotein cholesterol and other risk factors for coronary heart disease in female runners. *N Engl J Med* 334:1298-1303.

Wilmore, J.H., and Costill, D.L. 1994 *Physiology of sport and exercise*. Champaign, IL: Human Kinetics.

Young, D.R., Haskell, W.L., Jatulis, D.E., and Fortmann, S.P. 1993. Associations between changes in physical activity and risk factors for coronary heart disease in a community-based sample of men and women: The Stanford five-city project. *Am J Epidemiol* 138:205-216.

11

CHAPTER

Nonsteroidal Anti-Inflammatory Drugs (NSAIDs) and Salicylates

■ *CASE*   Suzanne is 26 years old and exercises five or six days a week. Her friends think she overdoes it. She routinely runs more than 20 miles in a week, and she is an enthusiastic member of an aerobics class. Lately, her foot has been troubling her, but she is not about to stop her workouts. She asks you whether she should take aspirin, Advil, or Aleve for it—they all have such similar names that she is confused.

■ *COMMENT*   Many questions come to mind in Suzanne's case: Does she have a stress fracture? Could it be plantar fasciitis? These are conditions where rest or other nonpharmacologic modalities such as physical therapy may be indicated; taking an anti-inflammatory drug may suppress the symptoms without addressing the true cause. For simple myalgias or arthralgias, Suzanne could get the same degree of relief from any of the three drugs she mentions; they all have anti-inflammatory and analgesic properties. The difference is that Advil and Aleve are nonsalicylates. Aspirin is the least expensive, but it must be taken every 3-4 hours, while the other two drugs don't require such frequent doses. Unfortunately, all three drugs may cause gastrointestinal side effects, including gastropathy and dyspepsia. Besides taking anti-inflammatory analgesics, Suzanne should be encouraged to include some nonexercise days in each week (and perhaps convinced that this is okay for her well-being) and also to ice her foot after exercising.

Musculoskeletal injuries occur in young athletes as well as in older people. In general, the knee is the site of injury in younger athletes and is related to their running, fitness classes, and field sports. Some of the most common injuries in this age group are patellofemoral pain syndrome and stress fractures or periostitis. The foot is more often the source of problems in older subjects and is related to their playing racquet sports, walking, and engaging in low-intensity activities. Metatarsalgia, plantar fasciitis, and meniscal injury are more common in this older age group. Tendinitis occurs equally in both age groups (Matheson et al. 1989).

Younger and older individuals alike readily consume anti-inflammatory drugs to treat these muscle and joint problems. In a study of gastrointestinal (GI) bleeding in distance runners, more than half of the subject applicants had to be excluded because of regular aspirin use (Stewart et al. 1984). In the 1980s, some 14 million patients in the United States were taking nonsteroidal anti-inflammatory drugs (NSAIDs) regularly for symptoms of arthritis (Roth and Bennett 1987); roughly 80% of elderly ambulatory patients were using NSAIDs on a daily basis (Stewart, Hale, and Marks 1982). The number of prescriptions written for NSAIDs increased from 50 million annually in the mid-1980s (Roth and Bennett 1987) to roughly 70 million per year in the 1990s (Tamblyn et al. 1997). These figures are disturbing considering that potentially one-third of these prescriptions for NSAIDs in the elderly are inappropriate (Tamblyn et al. 1997). In addition, former prescription-only drugs, such as ibuprofen, ketoprofen, and naproxen, have since been reassigned to nonprescription, or over-the counter (OTC), status in the United States, which, combined with the aging of the population in general, makes it highly likely that the use of these drugs by the elderly will only increase (Helling et al. 1987; Hughes 1991; May et al. 1982; Phillips, Polisson, and Simon 1997). Because anti-inflammatory agents are widely used by both athletes and deconditioned people, it is important for athletic trainers, coaches, and all sports medicine personnel to understand how these agents work in all age groups.

Anti-Inflammatory Agents

There are many categories of anti-inflammatory drugs; only two of them—salicylates and nonsteroidal anti-inflammatory drugs—will be reviewed here. The term *nonsteroidal anti-inflammatory drugs* (NSAIDs) is somewhat of a misnomer. Not only does this group not include adrenal corticosteroids, but it also does not include the so-called disease-modifying agents. Corticosteroids and the disease-modifying agents are beyond the scope of this discussion. Analgesics such as acetaminophen and opiate agonists do not possess anti-inflammatory properties, and they, too, are not discussed. For the purposes of this discussion, salicylates will be thought of separately from the NSAIDs.

Aspirin is the most commonly used oral substance among the salicylates, although diflunisal is a more potent anti-inflammatory than aspirin. Aspirin, but not other salicylates, inhibits platelet aggregation and prolongs bleeding time; this may be due to its ability to acetylate proteins. Diflunisal and the nonacetylated salicylates appear to produce a lower incidence of gastropathy and to exert a less dramatic effect on platelet aggregation than does aspirin (Insel 1990).

Methyl salicylate is found in many topical OTC sport products. Methyl salicylate *should never be ingested* since it is extremely toxic; death has been reported even after topical use. All salicylates and NSAIDs are nonopiates and do not cause physical or psychological dependence. Tables 11.1 and 11.2 summarize the various agents.

Table 11.1   Availability and Duration of Action for Various NSAIDs

Generic name (trade name)	Duration	Rx or OTC
Diclofenac (Cataflam, Voltaren)	Short	Rx
Etodolac (Lodine)	Short	Rx
Fenoprofen (Nalfon)	Short	Rx
Flurbiprofen (Ansaid)	Short	Rx
Ibuprofen (Advil, Motrin, Nuprin)	Short	Rx, OTC
Indomethacin (Indocin)	Intermediate	Rx
Ketoprofen (Orudis, Actron)	Short	Rx, OTC
Ketorolac (Toradol)	Short	Rx
Mefenamic acid (Ponstel)	Short	Rx
Nabumetone (Relafen)	Long	Rx
Naproxen (Aleve, Naprosyn)	Intermediate	Rx, OTC
Oxaprozin (Daypro)	Long	Rx
Piroxicam (Feldene)	Very long	Rx
Sulindac (Clinoril)	Intermediate	Rx
Tolmetin (Tolectin)	Short	Rx

Adapted from Human Kinetics 1997.

Table 11.2   Salicylates

Acetylated salicylates	Topical salicylates
Aspirin (acetylsalicylic acid, ASA) (OTC)	Methyl salicylate[a] (Exocaine Medicated Rub, Exocaine Plus Rub) (OTC)
Salsalate (Disalcid) (Rx only)	
Non-acetylated salicylates	**Non-salicylates[b] (i.e., agents not hydrolyzed to salicylic acid)**
Choline salicylate (Arthropan) (OTC)	Diflunisal (Dolobid) (Rx only)
Choline-magnesium salicylate (Trilisate) (Rx only)	Salicylamide (ingredient in BC Powders and BC Tablets) (OTC)
Sodium salicylate (Rx only)	

[a] = Also available in combination with menthol in Flex-All Pain Relieving Gel, Heet, and various preparations of Banalg, Ben-Gay, Icy Hot, and Mentholatum.
[b] = These agents are mentioned here only for completeness since, due to their similar-sounding generic names, they may be mistaken for salicylates.

■ *NSAIDs vs. Glucosamine?*

In managing acute musculoskeletal injuries, the general approach of those in clinical medicine and those in sports medicine is to use anti-inflammatory agents such as ibuprofen or naproxen along with rest, ice, and compression. But for chronic overuse injuries, it might be logical to try to enhance the body's natural repair process. Supplements are becoming highly popular forms of self-treatment by the general public for a variety of conditions. But because these products are not regulated as drugs, product efficacy and purity are open to question.

One supplement that athletes may consider is glucosamine. Since this supplement has virtually no side effects, it seems that there might be a role for glucosamine in the management of athletes with chronic overuse joint (not muscle) injuries. Sold as a dietary supplement, glucosamine is not an herb. Rather, it is a naturally occurring 6-carbon amino sugar that is an essential building block for "ground substance," a component of cartilage matrix in human tissue. Limited clinical data indicate that glucosamine is actually superior to ibuprofen for the management of osteoarthrosis of the knee (Vaz 1982). Additional clinical data are needed to fully determine the role of glucosamine in sports medicine.

How Exercise Affects the Action of Anti-Inflammatory Agents

The effects of exercise on either the pharmacology or the pharmacokinetics of anti-inflammatory agents are largely unknown. Exercise training has been shown to affect platelet aggregation (Davis et al. 1990), but the combined effects of exercise and any of these drugs on platelet function is unclear.

It is worth noting an important issue regarding the pharmacokinetics of topical methyl salicylate. Percutaneous absorption of methyl salicylate is significantly enhanced by high ambient temperatures, and this absorption increases further when prolonged endurance exercise occurs at high ambient temperatures. In one study, 6 healthy males were exposed to temperatures of 22 and 40 °C while resting and while exercising at 30% $\dot{V}O_2$max. Six hours of bicycling at 30% $\dot{V}O_2$max in the 40 °C environment produced higher serum salicylate concentrations than during exercise at 22 °C or while resting at 40 °C (see figure 11.1;

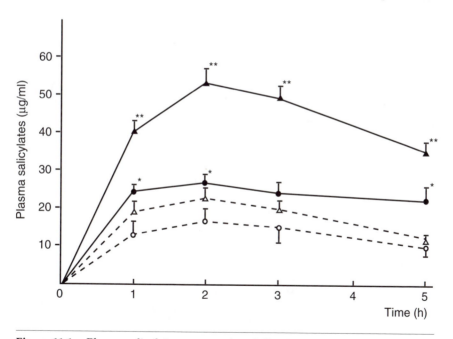

Figure 11.1 Plasma salicylate concentrations following percutaneous application of methyl salicylate. Mean ± *SEM* for 6 subjects. ○ = control conditions, rest at 22 °C; ● = rest at 40 °C; △ = exercise to 30% of $\dot{V}O_2$max, 45 min each hour, at 22 °C; ▲ = exercise at 40 °C. * = Significant differences ($p < 0.05$) compared to control; ** = significant differences ($p < 0.05$) compared with each of the other conditions.

Adapted from Danon, Ben-Shimon, and Ben-Zvi 1986.

Danon, Ben-Shimon, and Ben-Zvi 1986). This study called for the application of 5 g of methyl salicylate (no vehicle was used) to the chests and backs of the subjects. It is likely that athletes who use products containing methyl salicylate would apply it only to the affected muscle or joint; they probably would use a smaller quantity than the amount in this study. However, these products (see table 11.2 for topical products that contain methyl salicylate) are used multiple times per day. Therapeutic serum concentrations of salicylate in the treatment of rheumatic disease are generally considered to be in the range of 150–300 mcg/ml; the serum concentrations of salicylate in this study were substantially lower than that. Regardless, athletic trainers and athletes should realize that exercise in a hot environment substantially increases the cutaneous bioavailability of methyl salicylate. Topical application of ibuprofen (Campbell and Dunn 1994) and indomethacin (Akermark and Forsskahl 1990) have also been studied, and although they were superior to placebo, topical dosage forms of these drugs are not currently available in the United States.

How Anti-Inflammatory Agents Affect Exercisers

Because of the widespread use of anti-inflammatory agents by both deconditioned subjects and athletes, it is especially worthwhile to examine how these agents might modify the body's response to exercise.

Salicylates and NSAIDs inhibit the enzyme responsible for prostaglandin synthesis, cyclooxygenase (COX). Cyclooxygenase is an important enzyme in the synthesis of inflammatory prostaglandins from arachidonic acid. Inhibition of prostaglandin synthesis interferes with the inflammatory reaction. Figure 11.2 shows where salicylates and NSAIDs act in the biosynthetic pathway of prostaglandins. Inflammation is reduced, but because prostaglandins are also involved in fever and sensitizing nerves, these drugs also reduce fever and have analgesic properties. Recently, two forms of this enzyme, COX-1 and COX-2, were identified, and in 1999 specific inhibitors of COX-2 were marketed in the United States, specifically, celecoxib (Celebrex), meloxicam (Mobic), and rofecoxib (Vioxx). Specific COX-2 inhibitors appear to produce fewer adverse reactions compared to the older, nonspecific inhibitors.

Energy Metabolism

By disrupting oxidative phosphorylation, salicylates can cause life-threatening metabolic disturbances after toxic overdoses. This effect may not be relevant, however, when the salicylates are used intermit-

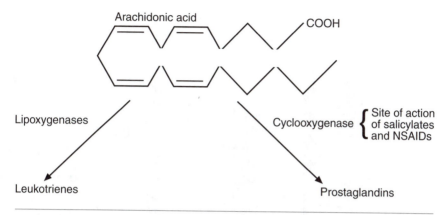

Figure 11.2   Biosynthesis of prostaglandins from arachidonic acid.

tently at therapeutic doses. DeMeersman, for example, studied the acute effects of a single dose of aspirin in males (1988a) and females (1988b) during 60 min of treadmill exercise at 50% $\dot{V}O_2$max and found no effect on glucose, insulin, or free fatty acid utilization. He concluded that single doses of aspirin should not affect glucoregulatory and counterregulatory metabolism during exercise. There are no data describing the effect of chronic salicylate consumption (i.e., a minimum of several days' consumption prior to exercise testing) on exercise physiology. More clinical research is needed to determine the effects of chronic aspirin ingestion on energy metabolism during sustained aerobic exercise.

Inflammatory Response

We know that aspirin and NSAIDs, by inhibiting COX, interfere with the inflammatory response. Nonsteroidal anti-inflammatory agents are effective in treating sprains and joint injuries, overuse injuries (such as tendinitis and bursitis), and strains and other types of muscle or soft-tissue injury (Hutson 1986; McLatchie et al. 1985; Moran 1991; Santilli, Tuccimei, and Cannistra 1980; Slatyer, Hensley, and Lopert 1997; Walker, VandenBurg, and Currie 1984). While it is beyond the scope of this book to discuss the clinical therapeutics of anti-inflammatory agents in sports medicine, this issue has been recently reviewed by Stanley and Weaver (1998).

Nonsteroidal anti-inflammatory agents are routinely used after competition or injury to suppress minor symptoms of muscle soreness and joint stiffness associated with overexertion. It is generally agreed that delayed onset muscle soreness after eccentric exercise peaks roughly at 2 to 3 days postexercise (Armstrong 1986; Clarkson and Newham 1995;

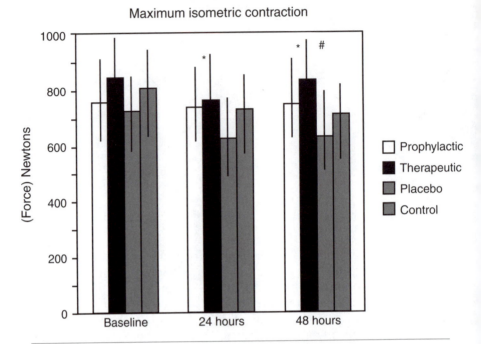

Maximum isometric contraction

Figure 11.3   Maximum isometric contraction of the quadriceps (expressed in Newtons) for the prophylactic, therapeutic, placebo, and control groups. Values are mean ± *SD*. * = Difference between the response of maximum knee extension isometric force (MVC) for prophylactic ibuprofen compared with the other treatments from baseline to 24 h and the response from 24 to 48 h compared with the placebo and control groups; # = difference between the response of MVC for therapeutic ibuprofen compared with the placebo and control from 24 to 48 h ($p < 0.05$).

Adapted from Hasson et al. 1993.

Miles and Clarkson 1994). Yet it is interesting to note that 24 h of low-dose ibuprofen, when initiated 4 h *before* the exercise bout, was superior to the same 24 h regimen initiated 24 h after exercise (see figure 11.3; Hasson et al. 1993). Oral diclofenac (Donnelly et al. 1988), oral ibuprofen (Hasson et al. 1993), and oral naproxen (Lecomte, Lacroix, and Montgomery 1998) have been found superior to placebo in reducing delayed-onset muscle soreness after eccentric exercise. Although effects on overall exercise performance were not assessed in these studies, maximum isometric force and peak quadriceps torque were found to be better in the active drug recipients than in subjects taking placebo. This was noted both when the oral NSAID was initiated before (Hasson et al. 1993) and after (Lecomte, Lacroix, and Montgomery 1998) the exercise bout. Other researchers, however, have not found oral ibuprofen to be

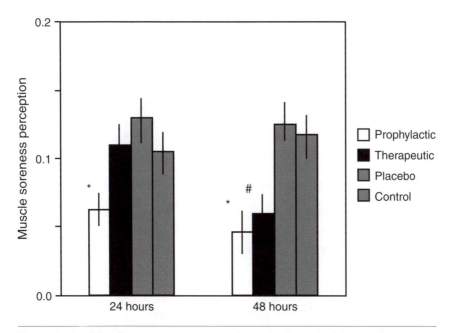

Figure 11.4   Muscle soreness perception (intensity × area) of the quadriceps.
Values are mean ± *SD*. * = Difference between prophylactic ibuprofen and the
other treatments at 24 h and placebo and control at 48 h; # = difference between
therapeutic ibuprofen and the placebo and control at 48 h (*p* < 0.05).
Adapted from Hasson et al. 1993.

better than placebo in this setting (Bourgeois et al. 1999; Donnelly,
Maughan, and Whiting 1990). It is not clear why nearly identical studies
produced these divergent observations. Even when NSAID treatment
has been shown to be beneficial in reducing symptoms of muscle
soreness, no effect on biochemical measurements of muscle injury (e.g.,
creatine kinase, CK) was seen (Hasson et al. 1993; Lecomte, Lacroix, and
Montgomery 1998).

Thus, while measurements of serum creatine kinase suggest that
NSAIDs do not modify exercise-induced muscle injury, some data
indicate that these drugs do provide a beneficial clinical effect (see figure
11.4). Whether the mechanism is anti-inflammatory or analgesic remains to be determined.

Adenosine

Nonsteroidal anti-inflammatory agents exert many other metabolic
effects. Their ability to potentiate adenosine is relevant to this discussion. Simpson and Phillis (1992) have reviewed the effects of adenosine

in exercise adaptation and concluded that adenosine is one of the mediators for improving aerobic capacity. Adenosine is an intermediate in the metabolism and synthesis of ATP and serves as a marker for energy metabolism. It has been shown to act as a vasodilator in most tissues, including brain, heart, and skeletal muscle, although more research is needed on the effects of adenosine on skeletal muscle vasodilation. Adenosine is also believed to stimulate glycogenolysis, participate in the activation of the sympathoadrenal response, and potentiate insulin-mediated myocardial glucose uptake (Simpson and Phillis 1992). Erythropoietin production by the kidney may also be controlled by adenosine. If adenosine does possess all these actions, one can easily see how it would exert ergogenic effects. Although it has not been directly demonstrated that NSAIDs increase adenosine levels, Simpson and Phillis (1992) suggest that at least some of them do. This theory remains unproved and requires more research in exercising humans.

How Anti-Inflammatory Agents Affect Exercise Performance

Salicylates, in toxic doses, can disrupt energy metabolism. NSAIDs, in general, can prevent delayed-onset muscle soreness, and they may potentiate adenosine, both of which might be beneficial. What, then, are the effects of these drugs on overall exercise and athletic performance? Regarding salicylates, aspirin does not affect exercise performance, but the data demonstrating this are limited and researchers have studied effects only from single doses. Roi and colleagues (1994) evaluated healthy, active subjects 30 min after the subjects ingested a single 1000 mg dose of aspirin; this team did not observe any statistically significant effects on cycle ergometer performance. Lisse and colleagues (1991), who looked at the effects of a single 650 mg dose on a 2 mi run 30 min after runners ingested aspirin, also found no effect (see figure 11.5). These small studies lend some assurance that aspirin does not affect aerobic performance. But they leave unknown whether detrimental effects of aspirin occur later than 30 min postingestion or whether daily, continuous ingestion or higher doses produce different results.

Because NSAIDs reduce postexercise muscle soreness, it is possible that this action represents an indirect ergogenic effect. Prophylactic ibuprofen significantly attenuated the decline in quadriceps isometric contraction as well as concentric and eccentric torque at 24 h postexercise (Hasson et al. 1993). Perhaps an individual competing in the final stages of the decathlon, or someone running multiple heats of the 400 m on

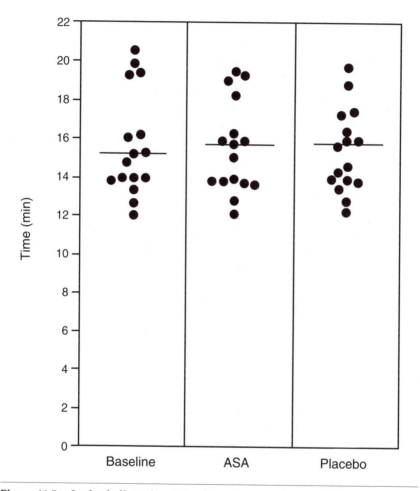

Figure 11.5 Lack of effect of aspirin (650 mg) on running performance. Each runner is represented by a point, and mean time for that series of runs is represented by the horizontal line.

Adapted from Lisse et al. 1991.

successive days, or someone playing a series of consecutive tennis matches might be able to improve their performances by taking NSAIDs. This intriguing possibility should be investigated.

Avoiding Potential Complications

Salicylates and nonsalicylate NSAIDs are well-known inhibitors of platelet aggregation. They also cause gastropathy, which can lead to GI bleeding and peptic ulcer, and they cause nephrotoxicity (Sandler, Burr, and Weinberg 1991). Each year, about 76,000 individuals are hospitalized from the effects of NSAIDs, and an estimated 7600 deaths occur as the result of individuals ingesting these agents (Tamblyn et al. 1997). Deaths due to NSAIDs are almost always seen in elderly subjects, particularly elderly females (Tamblyn et al. 1997), but even young athletes are not immune to the potential toxicity (Griffiths 1992). Exercise itself exerts various effects on platelet aggregation (Davis et al. 1990; Rauramaa et al. 1986). Thus, exercising while taking these drugs may produce additive effects.

Gastrointestinal Toxicity

One of the most recognized of all adverse drug reactions is gastropathy secondary to use of NSAIDs (Roth and Bennett 1987). Whether exercising while taking these drugs increases the risk, however, is unclear. Gastrointestinal bleeding (Stewart et al. 1984) and erosive gastritis (Cooper et al. 1987) have been reported in distance runners not taking aspirin or NSAIDs. Stewart and colleagues (1984) suggested that exercise induces GI bleeding by decreasing gut perfusion and that people who are deconditioned are more susceptible to this effect. If this is true, then encouraging the elderly to exercise could be detrimental, particularly since analgesic use is high in this population (May et al. 1982). Pahor and colleagues (1994) found, however, that the risk of severe GI hemorrhage was lower in elderly subjects who routinely exercised than in those who did not exercise (Pahor et al. 1994). This is hard to explain, considering the observations in marathon runners, and considering that fibrinolytic activity has been documented to increase moderately in the elderly in response to a 6-month intensive training program (Schuit et al. 1997).

How is it possible that exercise induces GI bleeding in distance runners, yet reduces the risk in the elderly? The answer probably lies in the frequency and intensity of exercise. After a competitive race, 83% of distance runners not taking aspirin or NSAIDs have an increase in detectable stool heme (Stewart et al. 1984), and the amount is clinically significant in roughly 20% of these individuals (Buckman 1984). Guaiac-positive stools were seen more often in younger and faster runners, suggesting that physiologic stress may be an important contributing factor (McMahon et al. 1984). If exercise causes detectable, though subclinical, GI blood loss among individuals who are not taking aspirin or NSAIDs, it is logical to conclude that the risk of GI bleeding increases in those who combine strenuous exercise with these drugs. In one small study of marathon runners (McMahon et al. 1984), however, no relationship was seen between use of these medications and GI bleeding. Thus, even though the limited data suggest that exercise intensity is a more critical risk factor for GI bleeding in elite runners than is NSAID use, the effects of NSAIDs should not be totally disregarded; their effects on the gastrointestinal system are well known. Finally, the marketing of NSAIDs that are specific inhibitors of COX-2 (e.g., celecoxib, meloxicam, rofecoxib) provides endurance athletes with an option when an anti-inflammatory drug is needed that has less potential for GI injury (see "COX-2 Inhibitors").

■ *COX-2 Inhibitors*

A new class of anti-inflammatory drug was introduced in 1999: COX-2 inhibitors. This name derives from the fact that these drugs are more selective in inhibiting type-2 cyclooxygenase (COX-2) than type-1 (COX-1). Most of the side effects of NSAIDs are due to inhibition of COX-1. Drugs in this class include celecoxib (Celebrex), meloxicam (Mobic), and rofecoxib (Vioxx). Initial clinical data do support the claim that these drugs cause less gastropathy than first-generation NSAIDs.

Nephrotoxicity

The nephrotoxicity of NSAIDs is well known. Nephrotoxicity has been reported in elderly subjects or patients with decreased renal perfusion (Heinrich 1983), but chronic renal toxicity has also been reported in a young, otherwise healthy athlete after taking ibuprofen regularly for several months (Griffiths 1992). Acute renal failure has been reported after running a marathon (Bar-Sela, Tur-Kaspa, and Eliakim 1979; Goldsmith 1984; MacSearraigh, Kallmeyer, and Schiff 1979; Seedat et al. 1989-90; Vitting, Nichols, and Seligson 1986). By inhibiting production of vasodilatory prostaglandins, aspirin and NSAIDs can augment exercise-induced reductions in renal blood flow and glomerular filtration rate (GFR) (Walker et al. 1994). Ibuprofen, a NSAID, impairs GFR more than acetaminophen during running while in a dehydrated state (Farquhar et al. 1999). Despite the fact that aspirin, ibuprofen, ketoprofen, and naproxen can be purchased without a prescription, exercisers should be encouraged not to overuse these drugs, particularly during prolonged endurance events.

NCAA and USOC Status

Neither aspirin, nonacetylated salicylates, nor nonsalicylate NSAIDs are banned from athletic competition. Athletes and their trainers should note, however, that some drug products combine these

Sport and Exercise Pharmacology

anti-inflammatory analgesics with other ingredients that are banned from use during competition. For example, Vicoprofen is a combination of ibuprofen with hydrocodone, an opiate agonist. Motrin IB Sinus contains ibuprofen with pseudoephedrine, a sympathomimetic.

Guidelines for Use

The anti-inflammatory agents discussed in this chapter do not appear to have ergogenic properties. While they are effective for the variety of aches and pains that occur with exercise, sports medicine professionals and the individuals who use these agents all should be aware of the potential toxicity of NSAIDs. Unfortunately, neither acetaminophen (Tylenol), tramadol (Ultram), or drugs of the opiate agonist class (e.g., codeine, hydrocodone) are viable alternatives, as these agents do not possess the anti-inflammatory properties of NSAIDs. Further, opiate agonists are banned substances. Finally, animal data indicate that acute exercise potentiates acetaminophen hepatotoxicity (Yoon, Kim, and Kim 1997), although physical training may minimize this risk (Lew and Quintanilha 1991). Here are several things to keep in mind:

- GI injury and GI bleeding can occur without symptoms, and (in athletes) mild anemia might be dismissed as "sports anemia" (i.e., pseudoanemia secondary to plasma volume expansion). Regular consumption of anti-inflammatory drugs should be discouraged. Ethanol increases the risk of NSAID-induced gastropathy.

- Some data indicate that beginning therapy with NSAIDs several hours before exercise may increase their anti-inflammatory efficacy. If competition cannot be endured without the use of these drugs, however, then perhaps it is time to rest!

- Despite the fact that aspirin, ibuprofen, ketoprofen, and naproxen can be purchased without a prescription, do not underestimate the potential toxicity of these drugs. Seedat and colleagues (1989-90) have cautioned against using NSAIDs during marathons and ultra-marathons. While use of NSAIDs may help prevent delayed-onset muscle soreness, these agents can increase the risk of nephrotoxicity after prolonged endurance exercise.

References

Akermark, C., and Forsskahl, B. 1990. Topical indomethacin in overuse injuries in athletes. A randomized double-blind study comparing Elmetacin with oral indomethacin and placebo. *Int J Sports Med* 11:393-396.
Armstrong, R.B. 1986. Muscle damage and endurance events. *Sports Med* 3:370-381.

Bar-Sela, S., Tur-Kaspa, R., and Eliakim, M. 1979. Rhabdomyolysis and acute renal failure in a marathon runner in Israel. *Isr J Med Sci* 15:464-466.

Bourgeois, J., MacDougall, D., MacDonald, J., and Tarnopolsky, M. 1999. Naproxen does not alter indices of muscle damage in resistance-exercise trained men. *Med Sci Sports Exerc* 31:4-9.

Buckman, M.T. 1984. Gastrointestinal bleeding in long-distance runners. *Ann Intern Med* 101:127-128.

Campbell, J., and Dunn, T. 1994. Evaluation of topical ibuprofen cream in the treatment of acute ankle sprains. *J Accid Emerg Med* 11:178-182.

Clarkson, P.M., and Newham, D.J. 1995. Associations between muscle soreness, damage, and fatigue. *Adv Exp Med Biol* 384:457-469.

Cooper, B.T., Douglas, S.A., Firth, L.A., Hannagan, J.A., and Chadwick, V.S. 1987. Erosive gastritis and gastrointestinal bleeding in a female runner. *Gastroenterol* 92:2019-2023.

Danon, A., Ben-Shimon, S., and Ben-Zvi, Z. 1986. Effect of exercise and heat exposure on percutaneous absorption of methyl salicylate. *Eur J Clin Pharmacol* 31:49-52.

Davis, R.B., Boyd, D.G., McKinney, M.E., and Jones, C.C. 1990. Effects of exercise and exercise conditioning on blood platelet function. *Med Sci Sports Exerc* 22:49-53.

DeMeersman, R. 1988a. The effects of acetylsalicylic acid upon carbohydrate metabolism during exercise. *Int J Clin Pharmacol Ther Toxicol* 26:461-464.

DeMeersman, R.E. 1988b. Thermal, ventilatory, and gluco-regulatory responses during exercise following short-term acetylsalicylic acid ingestion. *Int J Clin Pharmacol Res* 8:477-483.

Donnelly, A.E., Maughan, R.J., and Whiting, P.H. 1990. Effects of ibuprofen on exercise-induced muscle soreness and indices of muscle damage. *Br J Sports Med* 24:191-195.

Donnelly, A.E., McCormick, K., Maughan, R.J., Whiting, P.H., and Clarkson, P.M. 1988. Effects of a nonsteroidal anti-inflammatory drug on delayed onset muscle soreness and indices of damage. *Br J Sports Med* 22:35-38.

Farquhar, W.B., Morgan, A.L., Zambraski, E.J., and Kenney, W.L. 1999. Effects of acetaminophen and ibuprofen on renal function in the stressed kidney. *J Appl Physiol* 86:598-604.

Goldsmith, H.J. 1984. Acute renal failure after a marathon run. *Lancet* 1(8371):278-279.

Griffiths, M.L. 1992. End-stage renal failure caused by regular use of anti-inflammatory analgesic medication for minor sports injuries. A case report. *S Afr Med J* 81:377-378.

Hasson, S.M., Daniels, J.C., Divine, J.G., Niebuhr, B.R., Richmond, S., Stein, P.G., and Williams, J.H. 1993. Effect of ibuprofen use on muscle soreness, damage, and performance: A preliminary investigation. *Med Sci Sports Exerc* 25:9-17.

Heinrich, W.L. 1983. Nephrotoxicity of nonsteroidal anti-inflammatory agents. *Am J Kidney Dis* 2:478-484.

Helling, D.K., Lemke, J.H., Semla, T.P., Wallace, R.B., Lipson, D.P., and Cornoni-Huntley, J. 1987. Medication use characteristics in the elderly: The Iowa 65+ rural health study. *J Am Geriatr Soc* 35:4-12.

Hughes, G.R. 1991. The problems of using NSAIDs in the elderly. *Scand J Rheumatol Suppl* 91:19-25.

Hutson, M.A. 1986. A double-blind study comparing ibuprofen 1800 mg or 2400 mg daily and placebo in sports injuries. *J Int Med Res* 14:142-147.

Insel, P.A. 1990. Analgesic-antipyretics and anti-inflammatory agents: Drugs employed in the treatment of rheumatoid arthritis and gout. In *The pharmacological basis of therapeutics*, 8th ed., edited by A.G. Gil-man, T.W. Rall, A.S. Nies, and P. Taylor. New York: Pergamon Press.

Lecomte, J.M., Lacroix, V.J., and Montgomery, D.L. 1998. A randomized controlled trial of the effect of naproxen on delayed onset muscle soreness and muscle strength. *Clin J Sport Med* 8:82-87.

Lew, H., and Quintanilha, A. 1991. Effects of endurance training and exercise on tissue antioxidative capacity and acetaminophen detoxification. *Eur J Drug Metab Pharmacokinet* 16:59-68.

Lisse, J.R., Macdonald, K., Thurmond-Anderle, M.E., and Fuchs Jr., J.E. 1991. A double-blind, placebo-controlled study of acetylsalicylic acid (ASA) in trained runners. *J Sports Med Phys Fitness* 31:561-564.

MacSearraigh, E.T., Kallmeyer, J.C., and Schiff, H.B. 1979. Acute renal failure in marathon runners. *Nephron* 24:236-240.

Matheson, G.O., Macintyre, J.G., Taunton, J.E., Clement, D.B., and Lloyd-Smith, R. 1989. Musculoskeletal injuries associated with physical activity in older adults. *Med Sci Sports Exerc* 21:379-385.

May, F.E., Stewart, R.B., Hale, W.E., and Marks, R.G. 1982. Prescribed and nonprescribed drug use in an ambulatory elderly population. *South Med J* 75:522-528.

McLatchie, G.R., Allister, C., MacEwen, C., Hamilton, G., McGregor, H., Colquhuon, I., and Pickvance, N.J. 1985. Variable schedules of ibuprofen for ankle sprains. *Br J Sports Med* 19:203-206.

McMahon, L.F., Ryan, M.J., Larson, D.L., and Fisher, R.L. 1984. Occult gastrointestinal blood loss in marathon runners. *Ann Intern Med* 100:846-847.

Miles, M.P., and Clarkson, P.M. 1994. Exercise-induced muscle pain, soreness, and cramps. *J Sports Med Phys Fitness* 34:203-216.

Moran, M. 1991. Double-blind comparison of diclofenac potassium, ibuprofen and placebo in the treatment of ankle sprains. *J Int Med Res* 19:121-130.

Pahor, M., Guralnik, J.M., Salive, M.E., Chrischilles, E.A., Brown, S.L., and Wallace, R.B. 1994. Physical activity and risk of severe gastrointestinal hemorrhage in older persons. *JAMA* 272(8):595-599.

Phillips, A.C., Polisson, R.P., and Simon, L.S. 1997. NSAIDs and the elderly: Toxicity and economic implications. *Drugs Aging* 10:119-130.

Rauramaa, R., Salonen, J.T., Seppanen, K., Salonen, R., Venlalainen, J.M., Ihanainen, M., and Rissanen, V. 1986. Inhibition of platelet aggregability by moderate-intensity physical exercise: A randomized clinical trial in overweight men. *Circulation* 74:939-944.

Roi, G.S., Garagiola, U., Verza, P., Spadari, G., Radice, D., Zecca, L., and Cerretelli, P. 1994. Aspirin does not affect exercise performance. *Int J Sports Med* 15:224-227.

Roth, S.H., and Bennett, R.E. 1987. Nonsteroidal anti-inflammatory drug gastropathy. Recognition and response. *Arch Intern Med* 147:2093-2100.

Sandler, D.P., Burr, F.R., and Weinberg, C.R. 1991. Nonsteroidal anti-inflammatory drugs and the risk for chronic renal disease. *Ann Intern Med* 115:165-172.

Santilli, G., Tuccimei, U., and Cannistra, F.M. 1980. Comparative study with piroxicam and ibuprofen versus placebo in the supportive treatment of minor sports inuries. *J Int Med Res* 8:265-269.

Schuit, A.J., Schouten, E.G., Kluft, C., de Maat, M., Menheere, P.P., and Kok, F.J. 1997. Effect of strenuous exercise on fibrinogen and fibrinolysis in healthy elderly men and women. *Throm Haemost* 78(2):845-851.

Seedat, Y.K., Aboo, N., Naicker, S., and Parsoo, I. 1989-90. Acute renal failure in the "Comrades Marathon" runners. *Ren Fail* 11:209-212.

Simpson, R.E., and Phillis, J.W. 1992. Adenosine in exercise adaptation. *Br J Sports Med* 26:54-58.

Slatyer, M.A., Hensley, M.J., and Lopert, R. 1997. A randomized controlled trial of piroxicam in the management of acute ankle sprain in Australian regular army recruits. The Kapooka Ankle Sprain Study. *Am J Sports Med* 25:544-553.

Stanley, K.L., and Weaver, J.E. 1998. Pharmacologic management of pain and inflammation in athletes. *Clin Sports Med* 17:375-392.

Stewart, J.G., Ahlquist, D.A., McGill, D.B., Ilstrup, D.M., Schwartz, S., and Owen, R.A. 1984. Gastrointestinal blood loss and anemia in runners. *Ann Intern Med* 100:843-845.

Stewart, R.B., Hale, W.E., and Marks, R.G. 1982. Analgesic drug use in an ambulatory elderly population. *Drug Intell Clin Pharm* 16:833-836.

Tamblyn, R., Berkson, L., Dauphinee, W.D., Gayton, D., Grad, R., Huang, A., Isaac, L., McLeod, P., and Snell, L. 1997. Unnecessary prescribing of NSAIDs and the management of NSAID-related gastropathy in medical practice. *Ann Intern Med* 127:429-438.

Vaz, A.L. 1982. Double-blind clinical evaluation of the relative efficacy of ibuprofen and glucosamine sulphate in the management of osteoarthrosis of the knee in out-patients. *Curr Med Res Opin* 8:145-149.

Vitting, K.E., Nichols, N.J., and Seligson, G.R. 1986. Naproxen and acute renal failure in a runner. *Ann Intern Med* 105:144.

Walker, J.W., VandenBurg, M.J., and Currie, W.J. 1984. Differential efficacy of two non-steroidal anti-inflammatory drugs in the treatment of sports injuries. *Curr Med Res Opin* 9:119-123.

Walker, R.J., Fawcett, J.P., Flannery, E.M., and Gerrard, D.F. 1994. Indomethacin potentiates exercise-induced reduction in renal hemodynamics in athletes. *Med Sci Sports Exerc* 26:1302-1306.

Yoon, M.Y., Kim, S.N., and Kim, Y.C. 1997. Potentiation of acetaminophen hepato-toxicity by acute physical exercise in rats. *Res Commun Mol Pathol Pharmacol* 96:35-44.

12
CHAPTER

Nutritional Supplements

■ *CASE* You are reading an issue of *Money* magazine that contains an article on vitamins. It describes a personal trainer who consumes the equivalent of $19,000 annually in vitamins and supplements. His regimen includes L-carnitine 1500 mg/day, coenzyme Q-10 60 mg/day, chlorophyll 8050 mg/day, chromium picolinate 400 mcg/day, saw palmetto 120 mg/day, the herb *Pygeum africanum* 150 mg/day—and quite a bit more. You are astounded that people actually do this. Are all these supplements necessary to attain this level of fitness? You are even more amazed that this is reported in a financial magazine. Is the use of dietary supplements so widespread that magazines like this write articles about them?

■ *COMMENT* It is unfortunate that some people assume that nutritional supplements are necessary and readily endorse and recommend them to others. There is little evidence, after all, that consuming traditional vitamins in doses far beyond the recommended daily allowance benefits performance. Even less is known about the dietary supplements, also known as *nutraceuticals*, that many people ingest. Dietary supplements sold as nutraceuticals are not regulated by the FDA, and quality control, therefore, is not ensured as it is for prescription and even nonprescription drugs.

Interest among the general public in "nontraditional," or alternative, forms of health care surged in the mid-1990s. Not only patients seeking medical treatments but people wanting to enhance their athletic or exercise performance or physical appearance have expressed a pervasive interest in dietary supplements. In 1994, for example, Americans spent some $5 billion for vitamins and minerals (see Rock 1995), and in 1996, $3.2 billion was spent on herbal or alternative medicines (see McCann 1997). In 1999, herbal supplements have been estimated as a $4 billion industry (National Public Radio [NPR], *Morning Edition*, 2 April 1999). The FDA has recently estimated that there are 25,000-30,000 products available as dietary supplements (NPR, *Morning Edition*, 30 March 1999). Moreover, in the United States alone the market for these products is projected to exceed $12 billion by the year 2001 (Smith 1998), although some estimates project the total market for nutritional supplements has exceeded that figure already (Ritter 1999).

To satisfy this lucrative market, supplements are being heavily promoted. It seems every retailer wants a piece of the action. Since 1998, big drugmakers like Bayer and Warner-Lambert have introduced specific marketing lines of herbal products. General Nutrition Centers, which has long marketed many types of dietary supplements, stated in 1998 that the company planned to bring many new products to market, from pills to beverages to powders (Smith 1998). Even the widely circulated *Performance* catalog of bicycle gear in 1998 began offering nutritional supplements for sale! Following Mark McGwire's home-run record in 1998, ESPN began airing commercials for androstenedione, one of two supplements he admitted to using. (ESPN soon after pulled the commercial because of the outcry from high school and college athletic organizations; see McGraw 1998.)

It is clear there is demand for nutritional supplements among athletes, and endorsements of these supplements by muscular personal trainers only fuel this demand. At local-area races, supplement manufacturers hold expositions promoting their products. Representatives from these companies are quick to offer advice on why this or that particular ingredient is necessary, always with the underlying message (direct or implied) that it enhances performance. Unfortunately, the (mis)belief that these products are helpful is so widespread that roughly 35% of the money spent on vitamins and supplements buys products of no scientifically proved value (Rock 1995). Unfortunately, fewer than a dozen of more than 600 botanicals, or herbal supplements, commercially available in the United States have been subjected to controlled clinical trials (Rock 1995).

This chapter discusses some of the better recognized and controversial vitamins, minerals, and supplements that athletes and other individuals use. Creatine and caffeine are discussed in separate chapters.

Pharmaceutical or Nutraceutical?
The DSHEA Law of 1994

Most readers recognize the term *pharmaceuticals,* but may not be as familiar with the more recently coined *nutraceuticals. Pharmaceutical* describes the traditional prescription drugs and over-the-counter (OTC) medications that are routinely purchased at any pharmacy. Pharmaceuticals have recognized, FDA-approved uses—and they must pass through a lengthy research and evaluation process to obtain this endorsement. *Nutraceutical* is a term that was coined in the mid-1980s by Stephen D. Felice, MD, chairman of the Foundation for Innovative Medicine. A nutraceutical is any dietary or nutritional supplement that is being used for general health benefits. Note that even though both nutraceuticals and nonprescription pharmaceuticals are now commonly sold in pharmacies, these two general types of products are distinctly different.

The distinction between a nutraceutical and a nonprescription pharmaceutical arises not so much from what the compound *is,* but from *how it is marketed.* In 1994, Congress passed the Dietary Supplement Health and Education Act (DSHEA), which allowed manufacturers of dietary supplements to distribute their products without a prescription and, more importantly, outside the domain of the FDA. A nutraceutical does not have to be an herbal substance. The DSHEA law defines a dietary supplement as a food product that contains at least one of the following ingredients: vitamin, mineral, herb or botanical, amino acid, metabolite, constituent, or extract. Since these products were considered dietary supplements and not drugs, they were not required to undergo safety and efficacy review, as all OTC and prescription drugs must. The tradeoff was that manufacturers could not claim that their products "cure, mitigate, treat, or prevent" a specific disease; instead, they could only make general statements about what the product does. For example, a manufacturer might state, "Helps maintain cardiovascular health" or "Helps support the immune system." It could not state something like "Protects against cancer," and any mention of a specific disease state was prohibited.

Passage of the DSHEA law may make life simpler for supplement manufacturers, but it has created problems for consumers. First, the act permits a product to be marketed without any scientific research to back up even the general claims it makes, and second, it allows for labeling information to be made intentionally vague. Consumers are misled as a result. Many of them rely on advocates of supplements, such as clerks in health food stores or personal trainers interviewed in popular magazines, to help them make decisions about these products; as a result, they likely spend money unnecessarily.

Many athletes will try anything that they believe might boost performance. Consider the issue of Mark McGwire and the "supplement" androstenedione. Because androstenedione is marketed as a dietary supplement, and because its manufacturers do not make specific claims on their label about the pharmacology or medical use, this substance is free from FDA regulation. From a scientific standpoint, however, androstenedione is a metabolic intermediate between cholesterol and either testosterone or estrogen, depending on the sex of the individual who ingests it. Charles Yesalis, PhD, a noted authority on anabolic steroids, states that androstenedione has been shown to be anabolic in castrated dogs (Yesalis 1993), and there is no doubt in his mind that the "supplement" is actually an anabolic hormone (Ritter 1999), regardless of the fact that scientific data on this compound are limited. Thus, the classification of androstenedione (i.e., drug or dietary supplement) depends on who is looking at it (Yesalis 1999).

With the above issues in mind, several supplements will be discussed in this chapter. Due to the diversity of the products and the lack of data on many of them, each product will be discussed according to an overview, claimed benefits, clinical data, and conclusions.

DHEA and Androstenedione

Dehydroepiandrosterone (DHEA) and androstenedione are hormone precursors, or "prohormones." Dehydroepiandrosterone is a metabolic precursor for androstenedione, which, in turn, is converted into testosterone (see figure 12.1). Produced by the adrenal gland, DHEA is a precursor for both testosterone and estradiol. In addition, DHEA is physiologically active. But the degree of either the anabolic or androgenic effect of DHEA is highly variable from one individual to the next, due to intrinsic metabolism, genetics, sex, fitness level, age, or perhaps other factors (Johnson 1999). Androstenedione is synthesized in the testes, but it can also be derived from DHEA peripherally (Phillips 1996). Androstenedione is directly converted into testosterone. This latter step appears to be more important in females than in males (Mahesh and Greenblatt 1962); a large percentage (approximately 60%) of circulating testosterone in women is derived from androstenedione, whereas this conversion contributes minimally (less than 0.3%) to the total testosterone supply in males (Horton and Tait 1966). In females, while the rate of conversion of androstenedione to testosterone is greater, circulating testosterone levels are much lower than in males (Horton and Tait 1966).

Dehydroepiandrosterone was first identified in 1934, but only recently has it attracted attention from the clinical medicine and sports

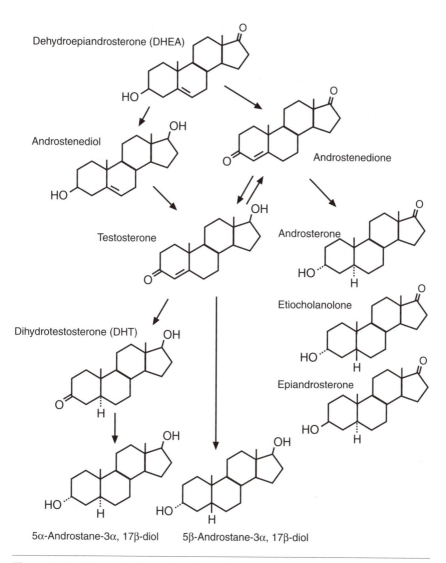

Figure 12.1   Biosynthetic relationships of androgens.
Adapted from Bowers 1998.

medicine communities. A half century after the discovery, in 1984, the
FDA banned its sale without a prescription because of concerns about
hepatotoxicity. Nevertheless, with the passage of the 1994 DSHEA
law, it is once again available, this time in health supplement stores! In
clinical medicine, DHEA is being studied for the management of
lupus. Investigators also are studying a synthetic version of DHEA,
known as "fluasterone," for medical purposes. As an androgen, DHEA

is relatively insignificant, due to its low potency and rapid hepatic clearance.

At one time, androstenedione was used by East German athletes as a nasal spray; in the United States, the substance is available as tablets and capsules. Commercial marketing of androstenedione in the United States occurred only recently, apparently, in 1996 when an Illinois chemist decided the German patent applied to only the intranasal dosage form. A recent review of anabolic agents in the sports medicine literature did not even mention androstenedione (Sturmi and Diorio 1998). Still more recently, national focus turned to androstenedione when baseball stars Mark McGwire and Jose Canseco claimed to have used it during the 1998 season (see Patrick 1998). MET-Rx Engineered Nutrition (a company in Irvine, California) even made plans to sell androstenedione chewing gum in 1999, predicting that the year's sales of androstenedione would exceed $100 million, a 10-fold increase over 1998 (McGraw 1998).

How Androstenedione and DHEA Affect Exercisers

Exercise intensity can influence endogenous production of androstenedione (Kuoppasalmi et al. 1980), but the meaning of these data are unclear. There is no evidence that androstenedione increases athletic performance, and the long-term effects of high-dose exogenous androstenedione are unknown at this time. Although the metabolic biochemistry of androstenedione is known (Phillips 1996; Ritter 1999), little clinical data are available on either its efficacy or its side effects.

Body Composition

Body composition did not differ between men receiving androstenedione 300 mg/day or placebo during an 8-week resistance training regimen (King et al. 1999). Dehydroepiandrosterone, in doses of 1600 mg/day for 4 weeks, had no effect on body weight, lean body mass, or on parameters of energy or protein metabolism in healthy males in one study (Welle, Jozefowicz, and Statt 1990), but was shown, at the same large dose, to reduce body fat and increase muscle mass in men in another study (Nestler et al. 1988). These data are very limited, and thus it is not possible to draw firm conclusions.

Testosterone Levels

Despite the belief by many athletes that androstenedione or DHEA boost testosterone levels, the available data make it difficult to draw firm conclusions on this issue. In a study of 19 untrained males, an 8-week regimen of androstenedione 100 mg three times per day combined with resistance training had no effect on serum free or total testosterone.

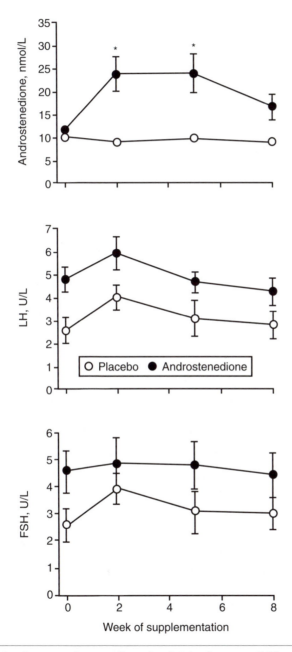

Figure 12.2 Serum androstenedione, luteinizing hormore (LH), and follicle-stimulating hormone (FSH) concentrations with 100 mg three times per day of androstenedione ($n = 9$) and placebo ($n = 10$). Values are mean ± *SEM*. * = Significant difference from time zero for androstenedione ($p < 0.05$).

Adapted from King et al. 1999.

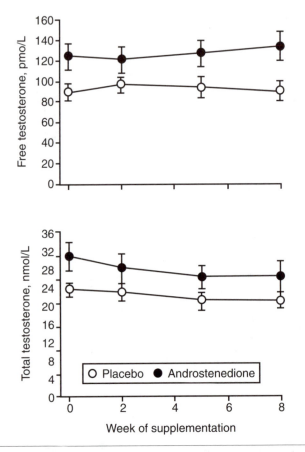

Figure 12.3   Serum free and total testosterone concentrations with 100 mg three times per day of androstenedione ($n = 9$) and placebo ($n = 10$). Values are mean ± *SEM*. Androstenedione had no effect on testosterone levels in males.

Adapted from King et al. 1999.

Estrone and estradiol concentrations, however, did increase (King et al. 1999; see figures 12.2, 12.3, and 12.4).

Leder and colleagues also studied androstenedione doses of 300 mg/day in young males and found, in contrast to the findings of King and associates, that testosterone concentrations did increase (Leder 2000). Leder's group administered androstenedione as a single dose, whereas King's group gave it as three divided doses.

Unpublished data from research conducted at Eastern Michigan University apparently shows that androstenedione can increase testosterone levels by 15%, but the investigators themselves admit that this is insignificant since exercise alone can boost testosterone levels by 25% (Ritter 1999). Lack of an increase in testosterone levels after ingesting androstenedione

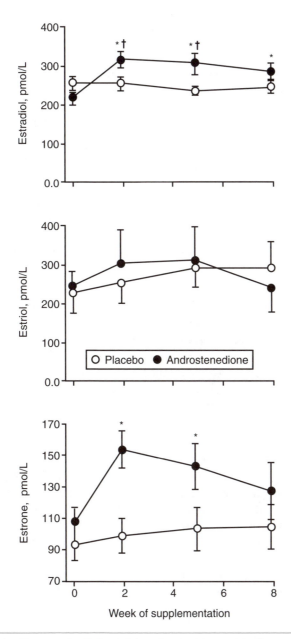

Figure 12.4 Serum estradiol, estriol, and estrone concentrations with 100 mg three times per day of androstenedione ($n = 9$) and placebo ($n = 10$). Values are mean ± *SEM*.

* = Significant difference from week zero for androstenedione ($p < 0.05$);

† = androstenedione significantly different from placebo ($p < 0.05$).

Adapted from King et al. 1999.

should not be surprising, really, since the conversion of androstenedione to testosterone in males is very slight (Horton and Tait 1966).

Regarding dehydroepiandrosterone (DHEA), urine testoterone: epitestosterone (T:E) ratios increased in one male subject after chronic doses of 50-150 mg/day for 6 months (Bowers 1999), but no increase was seen in three other male subjects after only 21 days of a similar dose. DHEA at doses of 1600 mg/day had no effect on either serum free or total testosterone levels in 5 other men (Nestler et al. 1988). Nevertheless, small quantities of DHEA are converted to testosterone as documented by using labeled DHEA (Dehennin et al. 1998) and by measuring urinary T:E ratios (Bowers 1999).

In females, however, serum testosterone concentrations have been shown to increase 60-90 min after single, oral doses of 100 mg of either DHEA or androstenedione; plasma testosterone rose 3-4 fold after androstenedione (Mahesh and Greenblatt 1962). These data, however, are four decades old and were obtained in only several subjects.

How Androstenedione and DHEA Affect Exercise Performance

Muscle strength, determined on eight different muscle groups, was not different in 19 men between those receiving androstenedione 300 mg/day or placebo during an 8-week resistance training regimen (King et al. 1999).

Considering how widely used the supplements androstenedione and DHEA are, there is an urgent need for better research than the data provided from these few studies of small numbers of subjects.

Avoiding Potential Complications

Data regarding toxicity after either short-term or long-term use of androstenedione are not available. In August 1998 General Nutrition Centers ordered its 3700 stores not to sell androstenedione because of uncertainty regarding its safety. The order may have been as much a reaction to public outcry over the inconsistent regulation of this supplement by the various sports governing bodies as evidence of true concern over the toxicity of androstenedione. Estrogen levels can increase in males who take androstenedione (King et al. 1999). Thus, this would predispose males to gynecomastia, testicular atrophy, and perhaps other long-term effects. In addition, since DHEA can compete with natural testosterone for receptor binding sites, testosterone production can be suppressed, and excess DHEA shunted to estrogen production. Even though testosterone levels do not appear to be affected significantly by androstenedione (at least in males with preexisting normal levels of testosterone), there have been reports of shipments of androstenedione actually containing as much as 50% testosterone (Ritter 1999).

Hepatotoxicity has been documented in animal studies of DHEA, as mentioned earlier. Finally, since DHEA is sold as a dietary supplement and not as a pharmaceutical drug, the FDA has no authority to ensure quality control. Thus, many products may not contain the amount of DHEA stated on their labels.

■ *NCAA and USOC Status*

Randy Barnes, an Olympic shot-putter, missed the 1992 Olympics because he tested positive for a banned substance. He admitted that he had used androstenedione, but felt victimized since the product can be purchased over the counter. Olympic swimmer and three-time gold medalist Michelle de Bruin (formerly Michelle Smith) was permanently banned from competition when a urine test turned up androstenedione.

Note: From *Times* [London], 13 June 1999.

Androstenedione increases the ratio of testosterone to epitestosterone. In 1997 the International Olympic Committee added androstenedione and DHEA to its list of banned substances under the category of androgenic-anabolic steroids. Both androstenedione and DHEA are banned by the NCAA and the USOC. In addition, the NFL, the International Tennis Federation, and the ATP currently ban androstenedione. Major League Baseball (MLB) and the NBA do not ban the substance, but if Mark McGwire attempted to play baseball in the Olympics, he would have to stop using androstenedione! In September 1998, the IOC announced that they would press MLB to also ban androstenedione (see AP, 15 September 1998). Paul Beeston, MLB president and CEO, stated that this issue would be addressed after the 1998 baseball season (AP, 10 September 1998). About the same time, in September 1998, New Jersey became the first state to introduce a bill for discussion that, if passed, would prohibit sale of androstenedione to minors.

In July 1999, Barry R. McCaffrey, director of the White House's Office of National Drug Control Policy, announced he was examining whether androstenedione could be classified as an anabolic steroid under the Anabolic Steroids Act (Ritter 1999). Unfortunately, to qualify, a substance must be shown to promote muscle growth, and so far that has not been demonstrated for androstenedione. There are data in animals, however, showing that androstenedione does possess physiologic actions similar to those possessed by testosterone (Villalba, Auger, and DeVries 1999), and some data exist to support the belief that androstenedione and DHGA can be converted to testosterone, at least in certain subjects.

Whether or not androstenedione is clearly a testosterone precursor may be less important to focus on than the fact that it has not been universally banned by athletic organizations. True androgenic-anabolic steroids (e.g., nandrolone, stanozolol, testosterone) are not only banned by all athletic organizations, but are prescription-only pharmaceuticals and are classified as controlled substances. In contrast, androstenedione and DHEA can be purchased by anyone, including adolescents! It is not surprising, therefore, that some athletes are confused about the legality of a given substance, particularly one that can be simultaneously regarded as a dietary supplement and a banned substance.

Finally, because both androstenedione and DHEA are endogenous substances, a urinary threshold concentration should be adopted. One set of investigators, based on limited research, has proposed a urinary concentration of 300 mcg/L of DHEA glucuronide or higher, but cautioned that detection of this metabolite would need to be performed within 8 h of ingestion (Dehennin et al. 1998). Apparently a threshold urine concentration has not yet been established for androstenedione.

Guidelines for Use

Olympic athletes face a lifetime ban for using androstenedione, whereas world-class athletes in non-Olympic competitions set records while freely admitting to using it. Sport governing bodies need to establish consistency, but this may not be easy to accomplish. Even baseball analysts do not see the dichotomy; ESPN's Joe Morgan, for example, stated that he does not see anything wrong with McGwire's use of androstenedione since it is not banned by MLB (Martzke 1998). We badly need clinical data on androstenedione's performance-enhancing potential. And the governing bodies of various sports must adopt a uniform policy about this agent.

Chromium

Chromium is an essential micronutrient. It is a mineral required in very small amounts, what is called a "trace element." Dietary sources of chromium include apples, asparagus, brewer's yeast, cheese, grains, meats, potatoes, raisins, and seafood. Nevertheless, most adults in the United States are deficient in chromium from dietary sources. The required daily amount (RDA) is 50-200 mcg daily. From a perspective of nutrition and metabolism, chromium is thought to potentiate the actions of insulin at the cellular level. Chromium stabilizes blood sugar (and, in turn, insulin output). Furthermore, since insulin is also involved in the uptake of amino acids by muscle cells, some athletes believe that chromium can improve protein synthesis and therefore may be anabolic. Carrying this theory further, increased uptake of amino acids by skeletal muscle cells should alter body mass and body composition.

How Chromium Affects Exercisers

Despite the importance of chromium to human nutrition and specific physiologic pathways, supplementing chromium beyond daily needs (Lefavi et al. 1992) provides little added benefit in sports. When 924 mcg/day of chromium picolinate was given to older men undergoing a 12-week resistance training program, no impact was seen on either glucose metabolism (Joseph et al. 1999) or on iron metabolism or hematologic indices (Campbell et al. 1997). A separate group of investigators, however, did observe a decrease in transferrin saturation with doses of chromium picolinate 170-180 mcg/day (Lukaski et al. 1996). The impact of this finding is uncertain.

Regarding effects on body composition, in general, chromium picolinate has been shown not to modify the changes seen in body composition in response to a resistance training regimen. This has been documented in young males (Hallmark et al. 1996); in older males (Campbell et al. 1997); in obese, active-duty Navy personnel (Trent and Thieding-Cancel 1995); and in collegiate wrestlers (Walker et al. 1998) (see table 12.1). In obese women, however, chromium picolinate supplementation without exercise induced a significant increase in body weight. Unexpectedly, exercise with chromium *nicotinate*, but not exercise with chromium *picolinate*, leads to significant weight loss in these obese women. No explanation was offered for this observation. Both supplements were administered in doses of 400 mcg/day (Grant et al. 1997).

Regarding the ergogenic potential of adding chromium supplements to an exercise regimen, it appears that, here again, chromium offers no benefit for either strength or performance. Several groups of investigators administered chromium picolinate in doses of 200 mcg/day combined with resistance training for roughly 3 months to test changes in strength among young males. No benefit of chromium was seen in either untrained young males (Hallmark et al. 1996) or in NCAA Division I wrestlers (Walker et al. 1998). Similarly, no improvements were seen in either muscle strength or power in older males, even when higher doses (i.e., 924 mcg/day) were administered (Campbell et al. 1997; Lukaski et al. 1996).

In conclusion, data indicate that chromium supplementation does not improve muscle size or strength. Chromium picolinate does not enhance the effects of exercise on body composition, but the response of obese females to the nicotinate form of chromium needs further investigation.

Avoiding Potential Complications

Chromium, like all heavy metals, is potentially nephrotoxic. The fact that the body absorbs chromium poorly is actually a blessing in disguise.

Table 12.1   Effects of Resistive Training and Chromium Supplementation on Body Composition

	Pre	Post
Cr³⁺ group		
Weight (kg)	81.6 ± 4.1	82.00 ± 4.2
Body fat (%)	19.8 ± 1.9	18.8 ± 2.0
LBM (kg)	64.8 ± 2.4	65.8 ± 2.4
Waist/hip	0.88 ± 0.01	0.88 ± 0.01
Skinfolds Σ 7 (mm)	140 ± 13	118 ± 13
Circumferences Σ 5 (cm)	74.6 ± 10.8	73.4 ± 11.1
P group		
Weight (kg)	80.5 ± 5.2	80.9 ± 4.9
Body fat (%)	20.0 ± 3.7	20.1 ± 3.4
LBM (kg)	63.0 ± 2.7	63.5 ± 2.7
Waist/hip	0.89 ± 0.02	0.88 ± 0.02
Skinfolds Σ 7 (mm)	153 ± 26	119 ± 17
Circumferences Σ 5 (cm)	74.6 ± 11.1	74.5 ± 10.7

Values are means ± SE. Cr^{3+} = chromium group; P = placebo group; LBM = lean body mass; waist/hip = waist to hip ratio; Σ 7 = sum of 7 skinfolds (triceps, chest, subscapular, abdominal, iliac, mid-axillary, thigh); Σ 5 = sum of 5 circumferences (biceps, chest, waist, hip, calf).

Adapted from Hallmark et al. 1996.

Chromium is produced in nicotinate and picolinate forms to improve oral bioavailability. The hexavalent form is *extremely nephrotoxic,* but this form is generally found only in industrial chemicals; the hexavalent form should never be ingested.

Most nutritional forms of chromium are the trivalent type. These appear to be safe if excessive doses are not consumed. However, one case has been reported of a woman who developed interstitial nephritis after ingesting chromium picolinate 600 mcg/day (12 times the RDA) for 6 weeks (Wasser, Feldman, and D'Agati 1997). A separate case report noted that a 24-year-old female bodybuilder developed diffuse myalgias and rhabdomyolysis after ingesting 1200 mcg chromium picolinate over 2 days. Her creatine kinase peaked at 30,200 units per liter, and she eventually recovered (Martin and Fuller 1998). Others have reported headaches, sleep disturbances, and mood disorders attributed to chromium use (Huzonek 1993; Schrauzer, Shrestha, and Arce 1992).

NCAA and USOC Status

Neither the NCAA nor the USOC has banned chromium as a substance for athletes to take before sports events.

Guidelines for Use

Campbell and Anderson (1987) showed that aerobic exercise accelerates the depletion of chromium. Considering this and the fact that most diets are deficient in chromium, chromium supplementation appears justified in *moderate doses* (e.g., 50-100 mcg/day). There is no reason to believe that these doses or higher doses are anabolic, however. In fact, higher doses may be nephrotoxic.

Coenzyme Q-10

Coenzyme Q-10 (also known as ubiquinone and as Co-Q10) is an antioxidant. Produced in the body, it also is found in small amounts in meat and some seafood; the typical adult diet contains roughly 3-5 mg per day (Weber, Bysted, and Holmer 1997). Coenzyme Q-10 was isolated in pure form in 1957. It is a carrier for two-electron transfer within the mitochondrial membrane, and it is vital for energy production. It seems to act like a free radical scavenger or a membrane stabilizer (or both) against oxidative stress (Greenberg and Frishman 1988). There are no data that demonstrate that coenzyme Q-10 promotes or improves oxygen utilization by cardiac myocytes. Although its role is being studied in clinical medicine for ischemic heart disease, congestive heart failure, and drug-induced cardiotoxicity, at this time it can be regarded only as an experimental agent for these uses.

How Coenzyme Q-10 Affects Exercisers

Several studies have been published regarding the effects of the coenzyme Q-10 molecule in sports (Braun et al. 1991; Malm et al. 1997; Porter et al. 1995; Snider et al. 1992; Weston et al. 1997; Ylikoski et al. 1997). The dosage studied in these investigations ranged from a low of 1 mg/kg/day to a high of 300 mg/day. Administration of coenzyme Q-10 supplementation did not improve performance in elite cyclists (see Braun et al. 1991; Weston et al. 1997) or in elite triathletes (see Snider et al. 1992; Weston et al. 1997). Still, in one study of elite cross-country skiers, $\dot{V}O_2$max and exercise performance did improve after use of coenzyme Q-10 (Ylikoski et al. 1997). Two other groups of investigators studied untrained subjects. In one of the studies (Porter et al. 1995), the subjects reported a significant increase in "vigor," but $\dot{V}O_2$max was not changed.

In the other study (Malm et al. 1997), total work performed was actually lower in the coenzyme Q-10 group than in the placebo group.

It is unclear why coenzyme Q-10 improved performance only in cross-country skiers. The bioavailability of different product formulations may explain why separate investigations realized different results (Chopra et al. 1998). However, in the studies where significant increases in plasma levels of coenzyme Q-10 were documented, $\dot{V}O_2$max did not improve (Braun et al. 1991; Porter et al. 1995; Weston et al. 1997). Generally, all the investigators studied supranormal doses (relative to typical dietary intake) of coenzyme Q-10.

It is intriguing to speculate on the ergogenic potential of this compound. In the arena of clinical medicine, studies have shown that it is beneficial in patients who have had congestive heart failure (Morisco, Trimarco, and Condorelli 1993; Morisco et al. 1994) or muscular dystrophies (Folkers and Simonsen 1995). Literature reviews (see Greenberg and Frishman 1988, 1990) have suggested it is also beneficial in other aspects of cardiac disease. Children who have been treated with anthracycline-type antineoplastic drugs, which are well known to be cardiotoxic, develop abnormalities in oxygen uptake ($\dot{V}O_2$) measured during exercise that are attributed to a limited inotropic reserve (Johnson et al. 1997). Further, in mice exposed to doxorubicin, both exercise (Kanter et al. 1985) and pretreatment with coenzyme Q-10 (Combs et al. 1977) were found to minimize the cardiotoxic effects of the drug. The authors of both studies suggest that exercise and supplemental coenzyme Q-10 independently potentiate the antioxidant enzymes that are protective against cardiotoxicity from an anthracycline drug.

Guidelines for Use

Although data on coenzyme Q-10 are sketchy, this compound *might* have ergogenic effects, albeit in subjects with diminished cardiac reserve, although a recent study of patients with severe congestive heart failure showed that it offered no benefit (Watson et al. 1999). Thus, while coenzyme Q-10 supplements may offer nothing to elite athletes or otherwise healthy untrained individuals, they might be beneficial in recipients of anthracycline-type antineoplastic drugs who have diminished exercise capacity. Certainly, coenzyme Q-10 is worthy of further clinical investigation in this setting.

Sodium Bicarbonate

It has been proposed that intracellular and extracellular acidosis can contribute to fatigue. Acid-base alterations appear to be most dramatic during exercise that cannot be sustained for longer than 7 minutes (Linderman and Fahey 1991). Sodium bicarbonate ingested shortly before an endurance event is thought to be ergogenic by its neutralizing of accumulated lactic acid.

How Sodium Bicarbonate Affects Exercisers

Numerous investigators have examined the effects of increased buffer capacity on athletic performance (Bouissou et al. 1988; Iwaoka et al. 1989; Linderman and Fahey 1991). Linderman and Fahey (1991) reviewed the effects of sodium bicarbonate on athletic performance. In looking at 15 studies of sodium bicarbonate, they found that 6 showed a statistically significant benefit, 5 showed no benefit, and 4 did not assess the effects of bicarbonate on endurance. Interestingly, 5 of the 6 studies showing a benefit utilized higher doses of 300 mg/kg, whereas many of the other studies used lower doses; there may be a dose-related effect. Linderman and Fahey (1991) concluded that for activities lasting up to 7 minutes, sodium bicarbonate can enhance performance. Exercise beyond 7 minutes, resulting in exhaustion, means less reliance on glycolysis for energy; thus, it results in less lactate formation. For longer endurance events, a beneficial effect of sodium bicarbonate is not seen (Linderman and Fahey 1991). There may be a good explanation for this. Lactic acid generation is related to exercise intensity, but it might also be related to total muscle mass involved, and different levels of lactic acid at steady-state have been measured for different types of activities (see figure 12.5; Beneke and von Duvillard 1996).

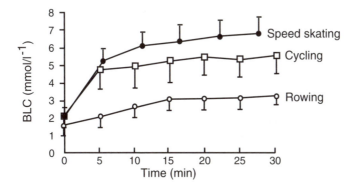

Figure 12.5   Blood-lactate concentration during maximal lactate steady state (MLSS) workload in rowing, cycling, and speed skating. All MLSS levels are significantly different (p 0.05).

Adapted from Beneke and von Duvillard 1996.

Avoiding Potential Complications

Keep in mind that oral sodium bicarbonate doses in the range of 300 mg/kg frequently cause gastrointestinal intolerance, which in and of itself may impair performance during endurance exercise. To satisfy a dose of 300 mg/kg, a 75 kg athlete would need to ingest as many as 35 tablets of 650 mg each.

NCAA and USOC Status

Neither the NCAA nor the USOC bans sodium bicarbonate or the related alkalinizing agent sodium acetate.

Guidelines for Use

Since enormous doses are required to achieve a beneficial effect, athletes interested in using sodium bicarbonate should test their tolerance before trying the substance during actual competition. In addition, sodium bicarbonate might not be ergogenic in events that are shorter than 1 minute or longer than 7 minutes, regardless of the dose ingested. Also, the half-life of sodium bicarbonate is very short. Thus, it is unlikely that ingesting it several hours prior to competition or ingesting it at the beginning of any event that lasts more than 2 to 3 hours would be beneficial. Finally, individuals should also consider the ethical issues surrounding use of an ergogenic substance, even if it is not classified as a banned one.

References

Beneke, R., and von Duvillard, S.P. 1996. Determination of maximal lactate steady state response in selected sports events. *Med Sci Sports Exerc* 28:241-246.

Bouissou, P., Defer, G., Guezennec, C.Y., Estrade, P.Y., and Serrurier, B. 1988. Metabolic and blood catecholamine responses to exercise during alkalosis. *Med Sci Sports Exerc* 20:228-232.

Bowers, L.D. 1999. Oral dehydroepiandrosterone supplementation can increase the testosterone:epitestosterone ratio. *Clin Chem* 45:295-297.

Braun, B., Clarkson, P.M., Freedson, P.S., and Kohl, R.L. 1991. Effects of coenzyme Q10 supplementation on exercise performance, VO_2max, and lipid peroxidation in trained cyclists. *Int J Sport Nutr* 1:353-365.

Campbell, W.W., and Anderson, R.A. 1987. Effects of aerobic exercise and training on the trace minerals chromium, zinc, and copper. *Sports Med* 4:9-18.

Campbell, W.W., Beard, J.L., Joseph, L.J., Davey, S.L., and Evans, W.J. 1997. Chromium picolinate supplementation and resistive training by older men: Effects on iron-status and hematologic indexes. *Am J Clin Nutr* 66:944-949.

Chopra, R.K., Goldman, R., Sinatra, S.T., and Bhagavan, H.N. 1998. Relative bioavailability of coenzyme Q-10 formulations in human subjects. *Int J Vitam Nutr Res* 68:109-113.

Combs, A.B., Choe, J.Y., Truong, D.H., and Folkers, K. 1977. Reduction by coenzyme Q10 of the acute toxicity of adriamycin in mice. *Res Commun Chem Pathol Pharmacol* 18:565-568.

Dehennin, L., Ferry, M., Lafarge, P., Peres, G., and Lafarge, J.P. 1998. Oral administration of dehydroepiandrosterone to healthy men: Alteration of the urinary androgen profile and consequences for the detection of abuse in sport by gas chromatography-mass spectrometry. *Steroids* 63:80-87.

Folkers, K., and Simonsen, R. 1995. Two successful double-blind trials with coenzyme Q10 (vitamin Q10) on muscular dystrophies and neurogenic atrophies. *Biochim Biophys Acta* 1271:281-286.

Grant, K.E., Chandler, R.M., Castle, A.L., and Ivy, J.L. 1997. Chromium and exercise training: Effect on obese women. *Med Sci Sports Exerc* 29:992-998.

Greenberg, S.M., and Frishman, W.H. 1988. Coenzyme Q-10: A new drug for myocardial ischemia? *Med Clin North Am* 72:243-258.

Greenberg, S.M., and Frishman, W.H. 1990. Coenzyme Q-10: A new drug for cardiovascular disease? *J Clin Pharmacol* 30:596-608.

Hallmark, M.A., Reynolds, T.H., DeSouza, C.A., Dotson, C.O., Anderson, R.A., and Rogers, M.A. 1996. Effects of chromium and resistive training on muscle strength and body composition. *Med Sci Sports Exerc* 28:139-144.

Horton, R., and Tait, J.F. 1966. Androstenedione production and interconversion rates measured in peripheral blood and studies on the possible site of its conversion to testosterone. *J Clin Invest* 45:301-313.

Huzonek, J. 1993. Over-the-counter chromium picolinate [Letter to the editor]. *Am J Psychiatry* 150:1560-1561.

Iwaoka, K., Okagawa, S., Mutoh, Y., and Miyashita, M. 1989. Effect of bicarbonate ingestion on the respiratory compensation threshold and maximal exercise performance. *Jap J Physiol* 39:255-265.

Johnson, D., Perrault, H., Fournier, A., Leclerc, J.M., Bigras, J.L., and Davignon, A. 1997. Cardiovascular responses to dynamic submaximal exercise in children previously treated with anthracycline. *Am Heart J* 133:169-173.

Johnson, R. 1999. Abnormal testosterone:epitestosterone ratios after dehydroepiandrosterone supplementation. *Clin Chem* 45:163-164.

Joseph, L.J., Farrell, P.A., Davey, S.L., Evans, W.J., and Campbell, W.W. 1999. Effect of resistance training with or without chromium picolinate supplementation on glucose metabolism in older men and women. *Metabolism* 48:546-553.

Kanter, M.M., Hamlin, R.L., Unverferth, D.V., Davis, H.W., and Merola, A.J. 1985. Effect of exercise training on antioxidant enzymes and cardiotoxicity of doxorubicin. *J Appl Physiol* 59:1298-1303.

King, D.S., Sharp, R.L., Vukovich, M.D., Brown, G.A., Reifenrath, T.A., Uhl, N.L., and Parsons, K.A. 1999. Effect of oral androstenedione on serum testosterone and adaptations to resistance training in young men. *JAMA* 281:2020-2028.

Kuoppasalmi, K., Naveri, H., Harkonen, M., and Adlercreutz, H. 1980. Plasma cortisol, androstenedione, testosterone and luteinizing hormone in running exercise of different intensities. *Scand J Clin Lab Invest* 40:403-409.

Leder, B.Z., Longcope, C., Catlin, D.H., Ahrens, B., Schoenfeld, D.A., Finkelstein, J.S.. 2000. Oral androstenedione administration and serum testosterone concentrations in young men. *JAMA* 283:779-782.

Lefavi, R.G., Anderson, R.A., Keith, R.E., Wilson, G.D., McMillan, J.L., and Stone, M.H. 1992. Efficacy of chromium supplementation in athletes: Emphasis on anabolism. *Int J Sports Nutr* 2:111-122.

Linderman, J., and Fahey, T.D. 1991. Sodium bicarbonate ingestion and exercise performance. *Sports Med* 11:71-77.

Lukaski, H.C., Bolonchuk, W.W., Siders, W.A., and Milne, D.B. 1996. Chromium supplementation and resistance training: Effects on body composition, strength, and trace element status of men. *Am J Clin Nutr* 63:954-965.

Mahesh, V.B., and Greenblatt, R.B. 1962. The in vivo conversion of dehydroepiandrosterone and androstenedione to testosterone in the human. *Acta Endocrinol* 41:400-406.

Malm, C., Svensson, M., Ekblom, B., and Sjodin, B. 1997. Effects of ubiquinone-10 supplementation and high intensity training on physical performance in humans. *Acta Physiol Scand* 161:379-384.

Martin, W.R., and Fuller, R.E. 1998. Suspected chromium picolinate-induced rhabdomyolysis. *Pharmacotherapy* 18:860-862.

Martzke, R. 1998. McGwire's enhancer use is foul talk, Morgan says. *USA Today,* 24 August.

McCann, B. 1997. Alternative medicine starting to penetrate hospital DURs. *Hospital Pharmacist Report,* December, 48-49.

McGraw, D. 1998. A pink viagra? Andro products target not only Mark McGwire wannabes but also older women. *US News & World Report,* 5 October.

Morisco, C., Nappi, A., Argenziano, L., Sarno, D., Fonatana, D., Imbriaco, M., Nicolai, E., Romano, M., Rosiello, G., and Cuocolo, A. 1994. Noninvasive evaluation of cardiac hemodynamics during exercise in patients with chronic heart failure: Effects of short-term coenzyme Q10 treatment. *Mol Aspects Med* 15(suppl):S155-S163.

Morisco, C., Trimarco, B., and Condorelli, M. 1993. Effect of coenzyme Q10 therapy in patients with congestive heart failure: A long-term multicenter randomized study. *Clin Investig* 71(8 suppl):S134-S136.

Nestler, J.E., Barlascini, C.O., Clore, J.N., and Blackard, W.G. 1988. Dehydroepiandrosterone reduces serum low density lipoprotein levels and body fat but does not alter insulin sensitivity in normal men. *J Clin Endocrinol Metab* 66:57-61.

Patrick, D. 1998. Androstenedione is well-known substance of strength. *USA Today,* 24 August.

Phillips, G.B. 1996. Relationship between serum dehydroepiandrosterone sulfate, androstenedione, and sex hormones in men and women. *Eur J Endocrinol* 134:201-206.

Porter, D.A., Costill, D.L., Zachwieja, J.J., Krzeminski, K., Fink, W.J., Wagner, E., and Folkers, K. 1995. The effect of oral coenzyme Q10 on the exercise tolerance of middle-aged, untrained men. *Int J Sports Med* 16:421-427.

Ritter, S.K. 1999. Faster, higher, stronger. *Chemical & Engineering News,* 6 September, 42-52.

Rock, A. 1995. Vitamin hype: Why we're wasting $1 of every $3 we spend. *Money,* September, 83-92.

Schrauzer, G.N., Shrestha, K.P., and Arce, M.F. 1992. Somatopsychological effects of chromium supplementation. *J Nutr Med* 3:42-48.

Smith, E.A. 1998. Nutraceutical future looks bright, says panel of experts. *Drug Topics*, 16 February, 24.

Snider, I.P., Bazzarre, T.L., Murdoch, S.D., and Goldfarb, A. 1992. Effect of coenzyme athletic performance system as an ergogenic aid on endurance performance to exhaustion. *Int J Sport Nutr* 2:272-286.

Sturmi, J.E., and Diorio, D.J. 1998. Anabolic agents. *Clin Sports Med* 17:261-282.

Trent, L.K., and Thieding-Cancel, D. 1995. Effects of chromium picolinate on body composition. *J Sports Med Phys Fitness* 35:273-280.

Villalba, C., Auger, C.J., and DeVries, G.J. 1999. Androstenedione effects on the vasopressin innervation of the rat brain. *Endocrinology* 140:3383-3386.

Walker, L.S., Bemben, M.G., Bemben, D.A., and Knehans, A.W. 1998. Chromium picolinate effects on body composition and muscular performance in wrestlers. *Med Sci Sports Exerc* 30:1730-1737.

Wasser, W.G., Feldman, N.S., and D'Agati, V.D. 1997. Chronic renal failure after ingestion of over-the-counter chromium picolinate. *Ann Intern Med* 126:410.

Watson, P.S., Scalia, G.M., Galbraith, A., Burstow, D.J., Bett, N., and Aroney, C.N. 1999. Lack of effect of coenzyme Q on left ventricular function in patients with congestive heart failure. *J Am Coll Cardiol* 33:1549-1552.

Weber, C., Bysted, A., and Holmer, G. 1997. Coenzyme Q10 in the diet: Daily intake and relative bioavailability. *Mol Aspects Med* 18(suppl):S251-S254.

Welle, S., Jozefowicz, R., and Statt, M. 1990. Failure of dehydroepiandrosterone to influence energy and protein metabolism in humans. *J Clin Endocrinol Metab* 71:1259-1264.

Weston, S.B., Zhou, S., Weatherby, R.P., and Robson, S.J. 1997. Does exogenous coenzyme Q10 affect aerobic capacity in endurance athletes? *Int J Sport Nutr* 7(3):197-206.

Yesalis, C.E. 1993. *Anabolic steroids in sport and exercise*. Champaign, IL: Human Kinetics.

Yesalis, C.E. 1999. Medical, legal, and societal implications of androstenedione use. *JAMA* 21:2043-2044.

Ylikoski, T., Piirainen, J., Hanninen, O., and Penttinen, J. 1997. The effect of coenzyme Q10 on the exercise performance of cross-country skiers. *Mol Aspects Med* 18(suppl):S283-S290.

IV
PART

Socially Used Drugs

13

CHAPTER

Caffeine

■ *CASE* Sarah has competed in several triathlons. Now she is getting even more serious and is seeking ways to improve her performance. A male friend, a fine athlete who has competed in triathlons for many years, encourages her to use caffeine. He thinks it will help her train harder and improve her race times. Sarah doesn't like how caffeine makes her feel, and, more importantly, wonders whether it really does enhance performance and is acceptable to use for that purpose.

■ *COMMENT* Caffeine has proven ergogenic effects, and its use is not banned from competition as long as concentrations in the urine do not exceed a predetermined limit. While these facts address her concerns, it would be wise to also explain to her that caffeine has diuretic properties and that, in turn, diuretics can exert ergolytic effects on endurance exercise. Despite the fact that individuals who are taking caffeine in low doses are not banned from competition (i.e., those who produce urine concentrations less than the maximum allowable concentration), Sarah might appropriately question the ethics of using caffeine to enhance her performance.

Caffeine long has been the most widely used drug in Europe and America (Curatolo and Robertson 1983). In fact, one clear reason why coffee is the world's most popular beverage is its caffeine content. However, because the physiologic response to caffeine differs from the response to coffee (Graham, Hibbert, and Sathasivam 1998), caffeine should not be considered synonymous with coffee. Caffeine is only one of more than a hundred chemicals found in coffee (Curatolo and Robertson 1983), which contains only some 2% caffeine (Graham, Hibbert, and Sathasivam 1998).

Caffeine is found in many other beverages; some soft drinks (e.g., Jolt, Surge, Mountain Dew) contain boosted amounts of caffeine. Surprisingly, even some brands of bottled water contain caffeine! Many sport products that are promoted as "energy" drinks contain caffeine among their ingredients: Red Bull Energy Drink, Spark Nutritional Beverage Mix, and many others. Of course, one should not overlook all the other potential sources of caffeine, such as teas and over-the-counter headache and antidrowsiness remedies. Caffeine makes frequent appearances in sports and exercise!

Thousands of scientific studies on caffeine have been published during the 20th century; hundreds of these studies have explored the effects of caffeine in sports and athletics. This chapter summarizes some of these data. Readers are also referred to reviews of caffeine by Curatolo and Robertson (1983); Graham, Rush, and van Soeren (1994); Nehlig and Debry (1994); and Williams (1991).

How Exercise Affects the Action of Caffeine

Caffeine is 99% bioavailable after oral ingestion. Plasma concentrations peak within 15 to 45 min after oral ingestion, although some metabolic effects may not reach their maximum until several hours later. Caffeine is almost entirely metabolized by the mixed-function oxidase system in the liver; only 0.5% to 3.5% of a dose is excreted unchanged in the urine. It appears that single doses in the range of 3 to 5 mg/kg can saturate this hepatic metabolic pathway (Graham and Spriet 1995). The elimination half-life of caffeine has been reported to be 3.0 to 7.5 h in nonexercising adults (Curatolo and Robertson 1983), but the time is affected by exercise, obesity, and sex.

Caffeine is a "flow-limited" drug (Somani et al. 1990). Exercise, by diverting blood flow away from the organs responsible for elimination, can inhibit the rate of elimination of flow-limited drugs. Sustained exercise decreases the systemic clearance and elimination rate of caffeine, and these effects are more pronounced in obese subjects, relative to lean ones (Kamimori et al. 1987). Paradoxically, Collomp and colleagues (1991) showed that caffeine's half-life did not increase during 60 min of cycling at 30% $\dot{V}O_2$max. These investigators proposed that exercise enhances the activity of hepatic microsomal enzymes enough to offset the flow-limiting effects of exercise. Regarding renal elimination, at rest males and females eliminate caffeine at equivalent rates when normalized to body weight. During sustained exercise at 50% $\dot{V}O_2$max, however, the elimination rate in females decreased fivefold; it decreased only twofold in males (Duthel et al. 1991). This has important implications for the use of urine tests to screen for caffeine abuse, discussed later.

Caffeine belongs to the group of drugs known as xanthines, which also includes theophylline. Both are cardiovascular stimulants, theophylline being the stronger of the two. These drugs can stimulate the heart both directly and by stimulating the release of catecholamines from adrenergic nerve terminals in the heart and the adrenal medulla. Positive inotropic and chronotropic effects are seen. Caffeine is a stronger central nervous system (CNS) stimulant than is theophylline; paradoxically, caffeine can induce bradycardia through its effects on vagal medullary centers. Caffeine can also increase the frequency of muscle contractions by liberating calcium. All of these actions can be observed at rest.

Caffeine stimulates epinephrine output to a greater degree when ingested as capsules compared to the ingestion of an equal quantity of caffeine from caffeinated coffee (Graham, Hibbert, and Sathasivam 1998). Increases in circulating epinephrine levels explain the "jittery" or nervous energy sensation we commonly associate with consuming caffeine-containing beverages. Both exercise and caffeine can independently increase epinephrine output (Wemple, Lamb, and McKeever 1997), but exercise appears to be the more dominant influence (see figure 13.1). In caffeine-naive individuals, resting epinephrine levels rise within 60 min of ingestion of a single dose of caffeine, and caffeine augments the epinephrine response to 1 h of exercise at 50% $\dot{V}O_2$max (Van Soeren et al. 1993). This treatment difference disappears after intense exercise, such as the Wingate sprint (Greer, McLean, and Graham 1998). In caffeine-tolerant subjects, however, caffeine does not augment the epinephrine response to exercise (Van Soeren et al. 1993). Nevertheless, an additive response may be clinically significant, considering that an exaggerated pressor response has been documented in subjects who exercise while taking caffeine (Pincomb et al. 1991).

How Caffeine Affects Exercisers

Tolerance to the effects of caffeine is well known. With routine (i.e., daily) use, the readily apparent adrenergic effects of caffeine diminish to the

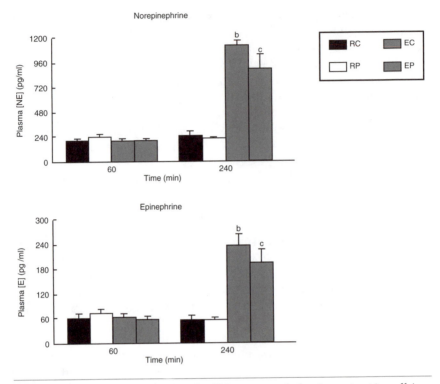

Figure 13.1 Effects of exercise and caffeine on catecholamine output in caffeine-naive subjects. Mean ± *SE* for norepinephrine and epinephrine. [b] EC vs. RC ($p <$ 0.01); [c] EP vs. RP ($p < 0.01$) ($n = 6$). RC = caffeine treatment at rest; RP = placebo treatment at rest; EC = caffeine treatment during exercise; EP = placebo treatment during exercise.

Adapted from Wemple, Lamb, and McKeever 1997.

point that chronic users can drink coffee even at night without having trouble falling asleep. When evaluating the effects of caffeine on individuals' physiology and performance, therefore, it is important to consider whether subjects are caffeine naive or caffeine tolerant.

Despite decades of research, investigators and sports medicine personnel still are uncertain of some of caffeine's effects. This is partly explained by the failure to distinguish acute effects (i.e., effects in caffeine-naive subjects) from chronic effects. Caffeine stimulates the CNS, enhances neuromuscular transmission, and improves skeletal muscle contractility (Nehlig and Debry 1994; Williams 1991). Acutely, caffeine increases systolic blood pressure (BP), and increases resting heart rate (HR). Nevertheless, complete tolerance to most, if not all, of these effects develops within several days of regular use (Curatolo and Robertson 1983). Some data suggest that caffeine increases epinephrine output in proportion to dose, but there does not appear to be any relationship between the resulting epinephrine levels and ergogenic effects on running performance (Graham and Spriet 1995). Some data indicate that the stimulatory effects of caffeine on epinephrine output is greater in trained subjects than in untrained subjects (LeBlanc et al. 1985). Interestingly, once exercise begins, epinephrine levels reflect the effects of exercise more than the effects of caffeine (Wemple et al. 1997). Variable effects of caffeine on norepinephrine output during exercise have been observed (see Graham and Spriet 1991, 1995).

Cardiovascular Effects

Caffeine's effect on HR may depend on when it was ingested. Generally, caffeine increases resting HR in caffeine-naive subjects (Curatolo and Robertson 1983). One study found, however, that neither resting nor exercise HRs were affected by a large (10 mg/kg), single dose of caffeine in caffeine-naive recreational cyclists who cycled to exhaustion (Flinn et al. 1990). In Flinn's study, the subjects were tested 3 h postdose. In still another study, no effect on exercise HR was seen when caffeine at 6 mg/kg was administered to caffeine-tolerant elite runners 60 min prior to treadmill running (Tarnopolsky et al. 1989). When hypertensive subjects were given 3.3 mg/kg caffeine (Sung et al. 1995), their resting HR decreased and their exercise HR increased, as compared to placebo. In this study, exercise began 40 min after the dose. Thus, the timing of measurements and the type of subjects studied can influence how investigators might interpret caffeine's effect on HR.

Caffeine was not found to affect cardiac output or stroke volume acutely in studies of either normotensive subjects (Sung et al. 1990) or of hypertensive subjects (Sung et al. 1995); there are no data on the chronic effects of caffeine on these cardiovascular parameters (Curatolo and Robertson 1983). Because of the development of tolerance, the effects of regular caffeine use on either cardiac output or stroke volume are probably minimal.

Sung and colleagues, on the other hand, found that single doses of caffeine (3.3 mg/kg) increased the BP response to exercise in both normotensive subjects (1990) and in hypertensive subjects (1995). Among the normotensive subjects, significantly more individuals in the caffeine group had systolic BPs greater than 230 mm Hg and diastolic pressures greater than 100 mm Hg *during maximal exercise* than in the placebo group (1990).

Renal Effects

For a detailed analysis of the combined effects of exercise and caffeine on renal physiology, we can turn to research conducted by Wemple, Lamb,

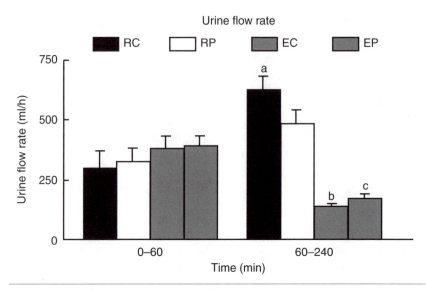

Figure 13.2   Effects of exercise and caffeine on urine flow rate. Mean ± *SE* for urine flow rate. [a]RC vs. RP ($p = 0.007$); [b]EC vs. RC ($p = 0.0000$); [c]EP vs. RP ($p = 0.001$) ($n = 6$). RC = caffeine treatment at rest; RP = placebo treatment at rest; EC = caffeine treatment during exercise; EP = placebo treatment during exercise.

Adapted from Wemple, Lamb, and McKeever 1997.

and McKeever (1997). Caffeine is well known to exert a moderate diuresis. Wemple and colleagues showed that although this effect occurs at rest, ingesting caffeine during prolonged endurance exercise does not augment exercise-induced fluid losses (see figure 13.2). Caffeine-naive subjects in the study consumed 8.7 mg/kg caffeine (about 490 to 680 mg total dose) over a period of 4 h while cycling at 60% $\dot{V}O_2$max. Since neither plasma vasopressin levels nor glomerular filtration rate (GFR) during exercise were affected by caffeine, the authors concluded that exercise-induced increases in catecholamine output constricts renal arterioles, reducing GFR and thereby limits the amount of filtrate that caffeine can act on to exert its diuretic effect (Wemple, Lamb, and McKeever 1997). Exercise-induced, insensible loss through sweat and respiration may also have decreased GFR. Thus, while ingesting caffeine at rest does induce a diuretic response, ingesting caffeine during exercise does not. Other investigators (Graham, Hibbert, and Sathasivam 1998) have reported similar observations.

Metabolic Effects

Acutely, caffeine can increase the basal metabolic rate. Some data (LeBlanc et al. 1985) indicate this effect is more pronounced in trained subjects; other data (Poehlman et al. 1985) indicate that the effect is greater in untrained subjects. As already mentioned, caffeine increases epinephrine concentrations, but this increase may not be linked to either the metabolic effects or the performance-enhancing effects seen with caffeine during exercise.

Earlier research indicated that caffeine stimulated lipolysis, with resting plasma levels of free fatty acids (FFAs) increasing 50-100% over baseline (Curatolo and Robertson 1983). Since a primary cause of fatigue during endurance exercise relates to depletion of muscle glycogen, the increased availability of FFAs may lead to a glycogen-sparing effect. Cleroux and colleagues (1989) demonstrated that lipolysis results from beta-adrenergic stimulation; specifically, adipose tissue lipolysis is controlled, in part, by beta-1 receptors, and skeletal muscle triglyceride breakdown is controlled exclusively by beta-2 receptors. Since caffeine stimulates epinephrine release—and because epinephrine is an agonist at both beta-1 and beta-2 receptors—it seems logical to conclude that caffeine's ergogenic properties are a result of its ability to enhance the breakdown of fats for energy, thereby sparing glycogen stores. However, a study by Graham, Hibbert, and Sathasivam in 1998 showed that neither glucose nor glycerol concentrations during treadmill exercise were significantly affected by caffeine in caffeine-naive elite runners. Further, reduction in glycolysis occurred only during the first 15 min of exercise, yet epinephrine levels remained high for the entire 90 min of exercise (Graham and Spriet 1991; Spriet et al. 1992). Ingesting three doses of caffeine during a 5-6 h, 40 km march did not influence performance during an exercise test conducted after the conclusion of the march; however, lactate levels were higher and RPE (ratings of perceived exertion) values were lower during the performance test in the group that received caffeine, suggesting that the individuals who received caffeine were able to exercise harder (Falk et al. 1989). Graham and Spriet (1995) concluded that increased epinephrine levels are not a prerequisite for caffeine's ergogenic action.

Nevertheless, caffeine clearly enhances fat oxidation during exercise, regardless of its effects on epinephrine levels. While the epinephrine response to caffeine wanes during chronic (i.e., several days to several weeks) use of caffeine, the beneficial effects of caffeine on fat oxidation persist (Bangsbo et al. 1992; Tarnopolsky et al. 1989). Pasman and colleagues in 1995 proposed that the effect of caffeine on fat oxidation is mediated via inhibition of adenosine receptors. Other investigators, however, found no relationship between caffeine dose, epinephrine levels, effects on FFAs, and performance (Graham and Spriet 1991). We may find explanations for these different findings by looking at when testing occurred in relationship to caffeine doses or at what intensity subjects were exercised.

When investigators have studied caffeine's effect on oxygen consumption, most of them have reported that the substance does not affect oxygen uptake ($\dot{V}O_2$). Gaesser and Rich, for example, in 1985 found that 5 mg/kg caffeine had no effect on either maximum or submaximum $\dot{V}O_2$ during cycling. Several years later, Graham, Sathasivam, and MacNaughton (1991) looked at the same amount of caffeine, 5 mg/kg, and found that it had no effect on $\dot{V}O_2$ of exercisers during 2 h of exercise in the cold. Tarnopolsky and colleagues (1989) made a similar study using 6 mg/kg caffeine, and found that amount had no effect on $\dot{V}O_2$ in subjects during 90 min of treadmill running at 70% $\dot{V}O_2$max.

Pulmonary Effects

Since both caffeine and theophylline are xanthines, it is not surprising that caffeine exerts some actions that are similar to those of theophylline. For example, both these xanthines exert protective effects in exercise-induced bronchoconstriction; caffeine at doses of 7 mg/kg was effective—but at doses of 3.5 mg/kg it was not (Kivity et al. 1990). In general, like theophylline, caffeine is a poor choice for this condition. In another study, single doses of 3.3 mg/kg caffeine increased tidal volume, increased alveolar ventilation, and decreased respiratory rate during treadmill walking. These effects occurred regardless of whether subjects were caffeine naive or caffeine tolerant (Brown et al. 1991). In addition to bronchodilatory effects, caffeine also stimulates ventilation centrally. D'Urzo and colleagues (1990) showed that caffeine 650 mg increased the chemosensitivity to CO_2 production during exercise below the anaerobic threshold. In doses of 7 mg/kg, caffeine affects other aspects of ventilatory and gas exchange during exercise (Powers et al. 1986). It is unclear, however, how these physiological effects impact exercise performance.

Neuromuscular Effects

Caffeine has been found to increase vigilance and decrease motor reaction time in response to both auditory and visual stimuli (Curatolo and Robertson 1983). However, despite its ability to enhance simple tasks (e.g., finger tapping a switch), caffeine may be detrimental in other tasks requiring fine motor coordination (e.g., archery, pistol shooting) or more complex skills (e.g., hitting a baseball, playing tennis). In one study of caffeine-naive college students, monosynaptic reflex response time was increased (i.e., an ergolytic action) by caffeine, but this study utilized large doses (6 mg/kg) of caffeine, and the degree of increase (23.8 milliseconds) is unlikely to be clinically significant in most athletes (Jacobson and Edwards 1990).

How Caffeine Affects Exercise Performance

You may recall that caffeine increases epinephrine output in proportion to dose, at least in caffeine-naive subjects (Graham and Spriet 1995). Unfortunately, there does not appear to be any relationship between the resulting epinephrine levels and ergogenic effects on running performance (Graham and Spriet 1995). But caffeine exerts metabolic effects, musculoskeletal effects, and CNS effects, and therefore may augment performance in other ways. Contrary opinions exist as to whether caffeine actually delays fatigue (Graham, Rush, and van Soeren 1994; Williams 1991). While caffeine serum concentrations peak within 1 h after ingestion, serum FFAs do not peak for 3 to 4 h after caffeine ingestion, which may explain some of the contradictory findings among the many studies of caffeine's effects on athletic performance (Flinn et al. 1990). Graham, Hibbert, and Sathasivam (1998) recently found that caffeine ingested as capsules improved treadmill running performance by 31% (compared with placebo). When subjects ingested the caffeine from coffee, however, no increase in performance was seen, despite a similar caffeine dose and equivalent caffeine plasma concentrations (see figure 13.3).

Other researchers have looked at specific activities in relation to consumption of caffeine. For example, Berglund and Hemmingsson (1982) conducted a study using subjects who participated in cross-country skiing. The skiers ingesting doses of 6 mg/kg produced a 1.7% improvement at an altitude of 300 m and a 3.2% improvement in performance at 2900 m. Other studies have looked at cyclists. Caffeine (10 mg/kg) was found to be ergogenic in caffeine-naive subjects when exercise testing involved cycling to exhaustion. During caffeine ingestion, the work completed and time to exhaustion were significantly increased. The study examined incremental cycling to exhaustion 3 h after ingestion of caffeine at 10 mg/kg (see table 13.1; Flinn et al. 1990). In another study (Spriet et al. 1992), single doses of 9 mg/kg caffeine administered 1 h prior to testing produced a 26.9% increase in cycling time in recreational cyclists.

These studies used large doses of caffeine. Since it is thought that doses of this magnitude may saturate metabolic pathways, Pasman and colleagues (1995) studied caffeine doses of 5, 9, and 13 mg/kg. All three doses were ergogenic in cycling to exhaustion at 80% Wmax, and no dose-response relationship was seen (see figure 13.4). The increase in cycling performance was about 27%. Others have confirmed an ergogenic effect of caffeine (5 mg/kg) during cycling at 85-90% Wmax (Trice and Haymes 1995). However, administering single doses of caffeine at 6 mg/kg 1 h prior to exercise testing did not improve peak power, average power, or rate of power loss during repeated 30 s Wingate exercise tests (Greer, McLean, and Graham 1998). Thus, it appears that

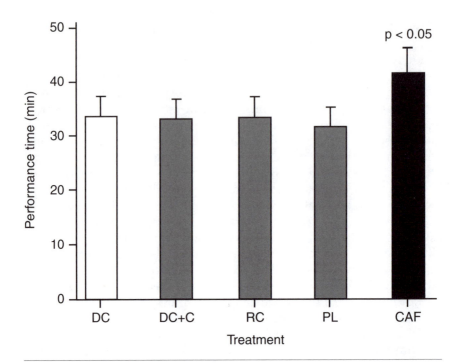

Figure 13.3 Effect of coffee and caffeine on submaximal running. Caffeine capsule test resulted in endurance being increased ($p < 0.05$) beyond that of the other four trials. There were no differences among the other trials. Increased endurance time after caffeine capsules meant that subjects were able to run an additional 2-3 km at the prescribed speed and slope. DC = decaffeinated coffee; DC + C = decaffeinated coffee plus caffeine capsules; RC = regular coffee; PL = placebo capsules; and CAF = caffeine capsules.

Adapted from Graham, Hibbert, and Sathasivam 1998.

Table 13.1   Effect of Caffeine on Times to Exhaustion and Work Done During Cycle Ergometry

	Time to exhaustion (min · sec)	Work completed (kilojoules)
Control	14.02 ± 3.1	164.3 ± 8.8
Placebo	14.85 ± 2.8	166.9 ± 7.7
Caffeine	17.52 ± 3.7*	206.4 ± 8.2*

*Significant difference from either the control or placebo measures ($p < 0.01$). Means ± SD.

Adapted from Flinn et al. 1990.

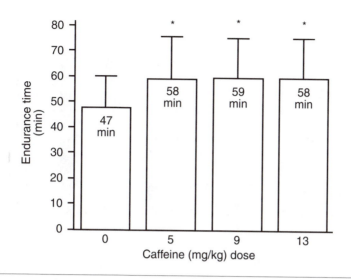

Figure 13.4 Endurance performance with different caffeine concentrations. The cycling time (minutes) is averaged for 9 subjects. The caffeine performances were significantly better than the placebo performance. No significant differences among the caffeine tests were found. * = $p < 0.05$ placebo vs. caffeine.

Adapted from Pasman et al. 1995.

caffeine is ergogenic in both prolonged and intense cycling, but not helpful for purely anaerobic levels of activity.

Graham and Spriet (1995) examined the impact of various doses of caffeine on running performance at 85% $\dot{V}O_2max$. Giving caffeine at single doses of 3 mg/kg and 6 mg/kg 1 h before running on a treadmill produced increases in performance of roughly 22% in elite, caffeine-naive runners with both doses. Administering doses of 9 mg/kg produced even greater improvements in running and cycling performance, at 85% $\dot{V}O_2max$ in another study (see figures 13.5 and 13.6; Graham and Spriet 1991). In yet another study, investigators found that doses of 4.45 mg/kg were also ergogenic on running at 85% $\dot{V}O_2max$, but only when the caffeine was ingested as capsules, not when ingested as coffee (Graham, Hibbert, and Sathasivam 1998) (see figure 13.3). A separate investigator found that caffeine 5 mg/kg administered 1 h before treadmill running at 125% $\dot{V}O_2max$ was also ergogenic in 9 well-trained males (Doherty 1998).

In 1991, Doubt and Hsieh concluded that caffeine 5 mg/kg during exercise in cold water (not actual swimming performance) had no beneficial effect on exercise physiology. Another study (Williams 1991) looked at issues of strength; despite the cellular effects of increased neuromuscular transmission and improved skeletal muscle contractility,

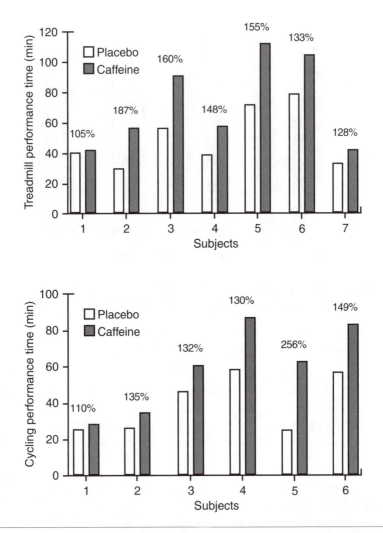

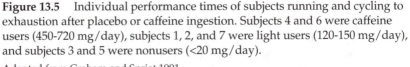

Figure 13.5 Individual performance times of subjects running and cycling to exhaustion after placebo or caffeine ingestion. Subjects 4 and 6 were caffeine users (450-720 mg/day), subjects 1, 2, and 7 were light users (120-150 mg/day), and subjects 3 and 5 were nonusers (<20 mg/day).

Adapted from Graham and Spriet 1991.

caffeine was not shown to improve muscular strength, maximum power output, or maximum voluntary contractions.

In summary, caffeine appears to offer ergogenic effects in prolonged endurance exercise but not during activities that require very short bursts of high-intensity effort. In that regard, caffeine is the opposite of agents like high doses of creatine and sodium bicarbonate, metabolic

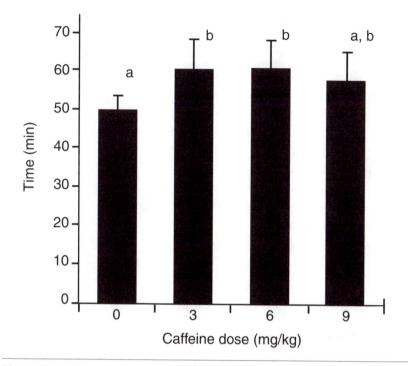

Figure 13.6   Exercise time during exercise to exhaustion. Data are mean data for exercise duration after placebo (0 mg/kg) or 3, 6, or 9 mg/kg of caffeine. Histogram bars with the same letter are data not significantly different from each other. Note that 0 and 3 mg/kg trials were significantly different despite lack of difference in plasma epinephrine and, conversely, that 0 and 9 mg/kg exercise times were not significantly different, although these trials had quite different plasma epinephrine data.

Adapted from Graham and Spriet 1995.

enhancers that are most ergogenic for short, high-intensity activity. For reasons that are unclear, caffeine ingested as capsules appears to elicit a greater ergogenic response than equal quantities ingested in the form of coffee. Graham, Rush, and van Soeren (1994) reviewed the various effects caffeine has on performance.

Avoiding Potential Complications

Exercisers may experience unpleasant effects while taking caffeine. Nausea is one example. When athletes ingest doses of 400 mg to 500 mg or higher, they risk experiencing nausea and abdominal discomfort. In one study, single doses of 9 mg/kg prevented one subject from

Table 13.2   Pros and Cons of Using Caffeine to Enhance Performance

Pros

  Increases aerobic endurance secondary to glycogen sparing effect.

  Facilitates voluntary reaction time.

  Improves alertness.

  At high doses, may prevent exercise-induced bronchoconstriction.

Cons

  Causes tremor; decreases hand steadiness.

  May cause tolerance and withdrawal symptoms.

  Banned substance if intake exceeds acceptable urinary limits.

  Lengthens monosynaptic reflex time.

  Has a diuretic effect if consumed several hours prior to exercise.

completing an exercise test due to gastrointestinal distress (Spriet et al. 1992).

A second problem is an exaggerated pressor response. Compared to placebo, caffeine increased the number of normotensive men who reached an abnormal exercise BP in a study conducted by Pincomb and colleagues (1991). Further, because caffeine possesses a diuretic action that can be detrimental to athletic performance, individuals should consume even small doses of it with caution, particularly during the several hours prior to endurance exercise. Falk and colleagues (1990), on the other hand, found that subjects could consume caffeine up to 2 h prior to exercise without augmenting their negative fluid balance during exercise.

Still another drawback to routine use of caffeine is that a withdrawal syndrome can occur after cessation of regular use (Silverman et al. 1992). Table 13.2 contains a summary of the pros and cons of using caffeine during athletic competition and physical exercise.

NCAA and USOC Status

According to the NCAA and USOC, caffeine is officially classified as a "restricted" substance and not a banned substance. Ethically, however, since beneficial effects on endurance exercise have been documented, caffeine can be considered a banned substance for use during competition. The IOC stipulates that any physiologic substance taken in abnormal quantity with the intention of artificially and unfairly increasing performance should be construed as doping (Williams 1994).

However, it is not simple to monitor use of caffeine. Single doses of caffeine at 9 mg/kg (i.e., doses in the range of 500-999 mg) or greater produce urine concentrations that exceed the USOC/IOC's and NCAA's acceptable limits, which are 12 mcg/ml and 15 mcg/ml, respectively (Graham and Spriet 1991). But this urinary concentration limit of 12 mcg/ml does not prevent athletes from obtaining benefits from caffeine. Doses of 3 to 6 mg/kg, which do not produce urine concentrations that would result in disqualification, have been found ergogenic (Graham and Spriet 1991, 1995; Pasman et al. 1995). Even higher doses of 9 mg/kg in trained competitive runners produced urinary caffeine concentrations of only 8.7 to 10.0 mcg/ml roughly 2 h after running or cycling to exhaustion (Graham and Spriet 1991). Caffeine doses of 5 mg/kg were as ergogenic as higher doses of 9 and 13 mg/kg doses, but the lower ones did not produce urine concentrations that exceeded the limit of 12 mcg/ml (Pasman et al. 1995). To put these doses into perspective, one Vivarin tablet contains 200 mg, one cup of coffee contains approximately 100 mg, and one 12 oz can of Coca-Cola contains approximately 45 mg caffeine (see table 13.3).

The flaw in relying on urine concentrations is that the urinary excretion of caffeine decreases during prolonged exercise (van der Merwe, Luus, and Barnard 1992), particularly in females (Duthel et al. 1991). At rest, only 0.5% to 3.5% of caffeine is excreted unchanged into the urine. In addition, detecting the decrease in caffeine elimination during exercise is confounded by the simultaneous decrease in urine volume during exercise. Van der Merwe, Luus, and Barnard (1992) found that despite a decrease in caffeine elimination of 49% during exercise, urinary caffeine concentrations during exercise and without exercise were nearly identical (see figure 13.7). Because of the influence of exercise and gender on the urinary excretion rate of caffeine, as well as the cultural differences in dietary intake of caffeine, Duthel and colleagues (1991) have argued against a fixed limit for urinary detection of caffeine.

Guidelines for Use

Caffeine is abundant in the diet and it is ergogenic; so sports medicine personnel frequently encounter situations where its use during competition raises questions. Here are some guidelines for individuals to follow, particularly in competition.

First, avoid routine use of caffeine. An individual can build tolerance to many of the effects of caffeine within several days. There is documentation that once such tolerance occurs, abrupt discontinuation of caffeine use can lead to a withdrawal syndrome, consisting of headaches and poorer performance.

Table 13.3   Amount of Caffeine in Frequently-Used Commercial Products and Their Equivalents in Urine Within 2-3 Hours

Product	Amount/ dose	Equivalence in urine within 2-3 hours
Decaffeinated coffee	2.0-3.0 mg	0.03-0.04 mcg/mL
1 cup regular coffee	100.0 mg	1.50 mcg/mL
5 oz instant tea	28.0 mg	0.42 mcg/mL
5 oz brewed tea	20.0-110.0 mg	0.30-1.60 mcg/mL
12 oz Coca-Cola, Diet Coke	45.6 mg	0.68 mcg/mL
12 oz Dr. Pepper	39.6 mg	0.59 mcg/mL
12 oz Pepsi, Diet Pepsi	36.0 mg	0.54 mcg/mL
12 oz Mountain Dew	55.0 mg	0.85 mcg/mL
12 oz Jolt Cola	90.0 mg	1.35 mcg/mL
12 oz Red Bull	115.0 mg	1.73 mcg/mL
1 oz milk chocolate	6.0 mg	0.08 mcg/mL
1 oz bittersweet chocolate	20.0 mg	0.30 mcg/mL
1 oz baking chocolate	26.0 mg	0.40 mcg/mL
1 No Doz	100.0 mg	1.50 mcg/mL
1 Vivarin	200.0 mg	3.00 mcg/mL
1 Anacin	32.0 mg	0.48 mcg/mL
1 Excedrin	65.0 mg	0.97 mcg/mL
1 Midol	32.4 mg	0.48 mcg/mL

Adapted from Fuentes, R.J. 1999.

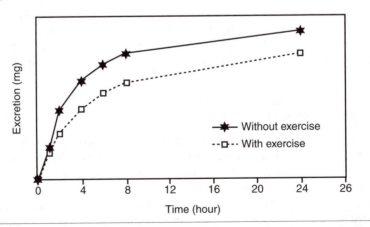

Figure 13.7   Cumulative urinary caffeine excretion (mg) during treadmill running in endurance-trained athletes. Mean values ($n = 9$).

Adapted from van der Merwe, Luus, and Barnard 1992.

Caffeine has ergolytic properties as well as ergogenic ones. More specifically, the ergolytic properties include diuretic actions, a detrimental effect on hand steadiness, and possibly a detrimental effect on reaction time.

Because of the potential for an increased pressor response, many individuals under the care of physicians should avoid ingesting caffeine prior to exercising.

References

Bangsbo, J., Jacobsen, K., Nordberg, N., Christensen, N.J., and Graham, T. 1992. Acute and habitual caffeine ingestion and metabolic responses to steady-state exercise. *J Appl Physiol* 72:1297-1303.

Berglund, B., and Hemmingsson, P. 1982. Effects of caffeine ingestion on exercise performance at low and high altitudes in cross-country skiers. *Int J Sports Med* 3:234-236.

Brown, D.D., Knowlton, R.G., Sullivan, J.J., and Sanjabi, P.B. 1991. Effect of caffeine ingestion on alveolar ventilation during moderate exercise. *Aviat Space Environ Med* 62(9 pt 1):860-864.

Cleroux, J., Van Nguyen, P., Taylor, A.W., and Leenen, F.H.H. 1989. Effects of beta-1 vs. beta-1 plus beta-2 blockade on exercise endurance and muscle metabolism in humans. *J Appl Physiol* 66:548-554.

Collomp, K., Anselme, F., Audran, M., Gay, J.P., Chanal, J.L., and Prefaut, C. 1991. Effects of moderate exercise on the pharmacokinetics of caffeine. *Eur J Clin Pharmacol* 40:279-282.

Curatolo, P.W., and Robertson, D. 1983. The health consequences of caffeine. *Ann Intern Med* 98(pt 1):641-653.

Doherty, M. 1998. The effects of caffeine on the maximal accumulated oxygen deficit and short-term running performance. *Int J Sport Nutr* 8:95-104.

Doubt, T.J., and Hsieh, S.S. 1991. Additive effects of caffeine and cold water during submaximal leg exercise. *Med Sci Sports Exerc* 23:435-442.

D'Urzo, A.D., Jhirad, R., Jenne, H., Avendano, M.A., Rubinstein, I., D'Costa, M., and Goldstein, R.S. 1990. Effect of caffeine on ventilatory responses to hypercapnia, hypoxia, and exercise in humans. *J Appl Physiol* 68:322-328.

Duthel, J.M., Vallon, J.J., Martin, G., Ferret, J.M., Mathieu, R., and Videman, R. 1991. Caffeine and sport: Role of physical exercise upon elimination. *Med Sci Sports Exerc* 23:980-985.

Falk, B., Burstein, R., Ashkenazi, I., Spilberg, O., Alter, J., Zylber-Katz, E., Rubinstein, A., Bashan, N., and Shapiro, Y. 1989. The effect of caffeine ingestion on physical performance after prolonged exercise. *Eur J Appl Physiol* 59:168-173.

Falk, B., Burstein, R., Rosenblum, J., Shapiro, Y., Zylber-Katz, E., and Bashan, N. 1990. Effects of caffeine ingestion on body fluid balance and thermoregulation during exercise. *Can J Physiol Pharmacol* 68:889-892.

Flinn, S., Gregory, J., McNaughton, L.R., Tristram, S., and Davies, P. 1990. Caffeine ingestion prior to incremental cycling to exhaustion in recreational cyclists. *Int J Sports Med* 11:188-193.

Gaesser, G.A., and Rich, R.G. 1985. Influence of caffeine on blood lactate response during incremental exercise. *Int J Sports Med* 6:207-211.

Graham, T.E., Hibbert, E., and Sathasivam, P. 1998. Metabolic and exercise endurance effects of coffee and caffeine ingestion. *J Appl Physiol* 85:883-889.

Graham, T.E., Rush, J.W., and van Soeren, M.H. 1994. Caffeine and exercise: Metabolism and performance. *Can J Appl Physiol* 19:111-138.

Graham, T.E., Sathasivam, P., and MacNaughton, K.W. 1991. Influence of cold, exercise, and caffeine on catecholamines and metabolism in men. *J Appl Physiol* 70:2052-2058.

Graham, T.E., and Spriet, L.L. 1991. Performance and metabolic responses to a high caffeine dose during prolonged exercise. *J Appl Physiol* 71:2292-2298.

Graham, T.E., and Spriet, L.L. 1995. Metabolic, catecholamine, and exercise performance responses to various doses of caffeine. *J Appl Physiol* 78:867-874.

Greer, F., McLean, C., and Graham, T.E. 1998. Caffeine, performance, and metabolism during repeated Wingate exercise tests. *J Appl Physiol* 85:1502-1508.

Jacobson, B.H., and Edwards, S.W. 1990. Effects of ingested doses of caffeine on neuromuscular reflex response time in man. *Int J Sports Med* 11:194-197.

Kamimori, G.H., Somani, S.M., Knowlton, R.G., and Perkins, R.M. 1987. The effects of obesity and exercise on the pharmacokinetics of caffeine in lean and obese volunteers. *Eur J Clin Pharmacol* 31:595-600.

Kivity, S., Ben Aharon, Y., Man, A., and Topilsky, M. 1990. The effect of caffeine on exercise-induced bronchoconstriction. *Chest* 97:1083-1085.

LeBlanc, J., Jobin, M., Cote, J., Samson, P., and Labrie, A. 1985. Enhanced metabolic response to caffeine in exercise-trained human subjects. *J Appl Physiol* 59:832-837.

Nehlig, A., and Debry, G. 1994. Caffeine and sports activity: A review. *Int J Sports Med* 15:215-223.

Pasman, W.J., van Baak, M.A., Jeukendrup, A.E., and de Haan, A. 1995. The effect of different dosages of caffeine on endurance performance time. *Int J Sports Med* 16:225-230.

Pincomb, G.A., Wilson, M.R., Sung, B.H., Passey, R.B., and Lovallo, W.R. 1991. Effects of caffeine on pressor regulation during rest and exercise in men at risk for hypertension. *Am Heart J* 122(4 pt 1):1107-1115.

Poehlman, E.T., Despres, J.P., Bessette, H., Fontaine, E., Tremblay, A., and Bouchard, C. 1985. Influence of caffeine on the resting metabolic rate of exercise-trained and inactive subjects. *Med Sci Sports Exerc* 17:689-694.

Powers, S.K., Dodd, S., Woodyard, J., and Mangum, M. 1986. Caffeine alters ventilatory and gas exchange kinetics during exercise. *Med Sci Sports Exerc* 18:101-106.

Silverman, K., Evans, S.M., Strain, E.C., and Griffiths, R.R. 1992. Withdrawal syndrome after the double-blind cessation of caffeine consumption. *N Engl J Med* 327:1109-1114.

Somani, S.M., Gupta, S.K., Frank, S., and Corder, C.N. 1990. Effect of exercise on disposition and pharmacokinetics of drugs. *Drug Dev Res* 20:251-275.

Spriet, L.L., MacLean, D.A., Dyck, D.J., Hultman, E., Cederblad, G., and Graham, T.E. 1992. Caffeine ingestion and muscle metabolism during prolonged exercise in humans. *Am J Physiol (Endocrinol Metab)* 262(25):E891-E898.

Sung, B.H., Lovallo, W.R., Pincomb, G.A., and Wilson, M.F. 1990. Effects of caffeine on blood pressure response during exercise in normotensive healthy young men. *Am J Cardiol* 65:909-913.

Sung, B.H., Lovallo, W.R., Whitsett, T., and Wilson, M.F. 1995. Caffeine elevates blood pressure responses to exercise in mild hypertensive men. *Am J Hypertens* 8(12 pt 1):1184-1188.

Tarnopolsky, M.A., Atkinson, S.A., MacDougall, J.D., Sale, D.G., and Sutton, J.R. 1989. Physiological responses to caffeine during endurance running in habitual caffeine users. *Med Sci Sports Exerc* 21:418-424.

Trice, I., and Haymes, E.M. 1995. Effects of caffeine ingestion on exercise-induced changes during high-intensity, intermittent exercise. *Int J Sport Nutr* 5:37-44.

Van der Merwe, P.J., Luus, H.G., and Barnard, J.G. 1992. Caffeine in sport. Influence of endurance exercise on the urinary caffeine concentration. *Int J Sports Med* 13:74-76.

Van Soeren, M.H., Sathasivam, P., Spriet, L.L., and Graham, T.E. 1993. Caffeine metabolism and epinephrine responses during exercise in users and nonusers. *J Appl Physiol* 75:805-812.

Wemple, R.D., Lamb, D.R., and McKeever, K.H. 1997. Caffeine vs. caffeine-free sports drink: Effects on urine production at rest and during prolonged exercise. *Int J Sports Med* 18:40-46.

Williams, J.H. 1991. Caffeine, neuromuscular function and high-intensity exercise performance. *J Sports Med Phys Fitness* 31:481-489.

Williams, M.H. 1994. The use of nutritional ergogenic aids in sports: Is it an ethical issue? *Int J Sport Nutr* 4:120-131.

14
CHAPTER

Ethanol

CASE STUDY

■ *CASE*   Geoff, Terry, and Nigel are professional rugby players and routinely drink 6 to 8 large glasses of beer after their matches. Nonsmokers, they maintain excellent cardiovascular fitness with the amount of running they engage in during each game. Although medical experts consider moderate alcohol consumption to be beneficial for the cardiovascular system, can the alcohol these rugby players regularly ingest be harmful in these high amounts?

■ *COMMENT*   Whether alcohol (ethanol) is beneficial or detrimental for the cardiovascular system depends on the amount ingested, the type of alcoholic beverage consumed, and the age and fitness level of the person in question. In general, 1 or 2 drinks daily reduces the risk of coronary heart disease—compared with larger amounts or even total abstinence. This guideline applies mainly to subjects at risk for cardiovascular disease, however, and it may be irrelevant for those individuals who are physically very fit. An issue to consider with these rugby players is the fact that ethanol is a diuretic. In the course of a full rugby game, large quantities of body water can be lost through sweat and expired air, depending on ambient temperature. Consider also that cardiac arrhythmias have been associated with binge drinking. Water is what Geoff, Terry, and Nigel need after a game. Encourage these players to drink plenty of water during and after every game—and reduce (or moderate) their ethanol consumption.

Ethanol, or alcohol as it is more commonly referred to, is available in the form of beer, wine, and distilled spirits. Roughly 90% of the population drinks alcohol. Among college athletes, whom Stainback surveyed (1997), some 88% had consumed alcohol in the previous year; among professional athletes, 93% had consumed alcohol in the 30 days before the survey. Although most athletes avoid alcohol before competition, "postgame consumption" is commonplace in some groups. Kit Saunder, director of women's sports at the University of Wisconsin, reported that nearly a quarter of Big 10 coaches had found *excessive use* of alcohol by their teams. Further, she reported that 14% of high school coaches had helped female athletes obtain counseling for drinking problems (see table 14.1; Woolley and Fuentes 1999). The NFL has recognized alcohol as the drug most abused by football players. During training, male athletes consume between 0.5% and 4.0% of their total calories in the form of alcoholic beverages; the corresponding value for female athletes is 0.5% to 1.0% (Economos, Bortz, and Nelson 1993).

The link between alcohol and sports is clear and likely to continue. This relationship is perpetuated by the likes of tequila-sponsored professional volleyball tours, by ex-NFL players serving as spokesmen in beer commercials, and by the free dispensing of beer to participants after completion of running, biking, and triathlon events. Indeed, "sports bars" exist in every city.

We should distinguish, however, between different types of ethanolic beverages, because their effect on serum lipids is a medical issue. There is substantial evidence that moderate amounts (i.e., 1 to 2 drinks per day) of ethanol reduce the risk of cardiovascular mortality in those at risk

Table 14.1   Substance Abuse Patterns in College Athletes

Substance	Athletes using drug in previous year (%)
Alcohol	89
Caffeine	64
Major analgesics	34
Marijuana	28
Smokeless tobacco	28
Anabolic steroids	5
Cocaine/crack	5

Adapted from Wagner 1991.

(Doll et al. 1994; Fuchs, Stampfer, and Colditz 1995; Rimm et al. 1996). However, nonalcoholic red grape juice has been shown to reduce the susceptibility of low-density lipoprotein (LDL) to oxidation (Day et al. 1997). Thus, wine drinkers may be afforded health benefits that beer drinkers are not.

As with all medical research, one should be careful not to extrapolate data generated in older, sedentary individuals to younger, physically active subjects. For example, athletes are most likely to consume ethanol as beer, not wine (Woolley and Fuentes 1999). Also, it is likely that the beneficial effects of *regular exercise* on the cardiovascular system far outweigh the proposed beneficial effects of ethanol on the cardiovascular system. And the cardiovascular benefit of ethanol must be balanced against its *detrimental* cardiovascular effects (discussed later in this chapter). Breathing secondhand smoke, for example, and the sedentary aspect or style of casual ethanol consumption may well offset any minor beneficial effects of ethanol in those who do not exercise regularly.

These remarks so far pertain to discussing the medical aspects of ethanol in populations at higher risk for cardiovascular disease. But what are the effects with a population of healthy exercisers or athletes? Research has shown that 33% of collegiate athletes engage in binge drinking. In middle-aged men (mean age of 52 years), binge beer drinking has been associated with increased mortality (Kauhanen et al. 1997). What are the effects of ethanol on athletic performance and on athletes in general?

How Exercise Affects the Action of Ethanol

An abundant literature on the pharmacology and pharmacokinetics of ethanol exists, and there are excellent summaries by Reilly (1988) and more recently by Stainback (1997).

Reilly (1988) describes the pharmacokinetics of ethanol. To begin, ethanol is readily absorbed throughout the gastrointestinal (GI) tract since it does not require digestion. And regardless of how much ethanol is ingested, the body metabolizes only one "drink" per hour. Substantial differences exist, however, in how ethanol is distributed within the body. For example, if you give males and females an equal quantity of ethanol normalized to their body weight, ethanol blood concentrations will be higher in the females. In general, females have a higher percentage of body fat than do males, and ethanol does not distribute into fat stores as easily as other tissues. While ethanol clearance can be diminished in some disease states (e.g., severe liver disease) or by some drugs, no factors *accelerate* ethanol metabolism to any great degree. Giving an intoxicated person coffee, in other words, or having him take a cold shower accomplishes little.

Only limited data exist that describe the effects of exercise on the *pharmacokinetics* of ethanol. Human data show that muscular exercise does not affect ethanol metabolism, and aerobic exercise may slightly increase the rate of ethanol clearance (Schurch et al. 1982), if at all (Massicotte et al. 1993). Data obtained in rats indicate that aerobic exercise acutely elevates the clearance rate of ethanol and that 7 weeks of endurance training can alter the clearance rate of ethanol at rest (Ardies et al. 1989).

Ethanol has many *pharmacologic actions*, although a comprehensive discussion of these aspects is beyond the scope of this book (two helpful sources, again, are *Alcohol and Sport* by Robert D. Stainback, 1997, and the chapter by T. Reilly in *Drugs in Sport*, 1988). It is worth noting some of the cardiovascular and the psychologic and neurologic effects of exercise and ethanol. Acute ethanol ingestion causes cutaneous vessels to dilate, thus increasing heat radiation. Resting heart rate increases, as does resting blood pressure. Ethanol is a diuretic, and it induces a negative water balance along with an electrolyte loss. Thus, some of the effects of ethanol ingestion and exercise might be additive.

How Ethanol Affects Exercisers

In addition to affecting the central and peripheral nervous systems, ethanol can acutely elicit cardiovascular and metabolic effects. In general, nearly all of these actions are *ergolytic*. We can look at research on cardiovascular effects as well as metabolic effects, and on neurologic and psychologic influences as well as pulmonary ones.

Cardiovascular Effects

Data collected from normotensive humans indicate that acute ethanol ingestion stimulates postganglionic sympathetic nerve discharge (Grassi et al. 1989). The effects of ethanol on the sympathetic nervous system add to an already complex heart rate response to athletic training (Furlan et al. 1993). Acute ethanol ingestion causes a rise in blood pressure mediated by increased sympathetic stimulation. A pressor effect in response to acute ethanol ingestion has been documented in humans (Randin et al. 1995). Ethanol causes vasodilation of peripheral vessels, but it does not appear to affect muscle blood flow or oxygen uptake during exercise (Reilly 1988).

Sports medicine personnel should remember that ethanol is a diuretic. While many obvious reasons exist for discouraging ethanol ingestion prior to competition, any substance that accelerates fluid loss should be considered potentially ergolytic, particularly in events of sustained endurance. Diuretics, for example, have been shown to exert ergolytic effects on aerobic activity (Armstrong, Costill, and Fink 1985). Exercise-induced sweating and ethanol-induced diuresis can combine to cause plasma volume contraction.

Metabolic Effects

Regarding ethanol's effects on energy substrates, carbohydrate metabolism is affected more than is fat metabolism. Ethanol lowers resting muscle glycogen and decreases splanchnic glucose output, perhaps as a result of its ability to inhibit liver gluconeogenesis. Ethanol also is known to cause a pronounced decline in blood glucose levels and leg muscle glucose uptake during a 3 h run, but does not impair lipolysis or free fatty acid utilization during exercise (Reilly 1988). Alcohol dehydrogenase in the liver metabolizes ethanol to acetaldehyde, which, in turn, is metabolized to acetyl CoA. Acetyl CoA is metabolized to lactic acid via the citric acid cycle. The accumulation of lactic acid and the diversion of the citric acid cycle in favor of this pathway offer several explanations of how ethanol ingestion produces a decrease in aerobic capacity (see Woolley and Fuentes 1999).

Some athletes might believe that beer is a good postexercise beverage because it contains so many carbohydrate calories. While beer does contain carbohydrate calories, a 12 oz beer provides only 12 g of carbohydrate, and a 12 oz "light" beer contains only 5 g. Compare that to 12 oz of orange juice, which provides 38 g of carbohydrate (Economos, Bortz, and Nelson 1993). The diuretic actions of ethanol far outweigh any benefit gained from the carbohydrates it supplies.

Neurologic and Psychologic Effects

The mood-altering effects of ethanol are widely known. Ethanol suppresses inhibitions and makes individuals feel euphoric. However, it is a central nervous system (CNS) depressant, and it likely demotivates athletes from attaining supreme levels of effort. Other effects on the nervous system have been demonstrated. Ethanol can affect peripheral nerve function. It has been shown that ethanol increases the discharge rate of postganglionic sympathetic nerves (Randin et al. 1995). This is but one of at least two ways that ethanol exerts detrimental effects on hand-eye coordination. Ethanol can block nerve conduction, and, in clinical medicine, ethanol injected in close proximity to a nerve can cause nerve degeneration. While it is tempting to conclude that ingestion of ethanol prior to a strenuous athletic event might produce an analgesic effect that in turn could improve performance, in fact, the concentrations required to affect peripheral nerve function greatly exceed those required to cause euphoria and other central effects.

Pulmonary Effects

Acute ethanol ingestion exerts detrimental effects on ventilatory adaption. One study showed that at an altitude of 3000 m, P_aO_2 decreased and PCO_2 increased after ingestion of 50 g of ethanol. These observations were apparently due to a decrease in respiratory rate (Roeggla et al. 1995). This finding is important for recreational skiers; it has been documented that 64% of tourists drink ethanol at moderate altitudes (Honigman et al. 1993). It may also be important for elite skiers. Thus, detrimental effects of ethanol on ventilatory adaption and its effects on temperature regulation are two concerns related to ingestion of alcohol at altitude.

How Ethanol Affects Exercise Performance

There are probably more data describing the effects of ethanol on human performance than for any other drug discussed in this book. Much of this research has been conducted in automobile drivers and airline pilots. Regarding sports, while some aspects of ethanol ingestion might seem to be ergogenic, ethanol is mainly ergolytic. Although acute ethanol ingestion furnishes fluid and carbohydrate calories, these properties are offset by the diuretic effect. And while the effects on the nervous system may produce a sense of euphoria, which an individual may use (briefly) to delay the sensation of fatigue, these effects are very transient.

Even though task performance is impaired, subjects nevertheless perceive an improvement in performance shortly after they drink ethanol. The effects of ethanol on mood and cognitive ability are best summarized in table 14.2.

The accumulation of lactic acid (see earlier discussion) also contributes to a predictable ergolytic response. O'Brien (1993) has specifically reviewed the effects of ethanol on athletic performance. Looking first at aerobic performance, ethanol acutely impairs aerobic metabolism. This was revealed in rugby players, in whom a decrease in $\dot{V}O_2$max of 11.4% was seen. Anaerobic performance was unaffected (O'Brien 1993). In another study, alcohol ingestion significantly slowed sprinting and middle-distance running times at blood alcohol concentrations of only 50 to 100 mg/dl (McNaughton and Preece 1986). Ingestion of ethanol prior to exercise testing has also been shown to impair maximum work

Table 14.2   Blood Alcohol Level and Behavioral Effects

Present blood alcohol level	Average effects
0.02	Reached after approximately one drink; light or moderate drinkers experience some pleasant feelings (e.g., sense of warmth and well-being).
0.04	Most people feel relaxed, energetic, and happy. Time seems to pass quickly. Skin may flush, and motor skills may be slightly impaired.
0.05	More observable effects begin to occur. Individual may experience lightheartedness, giddiness, lowered inhibitions, and impaired judgment. Coordination may be slightly altered.
0.06	Further impairment of judgment; individual's ability to make rational decisions concerning personal capabilities is affected (e.g., driving a car). May become "a lover or a fighter."
0.08	Muscle coordination definitely impaired and reaction time increased; driving ability suspect. Heavy pulse and slow breathing. Sensory feelings of numbness in the cheeks, lips, and extremities may occur. Legally drunk in some states.
0.10	Clear deterioration of coordination and reaction time. Individual may stagger and speech may become fuzzy. Judgment and memory further affected. Legally drunk in all states.
0.15	All individuals experience a definite impairment of balance and movement. Large increases in reaction time.
0.20	Marked depression in motor and sensory capability; slurred speech, double vision, difficulty standing and walking may all be present. Decidedly intoxicated.
0.30	Individual is confused or stuperous; unable to comprehend what is seen or heard. May lose consciousness (pass out) at this level.
0.40	Usually unconscious. Alcohol has become deep anesthetic. Skin may be sweaty and clammy.
0.45	Circulatory and respiration functions are depressed and can stop altogether.
0.50	Near death.

Reprinted from: *Drugs: Facts, Alternatives, Decisions* (p. 171) by J.M. Corry and P. Cimbolic, 1985, Belmont, CA: Wadsworth Publshing Company. Copyright 1985 by Wadsworth Publishing Company. Reprinted with permission.

Table 14.3 Effects of Alcohol Treatments In Archers

Variables	Sober	Placebo	0.02% BAC	0.05% BAC
Arm steadiness: time off-target (s)	2.64 ± 0.89	3.05 ± 0.74	3.24 ± 1.01	8.17 ± 1.49
Isometric strength (kg)	55.4 ± 4.9	56.8 ± 3.8	54.9 ± 5.7	53.0 ± 7.9
Muscular endurance (s)	11.4 ± 2.1	12.0 ± 2.5	12.0 ± 2.0	10.8 ± 2.0
Reaction time (ms)	211 ± 6.5	209 ± 8.5	223 ± 9.6	226 ± 11.2

BAC = blood alcohol concentration.
Mean ± SD.
Data taken from Reilly, T., and Halliday, F. 1985. Influence of alcohol ingestion on tasks related to archery. *J Jum Ergol* 14:99-104.
Adapted from Reilly 1988.

during cycle ergometry (Bond, Franks, and Howley 1983) and to impair 5 mi treadmill run times (Houmard et al. 1987).

As for ethanol's effects on reflex time and coordination, the substance makes individuals feel as if their performance has improved when, in fact, it may actually have declined. Countless tests have demonstrated that ethanol impairs driving ability (see Moskowitz, Burns, and Williams 1985), reaction time, and hand-eye coordination. In very low concentrations, ethanol may actually improve hand steadiness (Koller and Biary 1984), but at all other concentrations, acute ethanol ingestion impairs judgment, reflexes, and coordination. Reilly and Halliday (1985) studied the effects of various concentrations of blood alcohol on arm steadiness in archers. Arm steadiness and reaction time were increasingly impaired as blood alcohol concentrations rose (see table 14.3).

Some data indicate that functional ability is impaired for up to 24 h after ethanol ingestion. Navy pilots drank enough ethanol to achieve a blood alcohol concentration of 100 mg/dl; they then were tested 14 h later. Their performance during simulated flights was significantly worse than that of pilots who had had no ethanol for 48 h (Yesavage and Leirer 1986).

In summary, most authorities have concluded that ethanol is not an ergogenic substance and, in fact, may actually be ergolytic. It can cause vasodilation, leading to hypothermia during cold-weather exercise; it can cause dehydration, which adversely affects endurance exercise (Armstrong, Costill, and Fink 1985). In fact, nearly every physiologic effect of ethanol is ergolytic, as this list of effects shows:

- Metabolic—impaired aerobic metabolism, impaired heat dissipation results if hypohydration occurs.
- Cardiovascular—diuretic action, electrolyte loss, impaired inotropic ability, heat loss in cold ambient temperatures secondary to cutaneous vasodilation.
- Neurologic—impaired reaction time, impaired judgment, impaired coordination.

Avoiding Potential Complications

Some of the complications of using ethanol while exercising have already been discussed: impaired ventilatory adaption at altitude, impaired endurance, and impaired hand-eye coordination. And various studies have proved there are additional risks of cardiac arrhythmias, nutritional imbalances, and drug interactions.

Ninety milliliters of 80-proof whiskey produced atrial and ventricular tachyarrhythmias in 10 of 14 subjects (mean age 57 years) with a history of chronic alcohol consumption and symptoms of palpitations (Greenspon and Schaal 1983). The association of cardiac arrhythmias with binge drinking has been termed "holiday heart syndrome." Alcohol also has an acute myocardial depressant effect (Lang et al. 1985).

Ethanol can accelerate the loss of important nutrients. It is well known that chronic alcoholics are deficient in B complex, vitamin C, potassium, and magnesium. Acute ethanol ingestion is likely to worsen nutrient loss, something that has been documented to occur in elite athletes independently of ethanol use. Ethanol injures the GI epithelial lining, leading to GI blood loss, a problem that exists among some marathon runners.

Ethanol possesses other actions that make it undesirable for use during athletic competition or sporting events. Its diuretic effects make it detrimental during exercise in warm, ambient temperatures, and its ability to induce cutaneous vasodilation make it harmful during exercise in cold temperatures. Ethanol ingestion prior to athletic competition may indeed affect temperature regulation. In addition, the combined effects of arteriolar vasodilation and plasma volume contraction make it likely that acute ethanol ingestion intensifies postexercise hypotension.

Ethanol interacts significantly with many other medications. Since ethanol is a CNS depressant, its ability to cause drowsiness can be additive with antihistamines, sedatives or tranquilizers, opiate analgesics, and some antidepressants. Because ethanol is irritating to the GI epithelium, it should not be used with aspirin, other NSAIDs, or corticosteroids. Since many individuals use analgesics and anti-inflammatory agents, they should be aware that many drug interactions occur with ethanol. Combining ethanol with acetaminophen can intensify acetaminophen-induced hepatoxic effects.

The long-term effects of chronic ethanol abuse are beyond the scope of this text, but are nonetheless important. The reader is referred to an excellent discussion by Woolley and Fuentes (1999). It should also be pointed out that chronic alcoholism has been linked to skeletal muscle myopathy and cardiomyopathy (Fernandez-Sola et al. 1994).

NCAA and USOC Status

The NCAA bans ethanol, or ethanol-containing medications, for riflery competition. The USOC reserves the right to test for the presence of ethanol in athletes.

Guidelines for Use

For serious athletes, there is no benefit to ingesting ethanol before, during, or after competition. Ethanol impairs performance and only worsens nutrient and total body water losses. Drinking while snow skiing would seem to be particularly bad, since ethanol impairs judgment, coordination, and reaction time; interferes with energy utilization; enhances heat loss due to cutaneous vasodilation; and impairs ventilation. Further, athletes should be discouraged from drinking for several days before competition.

While the medical community has demonstrated the beneficial effects of ethanol on the risk of coronary artery disease, it does not appear that modest ethanol ingestion by highly active adults further lessens their risk. For the deconditioned individual who is beginning to exercise, modest ethanol ingestion is probably acceptable, keeping in mind the risks associated with ventilatory adaption at altitude, nutrient loss, and GI injury, among others.

References

Ardies, C.M., Morris, G.S., Erickson, C.K., and Farrar, R.P. 1989. Both acute and chronic exercise enhance in vivo ethanol clearance in rats. *J Appl Physiol* 66:555-560.

Armstrong, L.E., Costill, D.L., and Fink, W.J. 1985. Influence of diuretic-induced dehydration on competitive running performance. *Med Sci Sports Exerc* 17:456-461.

Bond, V., Franks, B.D., and Howley, E.T. 1983. Effects of small and moderate doses of alcohol on submaximal cardiorespiratory function, perceived exertion and endurance performance in abstainers and moderate drinkers. *J Sports Med Phys Fitness* 23:221-228.

Corry, J.M., and Cimbolic, P. 1985. *Drugs: Facts, alternatives, decisions.* Belmont, CA: Wadsworth.

Day, A.P., Kemp, H.J., Bolton, C., Hartog, M., and Stansbie, D. 1997. Effect of concentrated red grape juice consumption on serum antioxidant capacity and low-density lipoprotein oxidation. *Ann Nutr Metab* 41:353-357.

Doll, R., Peto, R., Hall, E., Wheatley, K., and Gray, R. 1994. Mortality in relation to consumption of alcohol: 13 years' observations on male British doctors. *Br Med J* 309:911-918.

Economos, C.D., Bortz, S.S., and Nelson, M.E. 1993. Nutritional practices of elite athletes. *Sports Med.* 16:381-399.

Fernandez-Sola, J., Estruch, R., Grau, J.M., Pare, J.C., Rubin, E., and Urbano-Marquez, A. 1994. The relation of alcoholic myopathy to cardiomyopathy. *Ann Intern Med* 120:529-536.

Fuchs, C.S., Stampfer, M.J., and Colditz, G.A. 1995. Alcohol consumption and mortality among women. *N Engl J Med* 332:1245-1250.

Furlan, R., Piazza, S., Dell'Orto, S., Gentile, E., Cerutti, S., Pagani, M., and Malliani, A. 1993. Early and late effects of exercise and athletic training on neural mechanisms controlling heart rate. *Cardiovasc Res* 27:482-488.

Grassi, G.M., Somers, V.K., Renik, W.S., Abboud, F.M., and Mark, A.L. 1989. Effect of alcohol intake on blood pressure and sympathetic nerve activity in normotensive humans: A preliminary report. *J Hypertens Suppl* 7:S20-S21.

Greenspon, A.J., and Schaal, S.F. 1983. The "holiday heart": Electrophysiologic studies of alcohol effects in alcoholics. *Ann Intern Med* 98:135-139.

Honigman, B., Theis, M.K., Koziol-McLaine, J., Roach, R., Yip, R., Houston, C., Moore, L.G., and Pearce, P. 1993. Acute mountain sickness in a general tourist population at moderate altitudes. *Ann Intern Med* 118(8):587-592.

Houmard, J.A., Langenfeld, M.E., Wiley, R.L., and Siefert, J. 1987. Effects of the acute ingestion of small amounts of alcohol upon 5-mile run times. *J Sports Med Phys Fitness* 27:253-257.

Kauhanen, J., Kaplan, G.A., Goldberg, D.E., and Salonen, J.T. 1997. Beer binging and mortality: Results from the Kuopio ischaemic heart disease risk factor study, a prospective population based study. *Br Med J* 315:846-851.

Koller, W.C., and Biary, N. 1984. Effect of alcohol on tremors: Comparison with propranolol. *Neurology* 34:221-222.

Lang, R.M., Borow, K.M., Neumann, A., and Feldman, T. 1985. Adverse cardiac effects of acute alcohol ingestion in young adults. *Ann Intern Med* 102:742-747.

Massicotte, D., Provencher, S., Adopo, E., Peronnet, F., Brisson, G., and Hillaire-Marcel, C. 1993. Oxidation of ethanol at rest and during prolonged exercise in men. *J Appl Physiol* 75:329-333.

McNaughton, L., and Preece, D. 1986. Alcohol and its effects on sprint and middle-distance running. *Br J Sports Med* 20:56-59.

Moskowitz, H., Burns, M.M., and Williams, A.F. 1985. Skills performance at low blood alcohol levels. *J Stud Alcohol* 46:482-485.

O'Brien, C.P. 1993. Alcohol and sport: Impact of social drinking on recreational and competitive sports performance. *Sports Med* 15:71-77.

Randin, D., Vollenweider, P., Tappy, L., Jequier, E., Nicod, P., and Scherrer, U. 1995. Suppression of alcohol-induced hypertension by dexamethasone. *N Engl J Med* 332:1733-1737.

Reilly, T. 1988. Alcohol, anti-anxiety drugs and exercise. In *Drugs in sport*, edited by D.R. Mottram. Champaign, IL: Human Kinetics.

Reilly, T., and Halliday, F. 1985. Influence of alcohol ingestion on tasks related to archery. *J Hum Ergol* 14:99-104.

Rimm, E.B., Klatsky, A., Grobbee, D., and Stampfer, M.J. 1996. Review of moderate alcohol consumption and reduced risk of coronary heart disease: Is the effect due to beer, wine, or spirits? *Br Med J* 312:731-736.

Roeggla, G., Roeggla, H., Roeggla, M., Binder, M., and Laggner, A.N. 1995. Effect of alcohol on acute ventilatory adaptation to mild hypoxia at moderate altitude. *Ann Intern Med* 122:925-927.

Schurch, P.M., Radimsky, J., Iffland, R., and Hollmann, W. 1982. The influence of moderate prolonged exercise and a low carbohydrate diet on ethanol elimination on metabolism. *Eur J Appl Physiol* 48:407-414.

Stainback, R.D. 1997. *Alcohol and sport*. Champaign, IL: Human Kinetics.

Wagner, J.C. 1991. Enhancement of athletic performance with drugs: An overview. *Sports Med* 12(4):250-265.

Woolley, B.H., and Fuentes, R.J. 1999. Alcohol use and the athlete. In *Athletic drug reference '99*, edited by R.J. Fuentes and J.M. Rosenberg. Durham, NC: Clean Data.

Yesavage, J.A., and Leirer, V.O. 1986. Hangover effects on aircraft pilots 14 hours after alcohol ingestion: A preliminary report. *Am J Psychiatry* 143:1546-1550.

15

CHAPTER

Amphetamines and Cocaine

CASE STUDY

■ *CASE*   One cold winter morning, a 37-year-old man with a history of cardiomyopathy and intravenous drug abuse went jogging after his intranasal use of cocaine. He developed ventricular tachycardia and chest pain 30 minutes later. He was taken to the hospital, where ventricular tachycardia was converted to atrial fibrillation. Ultimately, it was determined he had suffered a small myocardial infarction. Several hours later, he also suffered a left hemispheric stroke. Is it that dangerous to exercise while using cocaine?

■ *COMMENT*   In a word, yes. Cocaine is an extremely powerful cardio-vascular stimulant. Its use results in acute increases in catecholamine output, with corresponding increases in blood pressure and heart rate. Of course, exercise causes the same physiologic response, so the double-product of heart rate times blood pressure can increase enormously.

Amphetamines became widely used by troops during World War II to increase their endurance and to combat fatigue. In the decades that followed, as "thin is in" took ever increasing hold on the public's mentality, amphetamines were prescribed for use as appetite suppressants. Unfortunately, subjects learned that they developed a tolerance to amphetamines, and the use of amphetamines as weight-loss agents declined in the 1970s. In the 1990s, methamphetamine ("crank") use rose again in the general public (Schermer and Wisner 1999).

Athletes began using amphetamines because they believed these agents would increase both mental and physical capacity. Surprisingly, however, most of the subjects in one small study could not even discern if they had received amphetamine or placebo (Domino et al. 1972). Officials first suspected amphetamine use by athletes during the 1952 Olympic Games. Amphetamine use was linked to the death of a cyclist during the 1960 Summer Games in Rome.

With regard to cocaine, surveys conducted in 1985 and 1989 showed that the use of cocaine by college athletes had dropped somewhat, from 17% to 5%, and NCAA surveys showed that by 1993 usage was down still further (Wagner 1991). According to a 1990 survey compiled by the Iowa High School Athletic Association, 3% of male high school athletes had used cocaine during the previous year. Cocaine use, judging simply by these numbers, is not as large a problem as ethanol abuse is in young athletes. Unfortunately, the potential sequelae and toxicities of cocaine are far greater, as indicated by the case study at the beginning of this chapter.

How Exercise Affects the Action of Cocaine and Amphetamines

We turn first to see how exercise affects the pharmacology and pharmacokinetics of cocaine and amphetamines. Cocaine exerts sympathomimetic effects by stimulating the release of norepinephrine and by inhibiting norepinephrine and dopamine re-uptake by presynaptic nerve terminals. The result is an increased concentration of norepinephrine within the synaptic junction. These effects appear within seconds to minutes after cocaine use, depending on the route of administration. They also wear off rapidly, due to cocaine's very short plasma elimination half-life (about 38 min). Chronic cocaine administration in animals has been shown to result in diminished levels of tyrosine hydroxylase, which is the rate-limiting step in the formation of dopamine (Di Paolo et al. 1989). It has been postulated that dopamine depletion leads to a heightened response to sympathetic stimuli.

Han and colleagues (1996) studied how exercise might affect the pharmacokinetics of cocaine. They administered intravenous (IV) cocaine to rats just prior to the animals' exercise and found that cocaine plasma concentrations were higher during exercise compared to values obtained at rest.

Amphetamine is one of the most potent of the sympathomimetic amines in its effects on the central nervous system (CNS). In successively higher doses, amphetamine stimulates the release of norepinephrine, dopamine, and 5-hydroxytryptamine (5-HT), respectively, from nerve terminals. Amphetamine stimulates the respiratory center, but normal doses do not typically increase respiratory rate or minute ventilation. By causing catecholamine release, amphetamines are indirect stimulants of alpha- and beta-adrenergic receptors peripherally. Chemically, amphetamine exists in both a levorotatory and a dextrorotatory form, and both these isomers are potentially ergogenic (Bhagat and Wheeler 1973). Commercial preparations, however, consist of either the racemic mixture (e.g., amphetamine) or the dextrorotatory form (e.g., dextroamphetamine [Dexedrine]). Methamphetamine (Desoxyn) is another form. Both dextroamphetamine and methamphetamine exert greater effects on the CNS and lesser effects on the periphery than does racemic amphetamine. Both amphetamines in general and cocaine cause the release of catecholamines, but cocaine appears to be much more potent in this regard since it can also prevent re-uptake of synaptic catecholamines. However, amphetamine in all its forms is much longer acting than cocaine.

How Cocaine and Amphetamines Affect Exercisers

Cocaine increases resting levels of epinephrine, norepinephrine, and dopamine (Conlee et al. 1991b). Both exercise and cocaine can independently increase circulating catecholamine levels. Yet in one study, when rats were exercised immediately after receiving IV cocaine, the rise in epinephrine and norepinephrine levels was far greater than the sum of each factor individually (Han et al. 1996). By enhancing adrenergic activity, cocaine can promote glycogenolysis. When cocaine is used just prior to aerobic exercise, blood glucose is significantly lower, compared with exercise without cocaine (Han et al. 1996). Conlee and associates (1991a) have shown that exercise-induced decreases in glycogen content in the white vastus lateralis muscle of rats were augmented by cocaine. Concomitant with the enhanced rate of glycogen depletion, endurance is reduced (Bracken et al. 1988).

Exercise-induced increases in corticosterone levels in rats are also augmented by cocaine (Conlee et al. 1991b). As predicted by its effects on catecholamines, cocaine increases resting heart rate (HR) and blood pressure (BP). It also augments the increases in HR and BP that occur in response to the stress associated with nonexertional tasks (Foltin et al. 1988). Furthermore, among the population of chronic cocaine smokers, maximal HR during graded cycle ergometry to exhaustion was lower, compared to nonsmokers (Marques-Magallanes et al. 1997).

People who take amphetamines experience a decreased sense of fatigue, increased BP and HR, redistribution of blood flow to skeletal muscles, and mobilization of energy substrates. Since amphetamines promote weight loss by suppressing hunger, athletes who use amphetamines regularly also risk depleting glycogen stores.

How Amphetamines and Cocaine Affect Exercise Performance

Scientists began studying the effects of amphetamine on performance as early as the mid-1940s, but reports of their studies at that stage were contradictory and inconclusive. Even a generation later, Bhagat and Wheeler (1973) and Gerald (1978) reported directly opposite effects of amphetamine on the exercise endurance in rats. When rats were forced to swim until exhaustion, high doses of amphetamine (i.e., 10 mg/kg or greater), but not low doses, were ergogenic (Bhagat and Wheeler 1973). When rats were run on a treadmill, duration improved with low doses, but it was worse (compared to saline administration) with high doses (Gerald 1978). These divergent results cannot be explained.

The first in-depth study of the effects of amphetamines on human performance was conducted by Smith and Beecher in 1959. They found that a dose of 14 mg/70 kg bodyweight given 2 to 3 h prior to testing improved performance in weight throwers by 3% to 4%, improved performance in runners by 1.5%, and improved performance in swimmers by 0.5% to 1.1%. These improvements, small as they are, can make a difference between finishing first or second at elite levels of competition. In 1972, Borg and colleagues exercised subjects on a cycle ergometer for ten 45 s periods. These researchers found that performance during the initial periods was worse after amphetamine sulfate 10 mg, but that performance during the latter periods was improved after amphetamine, compared to placebo (Borg et al. 1972). In nonfatigued normal volunteers, a single 10 mg oral dose of dextroamphetamine did not affect stationary hand tremor or steadiness, but did improve performance of a more complex motor task requiring greater sustained subject attention and cooperation (Domino et al. 1972).

Still later, Chandler and Blair (1980) performed a thorough assessment of the effects of amphetamine on several variables of athletic performance in college students. While they found that dextroamphetamine at a dose of 15 mg/70 kg increased time to exhaustion, they saw no effect on aerobic power. The effect on muscular strength was variable (see table 15.1 for additional results).

Only limited data exists showing the effects of cocaine on physical performance. Cocaine appears to exert ergolytic effects on endurance. After intraperitoneal administration of cocaine at a dose of 20 mg/kg, rats ran on a treadmill only 29 ± 11.6 min compared to rats that received saline injection and ran for 74.9 ± 16.5 min (Bracken et al. 1988).

When only well-designed studies are considered, there is no evidence that cocaine has any ergogenic properties. Subjects who are chronic cocaine smokers show a poorer exercise performance on a graded maximal cycle ergometry test compared with nonsmokers, even without any identifiable defects in pulmonary physiology (Marques-

Table 15.1 Physical and Physiological Performance Changes With the Use of Amphetamines

Variable	Placebo	Drug	Mean difference	% difference
Elbow flexion strength (newtons)	681	724	43	6.3
Knee extension strength (newtons)	1,264	1,550	286	22.6*
Leg power (watts)	623	642	19	3.0
Peak speed (s per 10 yd)	1.11	1.11	0	0.0
Acceleration for 30-yd run $(m \cdot s^{-2})$	2.89	3.00	0.11	3.8*
Aerobic power $(L \cdot min^{-1})$	3.96	3.97	0.01	0.3
Time to exhaustion (s)	427	446	19	4.4*
Peak lactate $(mmol \cdot L^{-1})$	13.3	14.4	1.1	8.3*
Maximum heart rate (beats per min^{-1})	191	195	4	2.1*

*Statistically significant difference indicating a better performance while on amphetamines.

Adapted from Chandler, J.V., and Blair, S.N. 1980. The effect of amphetamines on selected physiological components related to athletic success. *Med Sci Sports Exerc* 12:65-69.

Adapted from Chandler and Blair 1980. Reprinted from Wilmore and Costill 1999.

Magallanes et al. 1997). As for nonexertional forms of task performance, intranasal cocaine did not affect task performance, despite increasing HR and BP, in test subjects (Foltin et al. 1988).

Avoiding Potential Complications

The case study at the beginning of this chapter is no fiction. Many readers may be more familiar with the cases of the elite athletes Len Bias and Don Rogers, whose deaths in June 1986 were attributed to cocaine. Such cases should alert readers to the dangers of combining cocaine and exercise. Cocaine abuse has been associated with a variety of cardiovascular complications, including myocardial infarction and sudden death. The acute cardiovascular reactions to cocaine use should not be surprising, considering its ability to augment the activity of catecholamines. Presumably because of the alpha-adrenergic effects of norepinephrine on the peripheral vessels, cocaine has been associated with loss of distal pulses in a young adult (Young and Glauber 1947). Toxic doses of cocaine may precipitate exercise-induced heat stroke during exercise at elevated ambient temperatures (Lomax and Daniel 1993). Cardiac dysrrhythmias can develop in cocaine users during withdrawal (Nademanee et al. 1989).

Giammarco (1987) has proposed that the risk of cocaine-related death is higher among elite athletes than in the general population. When elite athletes ingest cocaine in doses high enough to produce seizures, because of their greater muscle mass they generate higher quantities of lactic acid; this, in turn, increases their risk of death from lactic acidosis (Giammarco 1987).

Used regularly, cocaine can produce other problems. When chronic cocaine abusers with left ventricular hypertrophy (LVH) are exercised on a treadmill, an exaggerated pressor response is seen (see figure 15.1; Cigarroa et al. 1992). An association between an exaggerated pressor response to treadmill exercise and LVH has also been demonstrated for normotensive men who are not cocaine abusers (Gottdiener et al. 1990). Because many elite athletes have LVH, the possibility of this exaggerated pressor response is another reason for them to completely avoid cocaine use prior to aerobic exercise. Chronic cocaine smokers also exhibit unique pulmonary pathology (Itkonen, Schnoll, and Glassroth 1984). Table 15.2 summarizes some of the toxicities of cocaine abuse.

Both cocaine and amphetamines have a high potential for causing physical and psychological dependence (the term "addiction" is an imprecise term, so it is not used in pharmacology). Although amphetamines do not cause the same degree of catecholamine potentiation as does cocaine, their effects last longer than those of cocaine. In addition,

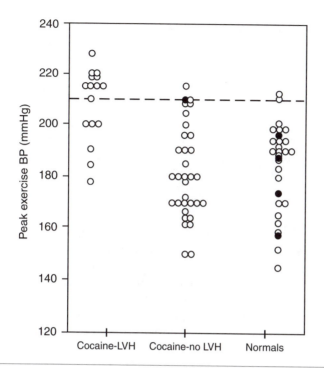

Figure 15.1 Plot showing the distribution of individual peak exercise systolic blood response in three different groups: cocaine abusers with left ventricular hypertrophy (LVH), cocaine abusers without LVH, and the control group. ● = individuals in the control group with echocardiographic LVH; BP = blood pressure.

Adapted from Cigarroa et al. 1992.

Table 15.2 Risks of Cocaine Use

Acute

Exaggerated pressor response

Peripheral ischemia

Cardiac arrhythmias

Seizures

Stroke

Hyperthermia

Sudden death

Decreased endurance

Psychosis

Chronic

Pulmonary pathophysiology (if smoked)

Paranoia and other personality changes

Physical and psychological dependence

Weight loss

some dosage forms of amphetamines are designed to be "sustained-release," making it possible for their effects to last still longer, up to 12 h. Many of the adverse effects of cocaine also apply to amphetamines.

NCAA and USOC Status

Cocaine in all forms is banned by both the USOC and the NCAA. In addition, pharmaceutical forms of cocaine are prescription drugs and are regulated as Schedule II controlled substances by the FDA. Amphetamine too is a banned substance and a Schedule II controlled substance.

Guidelines for Use

Amphetamines and cocaine are potentially toxic drugs. In addition, the FDA classifies both as controlled substances (category II). This means that possession of these substances without a valid prescription is a federal crime. For this reason, as well as the fact that they are banned substances during athletic competition, individuals should not use amphetamines and cocaine, especially in combination with sports and exercise.

References

Bhagat, B., and Wheeler, N. 1973. Effect of amphetamine on the swimming endurance of rats. *Neuropharmacology* 12:711-713.

Borg, G., Edstrom, C.G., Linderholm, H., and Marklund, G. 1972. Changes in physical performance induced by amphetamine and amobarbital. *Psychopharmacologica* 26:10-18.

Bracken, M.E., Bracken, D.R., Nelson, A.G., and Conlee, R.K. 1988. Effect of cocaine on exercise endurance and glycogen use in rats. *J Appl Physiol* 64:884-887.

Chandler, J.V., and Blair, S.N. 1980. The effect of amphetamines on selected physiological components related to athletic success. *Med Sci Sports Exerc* 12:65-69.

Cigarroa, C.G., Boehrer, J.D., Brickner, E., Eichhorn, E.J., and Grayburn, P.A. 1992. Exaggerated pressor response to treadmill exercise in chronic cocaine abusers with left ventricular hypertrophy. *Circulation* 86:226-231.

Conlee, R.K., Barnett, D.W., Kelly, K.P., and Han, D.H. 1991a. Effects of cocaine on plasma catecholamine and muscle glycogen concentrations during exercise in the rat. *J Appl Physiol* 70:1323-1327.

Conlee, R.K., Barnett, D.W., Kelly, K.P., and Han, D.H. 1991b. Effects of cocaine, exercise, and resting conditions on plasma corticosterone and catecholamine concentrations in the rat. *Metabolism* 40:1043-1047.

Di Paolo, T., Rouillard, C., Morissette, M., Levesque, D., and Bedard, P.J. 1989. Endocrine and neurochemical actions of cocaine. *Can J Physiol Pharmacol* 67:1177-1182.

Domino, E.F., Albers, J.W., Potvin, A.R., Repa, B.S., and Tourtellotte, W.W. 1972. Effects of d-amphetamine on quantitative measures of motor performance. *Clin Pharmacol Ther* 13:251-257.

Foltin, R.W., McEntee, M.A., Capriotti, R.M., Pedroso, J.J., and Fischman, M.W. 1988. Effects of cocaine, alone and in combination with task performance, on heart rate and blood pressure. *Pharmacol Biochem Behav* 31:387-391.

Gerald, M.C. 1978. Effects of (+)-amphetamine on the treadmill endurance performance of rats. *Neuropharmacology* 17:703-704.

Giammarco, R.A. 1987. The athlete, cocaine, and lactic acidosis: A hypothesis. *Am J Med Sci* 294:412-414.

Gottdiener, J.S., Brown, J., Zoltick, J., and Fletcher, R.D. 1990. Left ventricular hypertrophy in men with normal blood pressure: Relation to exaggerated blood pressure response to exercise. *Ann Intern Med* 112:161-166.

Han, D.H., Kelly, K.P., Fellingham, G.W., and Conlee, R.K. 1996. Cocaine and exercise: Temporal changes in plasma levels of catecholamines, lactate, glucose, and cocaine. *Am J Physiol (Endocrinol Metab)* 270(33):E438-E444.

Itkonen, J., Schnoll, S., and Glassroth, J. 1984. Pulmonary dysfunction in freebase cocaine users. *Arch Intern Med* 144:2195-2197.

Lomax, P., and Daniel, K.A. 1993. Cocaine and body temperature: Effect of exercise at high ambient temperature. *Pharmacology* 46:164-172.

Marques-Magallanes, J.A., Koyal, S.N., Cooper, C.B., Kleerup, E.C., and Tashkin, D.P. 1997. Impact of habitual cocaine smoking on the physiologic response to maximum exercise. *Chest* 112:1008-1016.

Nademanee, K., Gorelick, D.A., Josephson, M.A., Ryan, M.A., Wilkins, J.N., Robertson, H.A., Mody, F.V., and Intarachot, V. 1989. Myocardial ischemia during cocaine withdrawal. *Ann Intern Med* 111:876-880.

Schermer, C.R., and Wisner, D.H. 1999. Methamphetamine use in trauma patients: A population-based study. *J Am Coll Surg* 189:442-449.

Smith, G.M., and Beecher, H.K. 1959. Amphetamine sulfate and athletic performance. *JAMA* 170:542-557.

Wagner, J.C. 1991. Enhancement of athletic performance with drugs: An overview. *Sports Med* 12:250-265.

Young, D., and Glauber, J.J. 1947. Electrocardiographic changes resulting from acute cocaine intoxication. *Am Heart J* 34:272-279.

V
PART

Final
Thoughts

16

CHAPTER

Exercise: The Overlooked Prescription

■ *CASE*   You finish a long day of work and, while driving home, your mind wanders from the familiar landscape to some of the clients you saw today. Gordon, a black male executive with hypertension, is now taking your advice to exercise more. After his last appointment he started a running program. You counseled him on using diuretics while exercising, and he seemed to understand. His blood pressure is controlled nicely now, and you are thinking you might be able to terminate the diuretic, which should, in turn, further improve his exercise tolerance. Sally, an obese white female, has heeded your advice and enrolled in a water aerobics program. Although she still has a long way to go, she has already lost 22 pounds and her cholesterol profile is better. At her next visit, you are thinking you might assess her insulin levels to see if the weight loss and exercise has improved her insulin resistance. In any event, she is starting to develop a more positive image of herself, which may lead to improved dietary patterns. You feel good about how you are helping clients prevent serious health consequences. As you pull into the garage, you decide to go out for a jog.

In the preceding chapters, I have attempted to summarize the clinical data regarding issues that arise when medications are used during exercise. As was pointed out in the first part of the book, the use of drugs is pervasive in our society. Pharmaceutical companies are increasing their production of newer and more effective drugs, which makes it even more likely that individuals, particularly deconditioned ones, will be consuming some type of drug while exercising. If we are successful in getting more deconditioned subjects to exercise, then there will be questions about the safety of exercising while taking medications, and, for competitive athletes, the impact of the drug(s) on performance.

Concurrent with the increase in production of pharmaceuticals and nutraceuticals, some disease states, such as coronary artery disease (CAD), are not declining at a rate that would reflect the impact of these newer and more powerful drugs. Further, obesity has reached epidemic proportions in the United States (Mokdad et al. 1999). Obesity, in turn, causes secondary health problems, many of which are addressed pharmacologically. Exercise appears to be the overlooked prescription for many medical conditions. In this chapter, we will examine how exercise affects health and how we might best prescribe it more effectively.

Improving the Therapeutic Use of Exercise

Although messages that encourage regular exercise or physical activity now come at people from many directions, the vast majority of the population still does not exercise regularly (Pate et al. 1995). How much drug therapy could be avoided if exercise were a regular component in the lifestyle of most individuals?

Unfortunately, far too few adults exercise enough. From 1985 to 1991, the percent of subjects who were physically inactive remained at 24%, according to Public Health Service statistics (McGinnis and Lee 1995). A 1991 telephone survey summarizing the proportion of 87,433 adults who reported no leisure-time physical activity within the preceding month was published by the Centers for Disease Control (CDC) and the American College of Sports Medicine (ACSM) (Pate et al. 1995). In one demographic group, the prevalence of a sedentary lifestyle was as high as 48% (see table 16.1). Data from a similar 1994 random telephone survey revealed that the median rate of acceptable regular physical activity by state was 26.9%; the median value for no physical activity was 28.9% (CDC 1996). In every state surveyed, 60% of adults did not achieve the recommended amount of physical activity, and in half the states 73% were insufficiently active (CDC 1996). The mid-decade report on Healthy People 2000 (McGinnis and Lee 1995) showed that, although there is an observed positive trend for the proportion of adults who

Table 16.1   Adults Reporting No Leisure-Time Physical Activity Within the Last Month

Demographic group	Sedentary % (95% CI)
Sex	
Male	27.89 (27.18-28.60)
Female	31.48 (30.85-32.11)
Race	
White	27.75 (27.24-28.26)
Nonwhite	37.52 (36.27-38.77)
Age (y)	
18-34	23.77 (23.01-24.53)
35-54	29.50 (28.70-30.30)
55	38.00 (37.10-38.90)
Annual income ($)	
14,999	40.14 (39.06-41.22)
15,000-24,999	32.00 (30.90-33.10)
25,000-50,000	25.43 (24.63-26.23)
> 50,000	18.64 (17.60-19.68)
Education	
Some high school	48.06 (46.75-49.37)
High school/tech school graduate	33.57 (32.79-34.35)
Some college/college graduate	20.16 (19.55-20.77)

Data taken from the 1991 Behavioral Risk Factor Surveillance System, a population-based random-digit-dial telephone survey with 87,433 respondents aged 18 years and older from 47 states and the District of Columbia. Data are weighed, and point estimates and confidence intervals (CIs) are calculated using the SESUDAAN procedure to adjust for the complex sampling frame.

Adapted from R.R. Pate, M. Pratt, S.N. Blair, W.L. Haskell, C.A. Macera, C. Bouchard, D. Buchner, W. Ettinger, G.W. Heath, A.C. King, et al., 1995, "Physical activity and public health. A recommendation from the Centers for Disease Control and Prevention and the American College of Sports Medicine," *JAMA* 273 (5): 403.

exercise regularly, there has been no decline in the proportion of people who lead essentially sedentary lifestyles.

Pate and colleagues (1995) summarized data compiled by the U.S. Department of Health and Human Services. Thirty-eight percent of individuals aged 55 years and above had not exercised at least once in the prior month and thus were considered sedentary. The prevalence of individuals who had not exercised at least once within the previous month prior to being surveyed was directly associated with age and indirectly associated with annual income and education.

Exercise among children is also not being encouraged enough. In a 1990 survey of American high school youth, it was found that only 37% engaged in 20 min of vigorous physical activity 3 or more times per week. Forty-four percent of boys and 52% of girls were not even enrolled in physical education classes. Seventy percent of these same students reported watching television at least one hour per day, and 35% reported watching television three or more hours per day (Heath et al. 1994). Intervening in this sedentary activity has positive outcomes on body anthropometrics in children (Robinson 1999).

Medical Expenditures for Cardiovascular Disease

In the United States, cardiovascular disease is the highest cause of death in adults (see table 16.2). Some 700,000 patients are hospitalized each year with acute myocardial infarction, and roughly 400,000 to 500,000 people die every year from CHD. This represents about one-third of all deaths in adults. In economic terms, the annual cost of CHD is nearly $80 billion, which represents 15% of the annual health care budget in the United States (Hunink et al. 1997). Besides the cost of drug therapy for CHD, there are roughly 300,000 coronary bypass operations performed annually at a cost of $30,000 to $40,000 each.

Little change has been seen in the death rate from ischemic heart disease (see figure 16.1). From 1985 through 1995, deaths from cardio-vascular disease declined 22%; however, the actual number of deaths decreased only 2.8%. Clearly, cardiovascular diseases collectively represent the biggest health problem in the United States.

Considering the magnitude of cardiovascular disease in this country, it should not be surprising that cardiovascular agents occupy a promi-

Table 16.2   1996 Disease and Mortality Statistics

	Disease prevalence*	# deaths in 1996
Cardiovascular disease (all types)*	58,800,000	959,227
Coronary heart disease	12,000,000	476,124
Hypertension	50,000,000	41,634
Stroke	4,400,000	159,942
Cancer (all types)	N/A	544,728
HIV (AIDS)	N/A	32,655

*based on 1996 estimates.

Data taken from the American Heart Association web site, accessed January 23, 2000. http://www.americanheart.org/statistics/03cardio.html.

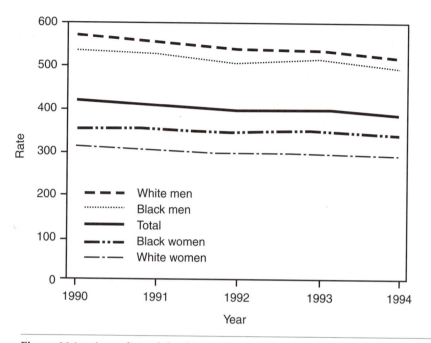

Figure 16.1 Age-adjusted death rate (per 100,000 population, adjusted to the 1980 U.S. standard population) of ischemic heart disease for adults aged 35 years, by race and sex, United States, 1990-1994. Data are presented only for blacks and whites because numbers for other racial/ethnic groups were too small for meaningful analysis.

Adapted from Centers for Disease Control and Prevention, 1997, "Trends in ischemic heart disease deaths—United States, 1990-1994," *Morbidity and Mortality Weekly Report* 46 (7): 147.

nent place when expenditures for various drug categories are compared. This drug group encompasses antihypertensives, antilipemics, antianginals, antiarrhythmics, and drugs for heart failure. Cardiovascular agents were the top drug category in terms of dollars spent in the first half of 1994 by HMOs and long-term care facilities; in hospitals they ranked fourth behind anti-infective agents, cancer and transplant drugs, and biotechnology drugs (Santell 1995). The sheer numbers of prescriptions filled for cardiovascular drugs (291.2 million in 1995) tells the story, and these prescriptions accounted for $10 billion in sales in retail pharmacies (Glaser 1996). This figure rose to $11.8 billion in 1997, according to independent research by Frost and Sullivan. In 1997, the drug category with the largest annual percent growth in use was cholesterol-reducing drugs (Gebhart 1998), a trend that likely reflects the aging of the general population and its sedentary habits.

What makes these statistics still more discouraging is that patients often do not take drugs as intended. One recent study found, for example, that only 52% of elderly patients who require lipid-lowering drugs actually continue to fill their prescriptions for these drugs after five years (Avorn et al. 1998). Problems with noncompliance have also been noted for antihypertensive drugs (Stephenson 1999), drugs for asthma (Yeung et al. 1994), and even drug therapy for hematologic malignancies (Levine et al. 1987). And there is this statistic: researchers at the University of Toronto determined that serious adverse drug reactions in the United States occurred in 6.7% of hospitalized patients. Of these, 106,000 (95% confidence interval, 76,000-137,000) resulted in death, making *adverse drug reactions* between the fourth and sixth leading cause of death in 1994, just behind heart disease, cancer, and stroke (Lazarou, Pomeranz, and Corey 1998). These statistics make one wonder if drug therapy is the best approach for treating some of these chronic diseases.

■ What's It Worth?

In 1995 $10 billion was spent on cardiovascular drugs in the United States. That same year, U.S. residents spent $3 billion on exercise machines.

Note: From *Dateline NBC,* 21 September 1996.

Treatment or Prevention?

Despite the availability of newer and better drugs and their increased use, cardiovascular disease does not seem to be lessening. But even if drug therapy could work miracles for this disease and other lifestyle-related illnesses, isn't it better to prevent a so-called preventable disease than to treat it with drugs? No matter how effective drugs become, addressing CHD with drug therapy still represents "treatment," an intervention initiated *after* the disease state has already become manifest. Indeed, statistics tell us that our current strategy of treating CHD is having little impact, despite the allocation and expenditures of billions of health care dollars.

The medical community does not sufficiently emphasize preventive medicine: it does not stress this approach enough in medical schools, and preventive therapy expenses are not reimbursed as readily as they should be. Alexander Leaf, MD, notes the following in an article published in the *Journal of the American Medical Association* in 1993: "Medicine traditionally stands on two pillars: prevention and cure. For the past century the profession has rallied almost exclusively under the banner of curative medicine. Preventive medicine has been largely relegated to the Public Health Service. Medical education provides minimal time and instruction in preventive medicine."

A growing amount of evidence supports the conclusion that exercise positively affects various disease states, including colon cancer, congestive heart failure, COPD (chronic obstructive pulmonary disease), coronary artery disease, diabetes mellitus, endometrial cancer, hyperlipidemia, hypertension, low back pain, obesity, osteoporosis, and stroke.

Several large studies published over the last dozen years have shown that leisure-time physical activity or improvements in physical fitness reduce the risk for cardiovascular disease in adults (Blair et al. 1995; Lakka et al. 1994; Leon et al. 1987; Morris et al. 1990; Young et al. 1993). Paffenbarger and colleagues have collected data from thousands of Cooper Clinic patients (see Farrell et al. 1998) and Harvard alumni (see Paffenbarger et al. 1986) that show exercise is inversely and independently associated with cardiovascular disease. Yet, as Leaf (1993) has pointed out, preventive approaches to care, such as cardiac rehabilitation programs, are largely excluded from reimbursement by insurers and by Medicare.

Also formal instruction in sports medicine or exercise physiology is not widely available in medical schools. Results of a survey of 92 medical schools published in 1988 revealed that only 38% offered such training (Whitley and Nyberg 1988). Members of the medical community often consider sports medicine issues to be primarily the domain of the orthopedist (Cantwell 1992), although general health issues (e.g., exercise) are common topics for family practitioners and internists. In addition, physicians are trained to focus on the patient's chief complaint rather than on disease risk (Scutchfield and Hartman 1995). In a study of Massachusetts primary care physicians surveyed in 1994, only 49% believed it was important for patients to engage in moderate daily physical activity (see figure 16.2), even though 89% agreed that educating patients about health-related risk factors is an important responsibility (Wechsler et al. 1996).

Moreover, important scientific papers published in major medical journals well into the 1990s continue to disregard exercise as a component of therapy for CHD. Several examples follow. When the MRFIT (Multiple Risk Factor Intervention Trial) study was published in November 1987, it showed that moderate exercise significantly lowers the risk of CHD and death (Leon et al. 1987). A decade later (and seven years after the creation of Healthy People 2000), a paper describing an elaborate computer model simulation that analyzed changes in mortality from CHD was published in the *Journal of the American Medical Association (JAMA)*. Although many important variables were evaluated in the computer model, *exercise was not one of them*. The contribution of exercise to this largely preventable disease was hardly discussed in the paper (Hunink et al. 1997). The authors simply admitted that exercise was a

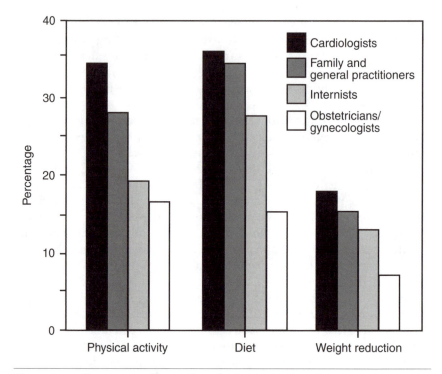

Figure 16.2   Percentage of general medical examinations that involved counseling, by physician specialty, United States, National Ambulatory Medical Care Survey, 1995.

Adapted from Centers for Disease Control and Prevention, 1998, "Missed opportunities in preventive counseling for cardiovascular disease—United States, 1995," *Morbidity and Mortality Weekly Report* 47 (5): 94.

possible "primary prevention effort" that may have played a role but was not included in their model, and this was the only mention they gave to exercise in the entire report!

In 1995, a major review of the relationship between cholesterol reduction and cardiovascular disease was published in the *New England Journal of Medicine* (Levine, Keaney, and Vita 1995); this review, too, did not discuss exercise as a potential treatment modality. In fact, the only mention of exercise was in a table comparing studies of various antilipemic therapies on cholesterol reduction where one study of combined diet-exercise was included. The following year a major review appeared in the *Annals of Internal Medicine* (Garber, Browner, and Hulley 1996), which discussed cholesterol screening in asymptomatic adults. Although the intent was not to focus on management, the paper did extensively review many randomized, controlled trials of cholesterol reduction and the associated morbidity and mortality of CHD. Exercise was not discussed anywhere in this review.

In 1998, a paper was published in *JAMA* that described the results of another 10-year model of CHD risk. This model was based on data from the Second National Health and Nutritional Examination Survey conducted from 1978 to 1982, when details regarding exercise may not have been available. The authors, however, in identifying limitations of their model, mention only "prophylactic aspirin therapy" as a variable that deserves consideration; they do not refer to exercise in their discussion (Avins and Browner 1998).

These important, recent papers followed no fewer than 43 epidemiologic studies conducted between 1950 and 1987 on the relationship between exercise and CHD (Powell et al. 1987). In fact, as early as 1977 Selvester, Camp, and Sanmarco had proposed that regular exercise could slow the development of atherosclerotic plaques in men. These findings were reproduced in monkeys that were fed an atherogenic diet (a study design that controlled for the variables that usually confound these types of studies in humans; see Kramsch et al. 1981). By 1984, Paffenbarger and colleagues (Paffenbarger et al. 1984; Paffenbarger and Hyde 1984), who had thoroughly investigated and written extensively on this topic, had published several comprehensive reviews of the inverse relationship between exercise and coronary heart disease. Their data were also published in the prestigious *New England Journal of Medicine* (Paffenbarger et al. 1986), several years prior to the more recent papers that omitted exercise from consideration. Similar inverse relationships between exercise and CHD risk have been described for women (Lapidus and Bengtsson 1986; Kokkinos, Holland, et al. 1995). Indeed, it is troubling that major reviews of cardiovascular disease state management continue to be published in the medical literature without discussing exercise. When a major scientific paper does not treat exercise as significant, it undermines the impact of the "pro-exercise" papers.

Becoming More Proactive in Recommending Exercise

There are three compelling basic reasons for physicians and other sports medicine personnel to become more proactive in urging individuals to exercise:

1. Regular exercise can reduce the need for drug therapy.
2. Obesity and cardiovascular disease are serious health problems, especially in the United States but also in other countries.
3. Sports medicine personnel have the ability to take advantage of the "teachable moment."

Reduce Need for Drug Therapy

First, I propose that regular exercise can alleviate the need for drug therapy in many individuals. Are there any data to support this possibility? Only two studies so far have directly examined the impact of regular exercise on the need for prescription medication. Although elderly subjects make up only about 12% of the United States population, they consume 25% of prescriptions. Some 60% to 78% of elderly subjects take at least one prescription drug (Chrischilles et al. 1992), and some of them take as many as 17 drugs concurrently (Helling et al. 1987). On the other hand, Fries and colleagues (1994) found that elderly runners consumed fewer medications than age-matched nonrunners. Kokkinos, Narayan, and colleagues (1995) found that both the dosage and the number of required antihypertensive drugs could be reduced in 10 of 14 black hypertensive males who rode an exercise bike regularly for 32 weeks, but no reductions in medication could be made in the control group that did not exercise. In 1995, more than 2.1 billion total prescriptions were dispensed in U.S. pharmacies (Glaser 1996), and the total prescription drug market rose from $27 billion in sales in 1988 to nearly $70 billion in 1996. Thus, the potential impact of regular exercise on prescription drug costs is enormous.

Exercise exerts a beneficial effect on many disease states, and the sad reality is that many forms of cancer and heart disease are lifestyle induced. Drug therapy for many chronic diseases could likely be reduced if more persons exercised. Increasing the amount of exercise, along with consuming a proper diet and quitting smoking, are probably the best actions individuals can take to improve their health (Paffenbarger et al. 1993, 1994). In one study, an improvement in fitness level produced a greater reduction in risk of death than other lifestyle changes, such as losing weight, lowering blood pressure, lowering cholesterol levels, or quitting smoking (Blair et al. 1995). We can only hope that this evidence, along with the efforts of sports medicine and other health professionals, will persuade increased numbers of deconditioned subjects to begin exercising regularly.

Fight Obesity

The second reason for becoming more proactive in encouraging exercise is obesity. Data from the Third National Health and Nutrition Examination Survey, conducted between 1988 and 1994, revealed a lack of exercise among youngsters, with a resulting increase in childhood obesity. While 80% of U.S. children reported performing three or more bouts of vigorous activity per week, 26% of them watched four or more hours of television daily. This group of children had greater body fat and greater body mass index than those who watched less than two hours per day (Andersen et al. 1998). Leisure time for many adolescents increasingly involves sedentary activity: watching television, playing video games, and using personal computers. It should be not surprising, then, that being overweight and obesity are so prevalent in our society.

Obesity is a major public health problem in North America. In the United States, according to a 1998 federal obesity guidelines report from the National Heart, Lung, and Blood Institute (NHLBI), an estimated 97 million adults are either obese or overweight; this represents 55% of the population (National Institutes of Health 1998). The percentage of the population that is obese has actually increased since the original development of the Healthy People 2000 recommendations (McGinnis and Lee 1995). In fact, the prevalence of obesity in the United States has been referred to as an "epidemic" (Mokdad et al. 1999). By contrast, the rate of mortality from AIDS, a more widely recognized epidemic, appears to be on the decline (see figure 16.3). Unfortunately, the general public seems much less aware of the obesity epidemic than the AIDS epidemic.

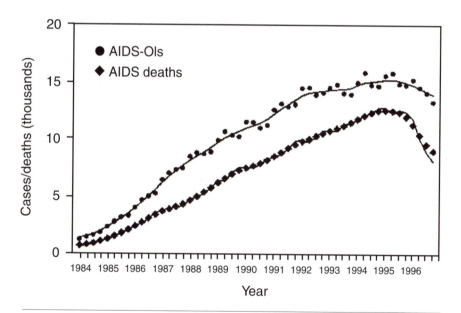

Figure 16.3   Estimated incidence of AIDS-opportunistic illnesses (AIDS-OIs) and estimated number of deaths among persons aged   13 years with AIDS (AIDS deaths), adjusted for delays in reporting, by quarter year of diagnosis/death, United States, 1984-1996. Points represent quarterly incidence; lines represent "smoothed" incidence. Estimates are not adjusted for incomplete reporting of AIDS cases.

Adapted from Centers for Disease Control and Prevention, 1997, "Update: Trends in AIDS incidence—United States, 1996," *Morbidity and Mortality Weekly Report* 46 (37): 862.

Obesity is a serious health concern because of its association with other major disease states. Obesity is associated with an increased risk for hyperlipidemias, gallbladder disease, sleep apnea, degenerative joint disease, hypertension and coronary heart disease, stroke, respiratory dysfunction, certain forms of cancer, and insulin resistance and diabetes mellitus (Must et al. 1999; Pi-Sunyer 1993; NIH 1998) (table 16.3). Recently, Bao and colleagues (1997) published data from the Bogalusa Heart Study, suggesting that the development of obesity in childhood is an ominous risk factor for cardiovascular disease in offspring of parents with coronary artery disease. The NHLBI, in cooperation with the National Institute of Diabetes and Digestive and Kidney Diseases (NIDDK) panel (see NIH 1998), concluded that

Table 16.3   Prevalence of Comorbidity by Obesity Class and Sex

Health condition	Under-weight	Normal	Over-weight	Obesity class 1**	Obesity class 2**	Obesity class 3**
Men (*n* = 6,987)						
Type 2 diabetes mellitus	4.69	2.03	4.93	10.10	12.30	10.65
Gallbladder disease	6.96	1.93	3.39	5.38	5.80	10.17
Coronary heart disease	12.45	8.84	9.60	16.01	10.21	13.97
High blood cholesterol level	6.66	26.63	35.68	39.17	34.01	35.63
High blood pressure	23.38	23.47	34.16	48.95	65.48	64.53
Osteoarthritis	0.39	2.59	4.55	4.66	5.46	10.04
Women (*n* = 7,689)						
Type 2 diabetes mellitus	4.76	2.38	7.12	7.24	13.16	19.89
Gallbladder disease	6.42	6.29	11.84	15.99	19.15	23.45
Coronary heart disease	12.07	6.87	11.13	12.56	12.31	19.22
High blood cholesterol level	13.36	26.89	45.59	40.37	40.96	36.39
High blood pressure	19.81	23.26	38.77	47.95	54.51	63.16
Osteoarthritis	7.79	5.22	8.51	9.94	10.39	17.19

Column group header: Weight status category*

*Estimates are weighted to account for the sample design. All data are percentages. Weight categories are based on the National Heart, Lung, and Blood Institute classification. **Class 1 = 30.0-34.9 BMI, class 2 = 35.0-39.9, class 3 = 40.0.

Adapted from Must et al. 1999.

- obesity is associated with increased morbidity and mortality;
- strong evidence exists indicating that weight loss in overweight and obese subjects decreases risk factors for diabetes mellitus and cardiovascular disease, decreases blood pressure, decreases triglycerides and increases HDL cholesterol, and decreases blood glucose;
- physical activity alone results in modest weight loss but also serves to help maintain weight loss; and
- exercise independently reduces cardiovascular disease risk.

Stefanick and colleagues (1998) showed that the combination of exercise with a low-fat diet was better than diet alone or exercise alone in reducing high-risk lipoprotein levels (see figure 16.4). But weight loss

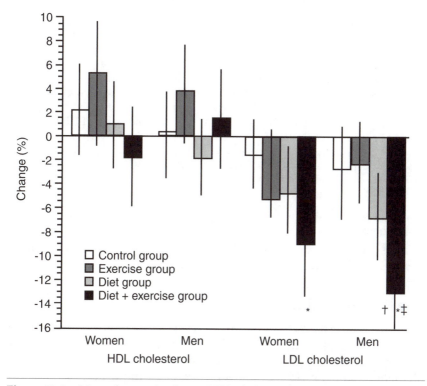

Figure 16.4   Mean changes in plasma HDL cholesterol and LDL cholesterol levels in four study groups at one year. Vertical lines represent 95% confidence intervals. * = $p < 0.05$ for the comparison with the control group; † = $p < 0.001$ for the comparison with the control group; ‡ $p < 0.001$ for the comparison with the exercise group.

Reprinted, by permission, from M.L. Stefanick, S. Mackey, M. Sheehan, N. Ellsworth, W.L. Haskell, and P.D. Wood, 1998, "Effects of diet and exercise in men and postmenopausal women with low levels of HDL cholesterol and high levels of LDL cholesterol," *New England Journal of Medicine* 339: 12-20.

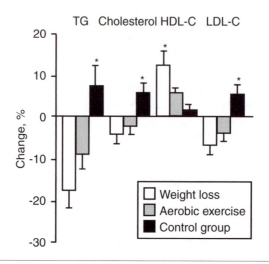

Figure 16.5 Comparisons of relative changes (postintervention to preintervention values) in plasma lipoprotein lipid concentrations with intervention in weight loss and aerobic exercise and at follow-up in sedentary, obese men. * = Significant difference at $p < 0.05$ (analysis of variance). Values are mean ± *SEM*. TG = triglycerides; HDL-C = high-density lipoprotein cholesterol; LDL-C = low-density lipoprotein cholesterol.

Adapted from L.I. Katzel, E.R. Bleecker, E.G. Colman, E.M. Rogus, J.D. Sorkin, and A.P. Goldberg, 1995, "Effects of weight loss vs. aerobic exercise training on risk factors for coronary disease in healthy, obese, middle-aged, and older men," *JAMA* 274 (24): 1918.

is still important also in reducing elevated lipids (see figure 16.5; Katzel et al. 1995).

Those in sports medicine are in the forefront of the clinical medicine community in recognizing the importance of exercise (see table 16.4).

Use the "Teachable Moment"

The third reason for us to feel compelled to become more proactive about exercise involves what is called the "teachable moment." Health care professionals, athletic trainers, others involved in sports medicine, and elementary and high school teachers all become important because they have the ability to influence behavior during teachable moments. Physicians, in particular, can have a dramatic effect on lifestyle behavior. For example, physician counseling sessions have had a significant beneficial impact on alcohol consumption in problem alcohol drinkers (Fleming et al. 1997). A meta-analysis of 74 studies of the effect of patient counseling on preventive behaviors revealed that it indeed was effective in changing behaviors. It is remarkable, however, that only one of the 74 studies was devoted to exercise counseling (Mullen et al. 1997).

Table 16.4 Percentage of Physicians Who Perceived Various Forms of Health-Promoting Behavior as "Very Important" for the Average Person, According to Survey Year

Desired behavior	1994 (n = 418)	1981 (n = 427)
Eliminate cigarette smoking	98*	93
Avoid using illicit drugs	85	N/A
Always use a seat belt when in a car	81*	62
Drink alcohol moderately or not at all	63*	46
Avoid foods high in saturated fats	55*	38
Avoid excess calories	52*	70
Engage in moderate daily physical activity	49	N/A
Eat a balanced diet	47*	58
Engage in aerobic activity at least three times a week	37*	27
Avoid undue stress	26	31
Have an annual physical examination	16	19
Decrease salt consumption	13*	40
Minimize sugar intake	6*	12
Have a baseline exercise test	3	6

*$p < 0.01$ by the z-test for the difference between the surveys.
The number of respondents varied slightly from question to question; not all respondents answered all questions. On a four-point scale, responses ranged from "very important" to "very unimportant."

Reprinted, by permission, from H. Wechsler, S. Levine, R.K Idelson, E.L. Schor, and E. Coakley, 1996, "The physician's role in health promotion revistited: A survey of primary care practitioners," *New England Journal of Medicine* 334: 997. Copyright © 1996 Massachusetts Medical Society. All rights reserved.

Although the U.S. Preventive Services Task Force (1996) recommends that physicians counsel patients on exercise routines, physician discussions of this type fall far short of the recommendations (Taira et al. 1997). Only about 30-40% of patients acknowledge that their physician counseled them about exercise (Galuska et al. 1999; Wee et al. 1999). When the issue of exercise does arise, physicians are more likely to discuss exercise with high-income patients than with low-income patients (Taira et al. 1997). One study found that simple two- to three-minute discussions of exercise advice, the distribution of an educational handout, and the promise of a follow-up phone call at one month by family medicine residents increased exercise (table 16.5; Lewis and Lynch 1993). A step in the right direction is the

Table 16.5   Advice Vs. No Advice: A Comparison of Changes in Exercise Frequency and Duration

	Change scores				
Change	Advice	n	No advice	n	p value
Minutes/session	27.46	66	−4.53	97	1.01
Times/week	0.68	69	0.35	100	0.37
Minutes/week	108.67	66	−23.70	97	0.01
Percentage exercising*	9.8	82	1.8	111	0.04

*Change scores represent difference between pretest and posttest. χ^2 used to compare percentages exercising at baseline ($p = 1.000$) and posttest ($p = 0.043$).

Adapted from Lewis and Lynch 1993.

appearance in some leading medical journals of papers that encourage physicians to urge their unfit patients to start a physical activity program (see Blair et al. 1995; Andersen et al. 1997; Fontanarosa 1999).

Of course, teachers and parents can also encourage meaningful changes in how children exercise. Results were published in 1996 of a three-year effort of an elementary school program modification combined with parental participation on the dietary and exercise patterns of third graders. Students who received the intervention program reported significantly more (58.6 min vs. 46.5 min, $p < 0.003$) daily vigorous activity than did controls (Luepker et al. 1996).

The ACSM together with the CDC published recommendations for physical activity for the general public (see Pate et al. 1995). After reviewing pertinent epidemiologic and clinical data, they concluded the following:

Every adult should accumulate 30 min or more of moderate-intensity physical activity on most, if not all, days of the week.

Moderate-intensity physical activity was defined as any bodily movement produced by skeletal muscles performed at an intensity of 3-6 METs (Pate et al. 1995).

Individuals say they do not exercise because of inclement weather, unsafe neighborhoods, lack of bicycle trails or walking paths, and so forth. These are issues the individual has little or no control over. Perhaps what is most important is for nonexercising adults to learn that vigorous, continuous exercise—the kind of exercise that causes

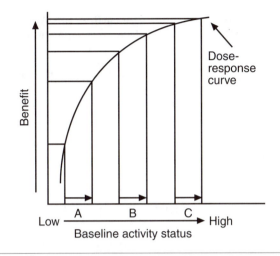

Figure 16.6 The dose-response curve represents the best estimate of the relationship between physical activity (dose) and health benefit (response). The lower the baseline physical activity status, the greater will be the health benefit associated with a given increase in physical activity (arrows A, B, and C). A = sedentary; B = moderately active; C = active.

Adapted from R.R. Pate, M. Pratt, S.N. Blair, W.L. Haskell, C.A. Macera, C. Bouchard, D. Buchner, W. Ettinger, G.W. Heath, A.C. King, et al., 1995, "Physical activity and public health. A recommendation from the Centers for Disease Control and Prevention and the American College of Sports Medicine," *JAMA* 273 (5): 404.

many individuals to lose their motivation to exercise—is not the type being promoted as necessary to achieve desired health benefits. Substantial health benefits can be obtained with "moderate" physical activity (see figure 16.6 and table 16.6). Clinical studies have shown that simply walking reduces the risk of cardiovascular disease (LaCroix et al. 1996) and is inversely associated with mortality (Hakim et al. 1998). Davison and Grant (1993) have reviewed the beneficial effects of walking.

Further, the health benefits of physical activity appear to accrue in approximate proportion to the total amount of physical activity performed. In this regard, the type of exercise is less important than the amount. Routine housework or some general home repairs qualify as moderate physical activity. Even an energy expenditure of as few as 200 calories per day is now considered enough to reap many of the health benefits once thought obtainable from only high-intensity exercise. Physicians and other health care professionals should become familiar with these recommendations so they can properly counsel deconditioned individuals who have questions about exercise. Additional recommendations are listed in table 16.6.

Table 16.6 Common Physical Activities for Healthy U.S. Adults by Intensity of Effort Required in MET Scores and Kilocalories per Minute

Light (< 3.0 METs or < 4 kcal · min⁻¹)	Moderate (3.0-6.0 METs or 4-7 kcal kcal · min⁻¹)	Hard/vigorous (> 6.0 METs or > 7 kcal · min⁻¹)
Walking, slowly (strolling) (1-2 mph)	Walking, briskly (3-4 mph)	Walking, briskly uphill or with a load
Cycling, stationary (< 50 W)	Cycling for pleasure or transportation (10 mph)	Cycling, fast or racing (> 10 mph)
Swimming, slow treading	Swimming, moderate effort	Swimming, fast treading or crawl
Conditioning exercise, light stretching	Conditioning exercise, general calisthenics	Conditioning exercise, stair ergometer, ski machine
—	Racket sports, table tennis	Racket sports, singles tennis, racketball
Golf, power cart	Golf, pulling cart or carrying clubs	—
Bowling	—	—
Fishing, sitting	Fishing, standing/casting	Fishing in stream
Boating, power	Canoeing, leisurely (2.0-3.9 mph)	Canoeing, rapidly (4 mph)
Home care, carpet sweeping	Home care, general cleaning	Moving furniture
Mowing lawn, riding mower	Mowing lawn, power mower	Mowing lawn, hand mower
Home repair, carpentry	Home repair, painting	—

Data from Ainsworth et al., Leon, and McCardle et al. The METs (work metabolic rate/resting metabolic rate) are multiples of the resting rate of oxygen consumption during physical activity. One MET represents the approximate rate of oxygen consumption of a seated adult at rest, or about 3.5 mL · min⁻¹ · kg⁻¹. The equivalent energy cost of 1 MET in kilocalories · min⁻¹ is about 1.2 for a 70-kg person, or approximately 1 kcal · kg⁻¹ · hr⁻¹.

Adapted from R.R. Pate, M. Pratt, S.N. Blair, W.L. Haskell, C.A. Macera, C. Bouchard, D. Buchner, W. Ettinger, G.W. Heath, A.C. King, et al., 1995, "Physical activity and public health. A recommendation from the Centers for Disease Control and Prevention and the American College of Sports Medicine," *JAMA* 273 (5): 404.

Guidelines for Physicians, Trainers, Teachers, and Parents

As individuals begin exercising again, there are concerns about the effects of exercise when taking medication, particularly in deconditioned subjects. Indeed, in the treatment of hypertension, some physicians recommend that patients have their blood pressure lowered to 180/105 with medication *before* embarking on an exercise program (Jacober and Sowers 1995). Some drugs that are widely used in clinical medicine, such as diuretics and beta-blockers, exert detrimental effects on an individual's potential duration of exercise. Occasionally, strenuous exercise during therapy with some drugs (e.g., some antilipemic drugs) can lead to adverse outcomes. As more deconditioned individuals begin exercising regularly, these types of problems are more likely to occur. So it is important that physicians consider the implications of combining exercise with medications. Here are some useful pointers to keep in mind for combining drug therapy with exercise.

For Physicians

You play a great role as a motivator, and should encourage exercise whenever appropriate. Review the goals of *Healthy People 2010* (published by the U.S. Public Health Service) as well as the conclusions from the CDC and ACSM regarding exercise recommendations and public health (Pate et al. 1995). Keep in mind that data about exercising while taking medication has not yet been studied well for many drugs. Even with a drug that may be effective in the treatment of a particular disease state (e.g., diuretics and beta-blockers as first-line therapy for the treatment of hypertension), you should remember to consider the medication's effects on exercise performance. Because exercise has such beneficial effects on many disease states and because persons who exercise regularly consume fewer medications, physicians should prescribe exercise as a treatment recommendation when and where appropriate. Perhaps this would lessen the reliance on drug therapy as the treatment of choice.

For Athletic Trainers

Note that physicians are not accustomed to recommending exercise as a treatment strategy for many disease states. Nor are they all that knowledgeable of the risks of combining exercise with medications. Many in our society regard physicians as having supreme knowledge on health issues, but the medical community *in general* is not well trained about exercise-related issues. In many cases, an athletic trainer is better suited to influence individuals' exercise patterns than is a physician.

Like physicians, however, you should review the goals of *Healthy People 2010* and the recommendations from the CDC and ACSM that have already been mentioned. Also, remember to consider the risks of exercising a client who is taking medications. Recognize that some drugs (e.g., caffeine, NSAIDs) can simultaneously exert beneficial and detrimental effects on exercise.

For Elementary School Teachers and Parents

You are in a wonderful position to influence the youngsters in your care. Encourage children to exercise and get physical activity every day. Conversely, discourage television watching and video game playing, and minimize the time that youngsters spend in front of the computer. Set a good activity model for them as well!

References

Andersen, R.E., Blair, S.N., Cheskin, L.J., and Bartlett, S.J. 1997. Encouraging patients to become more physically active: The physician's role. *Ann Intern Med* 127:395-400.

Andersen, R.E., Crespo, C.J., Bartlett, S.J., Cheskin, L.J., and Pratt, M. 1998. Relationship of physical activity and television watching with body weight and level of fatness among children. Results from the third national health and nutrition examination survey. *JAMA* 279:938-942.

Avins, A.L., and Browner, W.S. 1998. Improving the prediction of coronary heart disease to aid in the management of high cholesterol levels. *JAMA* 279:445-449.

Avorn, J., Monette, J., Lacour, A., Bohn, R.L., Monane, M., Mogun, H., and LeLorier, J. 1998. Persistence of use of lipid-lowering medications. *JAMA* 279:1458-1462.

Bao, W., Srinivasan, S.R., Valdez, R., Greenlund, K.J., Wattigney, W.A., and Berenson, G.S. 1997. Longitudinal changes in cardiovascular risk from childhood to young adulthood in offspring of parents with coronary artery disease. The Bogalusa Heart Study. *JAMA* 278:1749-1754.

Blair, S.N., Kohl, H.W., Barlow, C.E., Paffenbarger, R.S., Gibbons, L.W., and Macera, C.A. 1995. Changes in physical fitness and all-cause mortality. A prospective study of healthy and unhealthy men. *JAMA* 273:1093-1098.

Cantwell, J.D. 1992. The internist as sports medicine physician. *Ann Intern Med* 116:165-166.

Centers for Disease Control and Prevention. 1996. State-specific prevalence of participation in physical activity, 1994. *Morbid Mortal Wkly Rep* 45:673-675.

Chrischilles, E.A., Foley, D.J., Wallace, R.B., Lemke, J.H., Semla, T.P., Hanlon, J.T., Glynn, R.J., Ostfeld, A.M., and Guralnik, J.M. 1992. Use of medications by persons 65 and over: Data from the established populations for epidemiologic studies of the elderly. *J Gerontol Med Sci* 47:M137-M144.

Davison, R.C.R., and Grant, S. 1993. Is walking sufficient exercise for health? *Sports Med* 16:369-373.

Farrell, S.W., Kampert, J.B., Kohl, H.W., Barlow, C.E., Macera, C.A., Paffenbarger, R.S., Gibbons, L.W., and Blair, S.N. 1998. Influences of cardiorespiratory fitness levels and other predictors on cardiovascular disease mortality in men. *Med Sci Sports Exerc* 30:899-905.

Fleming, M.F., Barry, K.L., Manwell, L.B., Johnson, K., and London, R. 1997. Brief physician advice for problem alcohol drinkers. A randomized controlled trial in community-based primary care practices. *JAMA* 277:1039-1045.

Fontanarosa, P.B. 1999. Patients, physicians, and weight control. *JAMA* 282:1581-1582.

Fries, J.F., Singh, G., Morfeld, D., Hubert, H.B., Lane, N.E., and Brown, B.W. 1994. Running and the development of disability with age. *Ann Intern Med* 121:502-509.

Galuska, D.A., Will, J.C., Serdula, M.K., and Ford, E.S. 1999. Are health care professionals advising obese patients to lose weight? *JAMA* 282:1576-1578.

Garber, A.M., Browner, W.S., and Hulley, S.B. 1996. Cholesterol screening in asymptomatic adults, revisited. *Ann Intern Med* 124:518-531.

Gebhart, F. 1998. Annual Rx survey. The new golden age. *Drug Topics,* 16 March, 71-83.

Glaser, M. 1996. Annual Rx survey. *Drug Topics,* 8 April, 97-104.

Hakim, A.A., Petrovitch, H., Burchfiel, C.M., Ross, G.W., Rodriguez, B.L., White, L.R., Yano, K., Curb, J.D., and Abbott, R.D. 1998. Effects of walking on mortality among nonsmoking retired men. *N Engl J Med* 338:94-99.

Heath, G.W., Pratt, M., Warren, C.W., and Kann, L. 1994. Physical activity patterns in American high school students: Results from the 1990 youth risk behavior survey. *Arch Pediatr Adolesc Med* 148:1131-1136.

Helling, D.K., Lemke, J.H., Semla, T.P., Wallace, R.B., Lipson, D.P., and Cornoni-Huntley, J. 1987. Medication use characteristics in the elderly: The Iowa 65+ Rural Health Study. *J Am Geriatr Soc* 35:4-12.

Hunink, M.G.M., Goldman, L., Tosteson, A.N.A., Mittleman, M.A., Goldman, P.A., Williams, L.W., Tsevat, J., and Weinstein, M.C. 1997. The recent decline in mortality from coronary heart disease, 1980-1990. The effect of secular trends in risk factors and treatment. *JAMA* 277:535-542.

Jacober, S.J., and Sowers, J.R. 1995. Exercise and hypertension. *JAMA* 273:1965.

Katzel, L.I., Bleecker, E.R., Colman, E.G., Rogus, E.M., Sorkin, J.D., and Goldberg, A.P. 1995. Effects of weight loss vs. aerobic exercise training on risk factors for coronary disease in healthy, obese, middle-aged and older men. *JAMA* 274:1915-1921.

Kokkinos, P.F., Holland, J.C., Pittaras, A.E., Narayan, P., Dotson, C.O., and Papademetriou, V. 1995. Cardiorespiratory fitness and coronary heart disease risk factor association in women. *J Am Coll Cardiol* 26:358-364.

Kokkinos, P.F., Narayan, P., Colleran, J.A., Pittaras, A., Notargiacomo, A., Reda, D., and Papademetriou, V. 1995. Effects of regular exercise on blood pressure and left ventricular hypertrophy in African-American men with severe hypertension. *N Engl J Med* 333:1462-1467.

Kramsch, D.M., Aspen, A.J., Abramowitz, B.M., Kreimendahl, T., and Hood, W.B. 1981. Reduction of coronary atherosclerosis by moderate conditioning exercise in monkeys on an atherogenic diet. *N Engl J Med* 305:1483-1489.

LaCroix, A.Z., Leveille, S.G., Hecht, J.A., Grothaus, L.C., and Wagner, E.H. 1996. Does walking decrease the risk of cardiovascular disease hospitalizations and death in older adults? *J Am Geriatr Soc* 44:113-120.

Lakka, T.A., Venalainen, J.M., Rauramaa, R., Salonen, R., Tuomilehto, J., and Salonen, J.T. 1994. Relation of leisure-time physical activity and cardiorespiratory fitness to the risk of acute myocardial infarction in men. *N Engl J Med* 330:1549-1554.

Lapidus, L., and Bengtsson, C. 1986. Socioeconomic factors and physical activity in relation to cardiovascular disease and death: A 12 year follow up of participants in a population study of women in Gothenburg, Sweden. *Br Heart J* 55:295-301.

Lazarou, J., Pomeranz, B.H., and Corey, P.N. 1998. Incidence of adverse drug reactions in hospitalized patients. A meta-analysis of prospective studies. *JAMA* 279:1200-1205.

Leaf, A. 1993. Preventive medicine for our ailing health care system. *JAMA* 269:616-618.

Leon, A.S., Connett, J., Jacobs, D.R., and Rauramaa, R. 1987. Leisure-time physical activity levels and risk of coronary heart disease and death. The multiple risk factor intervention trial. *JAMA* 258:2388-2395.

Levine, A.M., Richardson, J.L., Marks, G., Chan, K., Graham, J., Selser, J.N., Kishbaugh, C., Shelton, D.R., and Johnson, C.A. 1987. Compliance with oral drug therapy in patients with hematologic malignancy. *J Clin Oncol* 5:1469-1476.

Levine, G.N., Keaney, J.F., and Vita, J.A. 1995. Cholesterol reduction in cardiovascular disease. *N Engl J Med* 332:512-21.

Lewis, B.S., and Lynch, W.D. 1993. The effect of physician advice on exercise behavior. *Prev Med* 22:110-121.

Luepker, R.V., Perry, C.L., McKinlay, S.M., Nader, P.R., Parcel, G.S., Stone, E.J., Webber, L.S., Elder, J.P., Feldman, H.A., Johnson, C.C., Kelder, S.H., and Wu, M. 1996. Outcomes of a field trial to improve children's dietary patterns and physical activity. The child and adolescent trial for cardiovascular disease. *JAMA* 275:768-776.

McGinnis, J.M., and Lee, P.R. 1995. Healthy People 2000 at mid decade. *JAMA* 273:1123-1129.

Mokdad, A.H., Serdula, M.K., Dietz, W.H., Bowman, B.A., Marks, J.S., and Koplan, J.P. 1999. The spread of the obesity epidemic in the United States, 1991-1998. *JAMA* 282:1519-1522.

Morris, J.N., Clayton, D.G., Everitt, M.G., Semmence, A.M., and Burgess, E.H. 1990. Exercise in leisure time: Coronary attack and death rates. *Br Heart J* 63:325-334.

Mullen, P.D., Simons-Morton, D.G., Ramirez, G., Frankowski, R.F., Green, L.W., and Mains, D.A. 1997. A meta-analysis of trials evaluating patient education and counseling for three groups of preventive health behaviors. *Patient Educ Couns* 32:157-173.

Must, A., Spadano, J., Coakley, E.H., Field, A.E., Colditz, G., and Dietz, W.H. 1999. The disease burden associated with overweight and obesity. *JAMA* 282:1523-1529.

National Institutes of Health, National Heart, Lung, and Blood Institute. 1998. *Obesity education initiative. Clinical guidelines on the identification, evaluation, and treatment of overweight and obesity in adults.* Bethesda, MD: National Institutes of Health.

Paffenbarger, R.S., and Hyde, R.T. 1984. Exercise in the prevention of coronary heart disease. *Prev Med* 13:3-22.

Paffenbarger, R.S., Hyde, R.T., Jung, D.L., and Wing, A.L. 1984. Epidemiology of exercise and coronary heart disease. *Clin Sports Med* 3:297-318.

Paffenbarger, R.S., Hyde, R.T., Wing, A.L., and Hsieh, C.C. 1986. Physical activity, all-cause mortality, and longevity of college alumni. *N Engl J Med* 314:605-613.

Paffenbarger, R.S., Hyde, R.T., Wing, A.L., Lee, I.M., Jung, D.L., and Kampert, J.B. 1993. The association of changes in physical-activity level and other lifestyle characteristics with mortality among men. *N Engl J Med* 328(8):538-545.

Paffenbarger, R.S., Kampert, J.B., Lee, I.M., Hyde, R.T., Leung, R.W., and Wing, A.L. 1994. Changes in physical activity and other lifeway patterns influencing longevity. *Med Sci Sports Exerc* 26(7):857-865.

Pate, R.R., Pratt, M., Blair, S.N., Haskell, W.L., Macera, C.A., Bouchard, C., Buchner, D., Ettinger, W., Health, G.W., King, A.C., et al. 1995. Physical activity and public health. A recommendation from the Centers for Disease Control and Prevention and the American College of Sports Medicine. *JAMA* 273(5):402-407.

Pi-Sunyer, F.X. 1993. Medical hazards of obesity. *Ann Intern Med* 119(7 pt 2):655-660.

Powell, K.E., Thompson, P.D., Caspersen, C.J., and Kendrick, J.S. 1987. Physical activity and the incidence of coronary heart disease. *Annu Rev Public Health* 8:253-287.

Robinson, T.N. 1999. Reducing children's television viewing to prevent obesity. *JAMA* 282:1561-1567.

Santell, J.P. 1995. Projecting future drug expenditures, 1995. *Am J Health-Syst Pharm* 52:151-163.

Scutchfield, F.D., and Hartman, K.T. 1995. Physicians and preventive medicine. *JAMA* 273:1150-1151.

Selvester, R., Camp, J., and Sanmarco, M. 1977. Effects of exercise training on progression of documented coronary arteriosclerosis in men. *Ann NY Acad Sci* 301:495-508.

Stefanick, M.L., Mackey, S., Sheehan, M., Ellsworth, N., Haskell, W.L., and Wood, P.D. 1998. Effects of diet and exercise in men and postmenopausal women with low levels of HDL cholesterol and high levels of LDL cholesterol. *N Engl J Med* 339:12-20.

Stephenson, J. 1999. Noncompliance may cause half of antihypertensive drug "failures." *JAMA* 282:313-314.

Taira, D.A., Safran, D.G., Seto, T.B., Rogers, W.H., and Tarlov, A.R. 1997. The relationship between patient income and physician discussion of health risk behaviors. *JAMA* 278:1412-1417.

U.S. Preventive Services Task Force. 1996. *Guide to clinical preventive services,* 2d ed. Alexandria, VA: International Medical Publishing.

Wechsler, H., Levine, S., Idelson, R.K., Schor, E.L., and Coakley, E. 1996. The physician's role in health promotion revisted: A survey of primary care practitioners. *N Engl J Med* 334:996-998.

Wee, C.C., McCarthy, E.P., Davis, R.B., and Phillips, R.S. 1999. Physician counseling about exercise. *JAMA* 282:1583-1588.

Whitley, J.D., and Nyberg, K.L. 1988. Exercise medicine in medical education in the United States. *Phys Sports Med* 16:93-100.

Yeung, M., O'Connor, S.A., Parry, D.T., and Cochrane, G.M. 1994. Compliance with prescribed drug therapy in asthma. *Respir Med* 88:31-35.

Young, D.R., Haskell, W.L., Jatulis, D.E., and Fortmann, S.P. 1993. Associations between changes in physical activity and risk factors for coronary heart disease in a community-based sample of men and women: The Stanford five-city project. *Am J Epidemiol* 138:205-216.

Additional Information Sources for Drugs and Exercise

Reviews From the Primary Literature

Bagatell, C.J., and Bremner, W.J. 1996. Androgens in men: Uses and abuses. *N Engl J Med* 334:707-714.

Bahrke, M.S., Yesalis, C.E., and Wright, J.E. 1990. Psychological and behavioural effects of endogenous testosterone levels and anabolic-androgenic steroids among males. A review. *Sports Med* 10:303-337.

Bahrke, M.S., Yesalis, C.E., and Wright, J.E. 1996. Psychological and behavioural effects of endogenous testosterone and anabolic-androgenic steroids. An update. *Sports Med* 22:367-390.

Caldwell, J.E. 1987. Diuretic therapy and exercise performance. *Sports Med* 4:290-304.

Clarkson, P.M, and Thompson, H.S. 1997. Drugs and sport. Research findings and limitations. *Sports Med* 24:366-384.

Fagard, R., Staessen, J., Thijs, L., and Amery, A. 1993. Influence of antihypertensive drugs on exercise capacity. *Drugs* 46(suppl 2):32-36.

Ghaphery, N.A. 1995. Performance-enhancing drugs. *Orthop Clin North Am* 26:433-442.

Haupt, H.A. 1989. Drugs in athletics. *Clin Sports Med* 8:561-582.

Hickson, R.C., and Kurowski, T.G. 1986. Anabolic steroids and training. *Clin Sports Med* 5:461-469.

Kindermann, W. 1987. Calcium antagonists and exercise performance. *Sports Med* 4:177-193.

Lowenthal, D.T., and Kendrick, Z.V. 1985. Drug-exercise interactions. *Ann Rev Pharmacol Toxicol* 25:275-305.

Macintyre, J.G. 1987. Growth hormone and athletes. *Sports Med* 4:129-142.

Nielsen, P., and Nachtigall, D. 1998. Iron supplementation in athletes: Current recommendations. *Sports Med* 26(4):207-216.

Rogol, A.D. 1985. Drugs to enhance athletic performance in the adolescent. *Semin Adolesc Med* 1:317-324.

Rosenbloom, D., and Sutton, J.R. 1985. Drugs and exercise. *Med Clin North Am* 69:177-187.

Smith, D.A., and Perry, P.J. 1992. The efficacy of ergogenic agents in athletic competition. Part I: Androgenic-anabolic steroids. *Ann Pharmacother* 26:520-528.

Smith, D.A., and Perry, P.J. 1992. The efficacy of ergogenic agents in athletic competition. Part II: Other performance-enhancing agents. *Ann Pharmacother* 26:653-659.

Somani, S.M., Gupta, S.K., Frank, S., and Corder, C.N. 1990. Effect of exercise on disposition and pharmacokinetics of drugs. *Drug Dev Res* 20:251-275.

Sports pharmacology. 1998. *Clin Sports Med* 17:211-396.

van Baak, M.A. 1988. Beta-adrenoceptor blockade and exercise. An update. *Sports Med* 5:209-225.

Wagner, J.C. 1991. Enhancement of athletic performance with drugs. An overview. *Sports Med* 12:250-265.

Williams, J.H. 1991. Caffeine, neuromuscular function and high-intensity exercise performance. *J Sports Med Phys Fitness* 31:481-489.

Williams, M.H. 1992. Ergogenic and ergolytic substances. *Med Sci Sports Exerc* 24(9 suppl):S344-S348.

Williams, M.H. 1994. The use of nutritional ergogenic aids in sports: Is it an ethical issue? *Int J Sport Nutr* 4:120-131.

Williams, M.H. 1998. Creatine supplementation and exercise performance: An update. *J Am Coll Nutr* 17:216-234.

Books

Fuentes, R.J., and Rosenberg, J.M. 1999. *Athletic drug reference '99*. Durham, NC: Clean Data, Inc.

Fuentes, R.J., Rosenberg, J.M., and Davis, A. 1996. *Athletic drug reference '96*. Durham, NC: Clean Data, Inc.

Lamb, D.R., and Williams, M.H, eds. 1991. *Ergogenics: Enhancement of performance in exercise and sport*. Ann Arbor, MI: Brown.

Mottram, D.R. 1988. *Drugs in sport*. Champaign, IL: Human Kinetics.

Reilly, T., and Orme, M., eds. 1997. *The clinical pharmacology of sport and exercise*. Amsterdam: Elsevier Science.

Ringhofer, K.R., and Harding, M.E. 1996. *Coaches guide to drugs and sport*. Champaign, IL: Human Kinetics.

Somani, S.M. 1996. *Pharmacology in exercise and sports*. Boca Raton, FL: CRC Press.

Stainback, R.D. 1997. *Alcohol and sport*. Champaign, IL: Human Kinetics.

Voy, R. 1991. *Drugs, sport, and politics*. Champaign, IL: Human Kinetics.

Wadler, G.I., and Hainline, B. 1989. *Drugs and the athlete*. Philadelphia: F.A. Davis Company.

Williams, M.H. 1997. *The ergogenics edge: Pushing the limits of sports performance*. Champaign, IL: Human Kinetics.

Williams, M.H., Kreider, R.B., and Branch, J.D. 1999. *Creatine: The power supplement*. Champaign, IL: Human Kinetics.

Yesalis, C.E., ed. 2000. *Anabolic steroids in sport and exercise (2nd ed)*. Champaign, IL: Human Kinetics.

About the Author

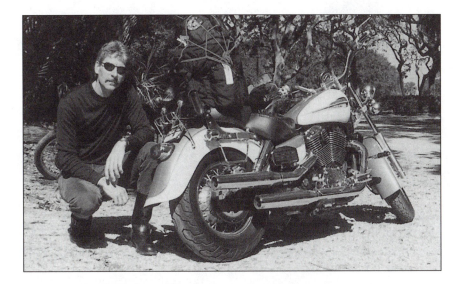

Author of more than a dozen research articles, **Stan Reents,** PharmD, is editor in chief of *Clinical Pharmacology,* an internationally acclaimed electronic drug reference for health care professionals.

Dr. Reents has been a certified personal trainer and has 14 years of experience as clinical pharmacist at hospitals in Illinois, Florida, and Missouri. He has taught pharmacology at the University of Florida, Purdue University, and the University of Illinois. He earned his PharmD from the University of the Pacific.

Dr. Reents lives in Tampa, Florida. He is an avid tennis player.